COPD CLINICAL PERSPECTIVES

Edited by **Ralph J. Panos**

COPD Clinical Perspectives
http://dx.doi.org/10.5772/57036
Edited by Ralph J. Panos

Contributors
Peter Lenz, Ralph J. Panos, Tomas Patrick Carroll, Emmet O'Brien, Noel G. McElvaney, Hatice Tel Aydın, Cormac McCarthy, Emer P. Reeves, David Bergin, Radostina Cherneva, Ognian Borissov Georgiev, Daniela Stoichkova Petrova, Emil Manov, Julia Petrova, Martín-Valero Rocio, Rodriguez-Martínez Mc, Cantero-Téllez R., Villanueva-Calvero E., Fernández-Martín F., William Eschenbacher

Published by InTech
Janeza Trdine 9, 51000 Rijeka, Croatia

Publishing Process Manager Iva Lipovic
Technical Editor InTech DTP team
Cover InTech Design team

First published July, 2014
Printed in Croatia

Additional hard copies can be obtained from orders@intechopen.com

COPD Clinical Perspectives, Edited by Ralph J. Panos
p. cm.
ISBN 978-953-51-1624-0

For EU product safety concerns:
IN TECH d.o.o., Prolaz Marije Krucifikse Kozulić 3, 51000 Rijeka, Croatia,
info@intechopen.com or visit our website at intechopen.com.

Meet the editor

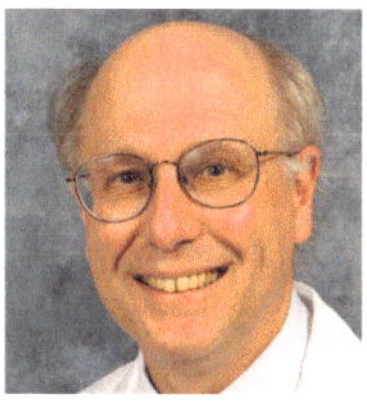

Ralph J. Panos is the Associate Chief of Medicine and Medical Director of the VISN 10 TeleICU at the Veterans Administration Medical Center in Cincinnati, Ohio. He is a Professor of Medicine and Associate Clinical Director in the Pulmonary, Critical Care, and Sleep Division at the University of Cincinnati College of Medicine. He graduated from the Brown University Program in Medicine, completed his internal medicine residency and chief residency at the University of Maryland, Baltimore, Maryland and his pulmonary fellowship at the University of Colorado, and National Jewish Hospital, Denver, Colorado. His major research interests are interstitial lung disease and chronic obstructive pulmonary disease.

Contents

Preface

When Iva Lipović, Publishing Process Manager from InTech, approached me several years ago to help edit a work on COPD, little did I know that it would be this long in the making. We have had a long and laborious road with many fits and starts but greatly appreciate the patience and perseverance of the authors and editors as this volume gradually took shape. Although greatly reduced from its initial expectations, this volume provides a succinct and concise overview of several key clinical perspectives on chronic obstructive pulmonary disease by an international group of experts.

In the first chapter, **Airflow Limitation and Spirometry** William L. Eschenbacher reviews the pathophysiology of airflow limitation, how obstruction is measured with spirometry, and technical aspects of pulmonary function testing. Next, Peter Lenz and Ralph J. Panos address the clinical and therapeutic differences between asthma and COPD in **Asthma and COPD: Overlapping Disorders or Distinct Processes?** The next two chapters explore the most common hereditary form of COPD, alpha-1-antitrypsin deficiency. Tomás P. Carroll, M. Emmet O'Brien, Laura T. Fee, Kevin Molloy, Blair Murray, Seshma Ramsawak, Oisín McElvaney, Catherine O'Connor, and Noel G. McElvaney provide a comprehensive overview of alpha-1-antitrypsin and review methods to improve screening studies in **Alpha-1-Antitrypsin Deficiency – A Missed Opportunity in COPD?** and in **Antiproteases as Therapeutics to Target Inflammation in Chronic Obstructive Pulmonary Disease** , Cormac McCarthy, Ciara A. O'Dwyer, David A. Bergin, Noel G. McElvaney and Emer P. Reeves review recent developments in protease:antiprotease biochemistry that have identified new therapeutic targets in the management of alpha-1-antitrypsin disease and COPD. The overlap syndrome, the presence of both obstructive sleep apnea and COPD, is an important clinical process with immense prognostic implications for patients and therapeutic decisions for providers. Radostina Vlaeva Cherneva, Ognian Borisov Georgiev, Daniela Stoichkova Petrova, Emil Ivanov Manov, Julia Ivanova Petrova review the pathophysiology of the overlap syndrome with an emphasis on oxygen radicals in **Sleep and Chronic Obstructive Pulmonary Disease- the Role of Oxidative Stress in Overlap Syndrome,** and Hatice Tel Aydin provides a broad overview of the clinical presentation and management approach to the patient with COPD and sleep apnea in **Chronic Obstructive Pulmonary Disease and Sleep Quality** . Finally, R. Martín-Valero, M.C. Rodríguez-Martínez, R. Cantero-Tellez, E. Villanueva-Calvero and F. Fernández-Martín review pulmonary rehabilitation, one of the most important therapies for COPD in **Advances in Comprehensive Pulmonary Rehabilitation for COPD Patients.**

I would like to thank the Editors at InTech and all of the authors for their energy and effort in producing this work. I would also especially like to thank my wife, Jean, for her infinite patience and tolerance that have allowed me to spend countless nights and weekends reading, editing, and revising this text to bring it to press.

Ralph J. Panos
[1] Department of Pulmonary,
Critical Care and Sleep Medicine,
University of Cincinnati Medical Center,
Cincinnati, Ohio, USA

[2] Pulmonary, Critical Care, and Sleep Medicine,
Cincinnati VAMC, Cincinnati, OH

Chapter 1

Airflow Limitation and Spirometry

William L. Eschenbacher

Additional information is available at the end of the chapter

http://dx.doi.org/10.5772/57549

1. Introduction

A patient with chronic obstructive pulmonary disease (COPD) may present with symptoms (dyspnea, cough, sputum production, chest tightness, wheezing, etc.) and appropriate history (cigarette smoking or occupational exposures). However, based on current accepted criteria established by professional societies, the diagnosis of COPD needs to be confirmed by the presence of airflow limitation as measured by spirometry testing. Unfortunately, as will be discussed in this report, the interpretation of spirometry testing that reveals airflow obstruction (a reduction in the FEV_1/FVC ratio) is an arbitrary metric for the presence of COPD.

As it is used, spirometry is one type of pulmonary function test that can measure the total amount of air that an individual can inhale and exhale and the speed or velocity with which the air moves. The test requires full cooperation of the individual performing the test, the supervision of a technician trained in this testing, and appropriate testing equipment (spirometer). The results of the testing session performed by the individual are reviewed to determine acceptable quality and repeatability before interpretation of the results can take place. Then the interpretation of airflow limitation can be made based upon the actual values of testing when compared to reference values for that individual.

2. Factors that contribute to maximal expiratory flow limitation

Expiratory flow rates from the lung have maximal values that cannot be exceeded in spite of increasing effort generated by the respiratory muscles of exhalation. The maximal flow that is achieved occurs close to total lung capacity and then decreases as lung volume (and in turn airway diameter) decreases until the lungs reach residual volume. This expiratory flow rate is affected by the elastic recoil of the lung and airway diameter. Expiratory flow limitation can be explained in its simplest terms by a gas flowing through a collapsible tube. In the examples below, the lungs and conducting airways can be represented by a balloon for the alveolar spaces with a single tube as the conducting airways.

At rest (Figure 1), there is a balance between the negative pleural pressure (caused in turn by the outward elastic recoil of the chest wall) that is exerting a force to distend the lungs and alveolar spaces and the elastic forces of the lung parenchymal structures that are causing the alveolar spaces to collapse. As a result of the equal forces, the alveolar pressure is zero and there is no pressure gradient to cause air to be exhaled. In terms of lung volume status, this balance between the outward chest wall force and the inward pulmonary parenchymal forces is the functional residual capacity (FRC).

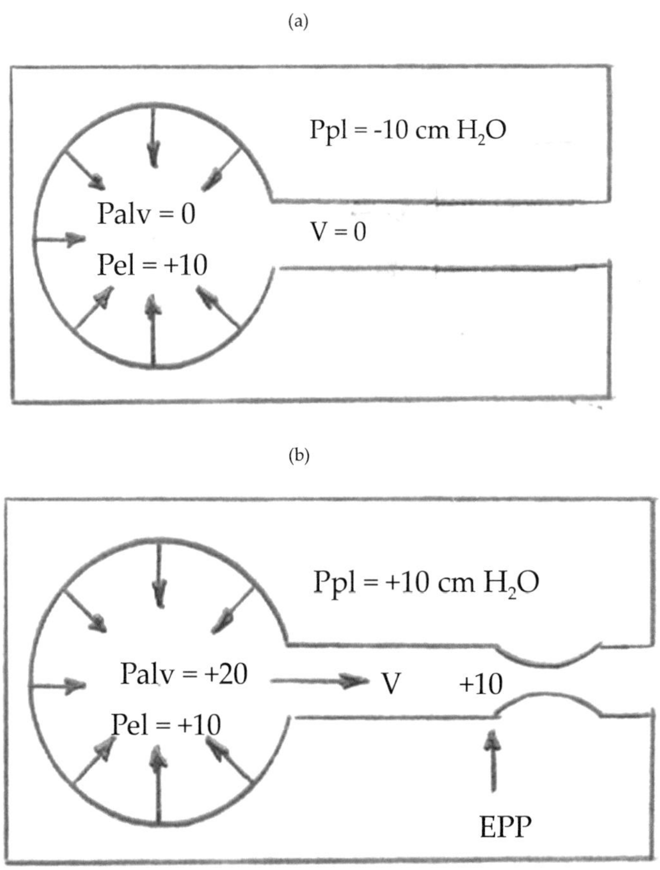

Figure 1. (a) Ppl=pleural pressure, Pel is the elastic recoil pressure of the lung, Palv is the resulting alveolar pressure which is a combination or balance between the elastic force which is attempting to collapse the alveolar space and the pleural pressure that is attempting to expand the alveolar space. Under these conditions, there is no flow rate of air since there is no pressure gradient from the alveolar space to the outside. (b) Force applied by respiratory muscles results in positive intrapleural pressure which when added to elastic recoil pressure of the parenchyma leads to positive intra-alveolar pressure which in turn creates a positive pressure gradient so that expiratory flow of air can occur.

When the expiratory respiratory muscles are activated, there is in an increase in the pleural pressure from-10 cmH_2O to+10 cmH_2O (Figure 2). This external pressure on the alveolar spaces is then in addition to the elastic force of the parenchymal structures to create a positive alveolar pressure of+20 cmH_2O. There is now a pressure gradient from the alveolar space to the outside of the lungs and as a result, air flow occurs. Because of the resistive forces in the airways, there will be a decrease in this driving pressure along the airway until a point is reached where the pressure within the airway is matched by the surrounding pleural pressure. This is referred to as the equal pressure point. The equal pressure point is defined physiologically and not anatomically and, for any individual, the anatomic location of the EPP may change with time based upon airway tone and other factors.

If the airway at this equal pressure point is in the larger airways/bronchi where cartilaginous support exists there would not be collapse of the airways. However, if this equal pressure point occurs closer to the alveolar spaces in smaller non-cartilaginous airways, then compression and collapse of the airway may occur. In either case, the expiratory flow rate is determined primarily by the elastic recoil pressure which in part determines the pressure gradient from the alveolar spaces to the outside and by the resistive elements of the airways which determine the pressure drop as flow occurs along the airways. Increasing the respiratory force generated by the expiratory respiratory muscles has little direct effect on most of the airflow during exhalation from total lung capacity to residual volume. In that regard, the expiratory flow is limited.

3. Anatomic location of airway resistance

As stated, the pressure drop when flow occurs during exhalation is determined by the presence of resistive forces within the airways. Airway resistance in turn depends on the flow pattern of the exhaled air (laminar vs turbulent flow), as well as the number and diameter of the airways which in turn determines the total cross-sectional area of the airways from the smallest airways to the major airways (bronchi and trachea). Because the airways divide again and again from the major airways, the number of smaller airways at the terminus of the conducting airways (0.6 mm) is over 40-60,000 in a normal individual so that the cross-sectional area is increased from 2.5 cm^2 at the trachea to 180 cm^2 at the level of these smaller airways.

Studies have shown that the airways < 2mm only contribute < 20% of the total airways resistance during expiratory flow. However, in the presence of COPD, that value has been shown to increase by 4-40 fold [1]. The question has been whether in COPD, the increase in resistance is due to a loss or destruction of these smaller airways or to a narrowing of these airways by disease. More recent studies using multidetector computed tomography (MDCT) and micro-CT imaging have shown that there is a combination of both a decrease in the number of the smaller airways due to destruction and also a reduction the airway diameter of these airways due to disease [1].

In summary, the factors that result in expiratory flow are 1) the elastic recoil of the lungs which is greater at higher lung volumes (highest at total lung capacity and decreases as exhalation occurs) and 2) resistive elements of the airways (lowest at total lung capacity and increases as exhalation occurs) that determine the pressure drop as airflow occurs along the airway. In COPD, both of these factors can be affected. The elastic recoil of the lungs can be reduced in COPD if there is evidence of emphysema that results in destruction of parenchymal tissue and the elastic forces that cause the lungs to collapse. Also, in COPD with loss of the number of airways and reduction in airway diameter due to disease, the resistive elements are increased with a greater pressure drop for any given flow rate along the airways. Also, the loss of supporting forces with emphysematous changes will also reduce the stiffness of the airways resulting in airway collapse with movement of the equal pressure point closer to the alveolar spaces.

The hallmark of airflow limitation is reduced maximal expiratory flow rates as measured by spirometry. The pathological changes in the lungs that result in the reduced expiratory flow rates are 1) increased flow resistive properties of the airways (as in chronic bronchitis) and 2) reduced elastic recoil of the lung (as in emphysema). In COPD, the airways can be narrowed as a result of inflammatory changes and smooth muscle hypertrophy in the airway wall and increased amount of mucous and inflammatory material within the airway lumen. There is increased resistance to airflow as a result of the narrowed airway leading to reduced flow rates for the same driving pressure that is generated to cause expiratory flow. In addition, loss of parenchymal tissue with emphyematous changes can reduce the support of airway walls contributing to airway narrowing and increased airway resistance. Also, the emphysematous changes reduce the elastic recoil and in turn the pressure gradient that is in part responsible for the generation of the expiratory flow rates. The contribution of these separate pathological changes has been studied extensively to determine the location of the greatest effect on reduced expiratory flow rates. The specific mechanisms involved are complex and have been the subject of extensive physiological research. It is sufficient to say that the clinically relevant measurement of maximal expiratory flow rates by spirometry is thought to be an appropriate measurement used to evaluate the reduction in flow rates that is the hallmark of and confirms the diagnosis of COPD.

4. Role of spirometry in identifying the presence of airflow limitation or obstruction in COPD

Spirometry testing has been used to confirm the presence of airflow limitation or obstruction in COPD but the testing must be performed correctly. Spirometry testing must be done according to established guidelines [2,3] to ensure adequate quality of test results. This means that the equipment (spirometers) used must meet basic requirements [2] and the technicians performing the testing should have completed appropriate training that includes courses such as those that use the National Institute for Occupational Safety and Health (NIOSH) Spirometry Training Guide. Also, as part of the ongoing testing process, spirometry results will be reviewed with feedback to the technicians to ensure continued adequate quality of results. Testing is performed for the individual patient until three acceptable maneuvers are obtained

http://dx.doi.org/10.5772/57549

with the necessary evidence for repeatability. The testing is done both at baseline and after the administration of a bronchodilator (post-bronchodilator results).

Once testing is completed, the spirometry test results for that individual (specifically the forced expiratory volume in one-second (FEV_1), forced vital capacity (FVC) and the ratio of those two values FEV_1/FVC) are compared to predicted values based on established reference equations [4].

The results of spirometry testing can be shown both in graphical format and by numerical results in tabular format (Table 1). Airflow limitation or obstruction as identified by spirometry is shown in Figures 2a, 2b, 3a and 3b.

(a)

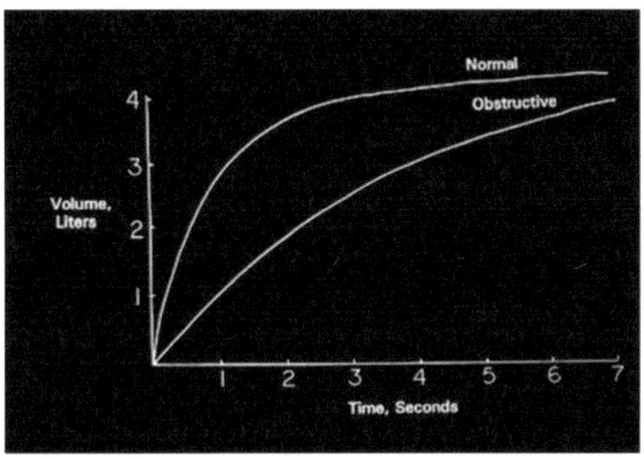

(b)

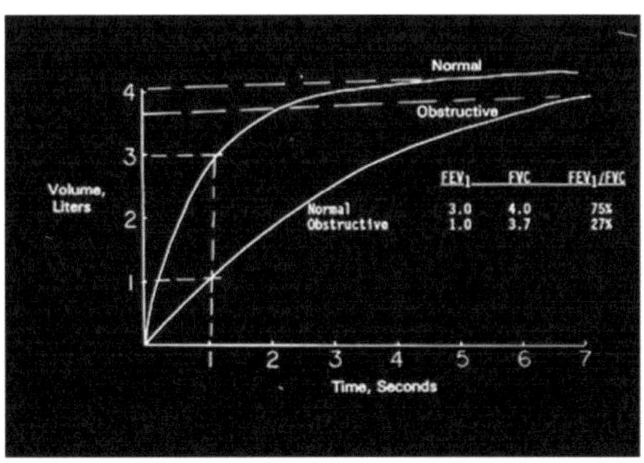

Figure 2. (a) Volume-time relationship from spiromtery testing for exhaled air in a normal individual and an individual with airflow obstruction (obstructive). Volume of exhaled air is in liters and time of exhalation in seconds. Note in airflow obstruction the volume of air exhaled at any time point is reduced compared to the exhaled air for the normal individual. (b) Calculation of the values of spirometry testing for a normal individual and an individual with airflow obstruction (obstructive). FEV_1 refers to the forced expiratory volume in one second and FVC refers to the forced vital capacity. The parameter that best describes the presence of airflow obstruction is a reduction in the ratio of FEV_1 to FVC as shown here: 27% for the ratio in the individual with airflow obstruction vs. 75% for the ratio for the normal individual.

4.1. Spirometry volume-time tracings

The results of a spirometry testing maneuver can be displayed as a volume-time tracing as shown in Figures 2a and 2b. After the individual has inhaled deeply to maximal inhaled volume (total lung capacity), he or she is asked to exhale forcefully and maximally without hesitation and told to keep exhaling until told to stop. The resulting tracing demonstrates the exhaled volume in liters against the time of exhalation in seconds. (Figures 2a and 2b) For a normal individual, the volume of air that is exhaled in the first second (Forced Expiratory Volume in 1 second or FEV_1) is usually about 70-80% of the total amount of air that can be exhaled (total amount of exhaled air is called the Forced Vital Capacity or FVC). It is that ratio of FEV_1/FVC when reduced that determines if airflow limitation is present. As shown in the example in Figures 2a and 2b, the normal individual has a ratio of FEV_1/FVC of 3.0 liters to 4.0 liters (3/4 or 75%) whereas the other individual with airflow obstruction or limitation has a ratio of FEV_1/FVC of 1.0 liters to 3.7 liters (1/3.7 or 27%). A reduced FEV_1/FVC ratio is the criterion for the intepretation of airflow obstruction.

4.2. Spirometry flow-volume tracings

In addition to displaying the results of spirometry as volume-time tracings, the same results can be expressed or displayed as flow-volume tracings or loops with both expiratory limbs and inspiratory limbs being displayed (Figures 3a and 3b). This additional information can be useful for evaluation of the actual expiratory flow rates achieved with spirometry and is also useful for the technician and the reviewer of spirometry testing to determine if the testing maneuvers are acceptable without errors. Errors that can occur with spirometry testing can be at the beginning of the maneuver (hesitancy, cough, sub-optimal effort, etc.) or at the end of the test (did not exhale completely).

Another example of spirometry test results is shown in Table 1 for a different individual with baseline testing and testing again after the administration of the one-time use of a bronchodilator.

Patient: BS2	**Age: 72**	**Height: 69 inches**		**Weight: 231 pounds**	**Sex: Male Race: Caucasian**		
		Baseline				**Post-Bronchodilator**	
	Actual	**Predicted**	**%Pred**	**LLN**	**Actual**	**%Pred**	**%Change**
FVC, L	2.05	4.18	49	3.27	2.23	53	8
FEV_1, L	1.11	3.05	36	2.27	1.19	39	7
FEV_1/FVC, %	54	73		63	53		
$FEF_{25-75\%}$, L/sec	0.48	2.28	21	0.73	0.61	27	26

FVC: Forced vital capacity; FEV_1: Forced Expiratory Volume in 1 second, $FEF_{25-75\%}$: Forced Expiratory Flow rates between 25 and 75% of vital capacity.

Table 1. The numerical results of spirometry testing for a patient with airflow obstruction

http://dx.doi.org/10.5772/57549

(a)

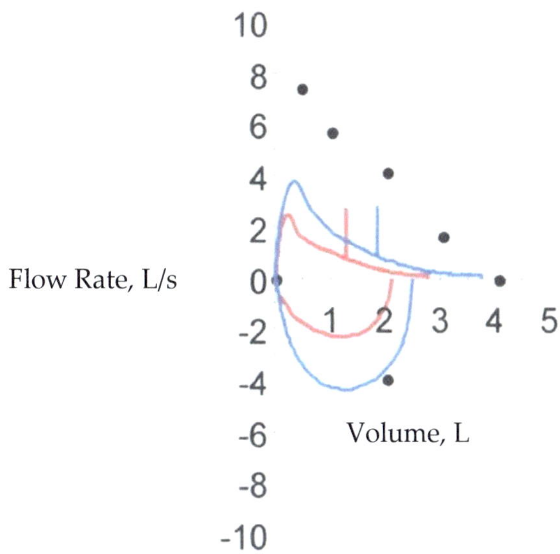

(b)

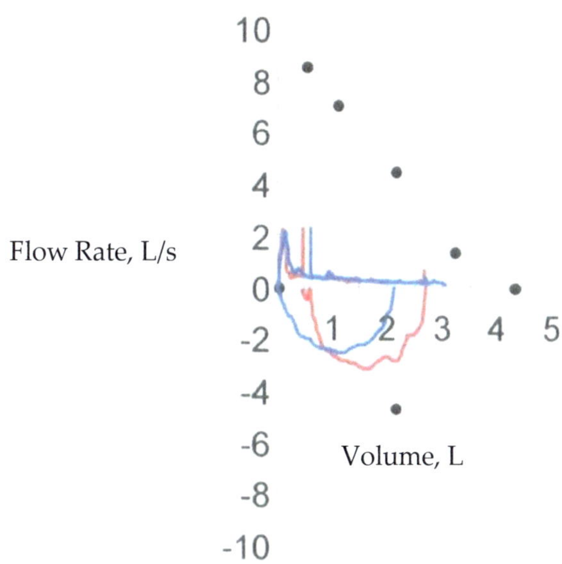

Figure 3. (a) and (b) Representations of airflow obstruction using flow vs. volume relationships. Flow of exhaled and inspired air in liters/second and volume of air exhaled and inhaled in liters. The red line refers to the baseline measurement of spirometry testing and the blue line represents the results after a bronchodilator has been given to the individual. The points refer to predicted values for the individual. (a) these figures shows an individual who has airflow obstruction of moderate severity. (b) these figures show an individual who has airflow obstruction that is very severe.

4.3. Definition of airflow limitation by spirometry

As mentioned, the determination of airflow limitation by spirometry depends on the criterion of a reduced FEV_1/FVC ratio. The specific definition of the actual criterion for airflow limitation or airflow obstruction has been a point of discussion based upon different statements from professional groups. Clinical guidelines for COPD disease management include the Global Initiative for Chronic Obstructive Lung Disease (GOLD) [5], the VA/DoD Clinical Practice Guideline for Management of Outpatient Chronic Obstructive Pulmonary Disease [6], and the American Thoracic Society/European Respiratory Society Standards for the Diagnosis and Management of Patients with COPD [7]. These three guidance documents have recommended being more inclusive for identifying individuals who may have COPD and have proposed that the presence of airflow limitation exists when the post-bronchodilator FEV_1/FVC ratio is < 0.70. These guidelines acknowledge that this approach may be overly sensitive and include older individuals who are normal but who have an FEV_1/FVC ratio that is < 0.70. Other guidance documents are based on a statistical approach for the interpretation of airflow limitation using reference equations which in turn are based on population studies. The ATS/ERS document on Interpretative Strategies for Lung Function Tests [2] states that the presence of an obstructive ventilatory defect exists when the FEV_1/FVC ratio is below the 5th percentile of its predicted value, a value referred to as the lower limit of normal or LLN for that ratio based on the chosen reference values. The most recent revised GOLD guidance [5] does acknowledge that the LLN values are based on a normal distribution and that the use of a fixed ratio of 0.70 will result in more frequent diagnosis of COPD in the elderly. This problem of the difference between using a fixed cutoff of 70% for the ratio of FEV_1/FVC compared with using the LLN for this ratio is illustrated in Figure 4. Younger individuals with an FEV_1/FVC above 70% but below the LLN would be classified as no airflow obstruction by use of a 70% cutoff but would be interpreted as airflow obstruction by use of the LLN (false negatives). On the other hand, older individuals with FEV1/FVC ratios below 70% but above the LLN would be classified as having airflow obstruction by the use of a 70% cutoff but would have no airflow obstruction by use of the LLN (false positives).

Post-bronchodilator spirometry test results can be used for the determination of airflow limitation recognizing that as many as 50% of patients with COPD will have a significant response to the one-time use of a bronchodilator (at least a 12% increase and a 200ml absolute increase in FEV_1 or FVC). The use of post-bronchodilator results is consistent with the aforementioned clinical guidance documents [4,5,6].

Once airflow limitation is determined to be present, the severity of limitation is then assessed based on the FEV_1 % of predicted value. Using the ATS/ERS guidelines for Interpretative Strategies for Lung Function Tests [2], the following severity categories are used:

Mild obstruction: FEV_1% predicted > 70% (which means the actual value measured is greater than 70% of the predicted value which in turn is based on the patient's age, height and gender with correction for race as appropriate).

Moderate obstruction: FEV_1% predicted <69% but > 60%

Moderately Severe obstruction: FEV_1% predicted <59% but > 50%

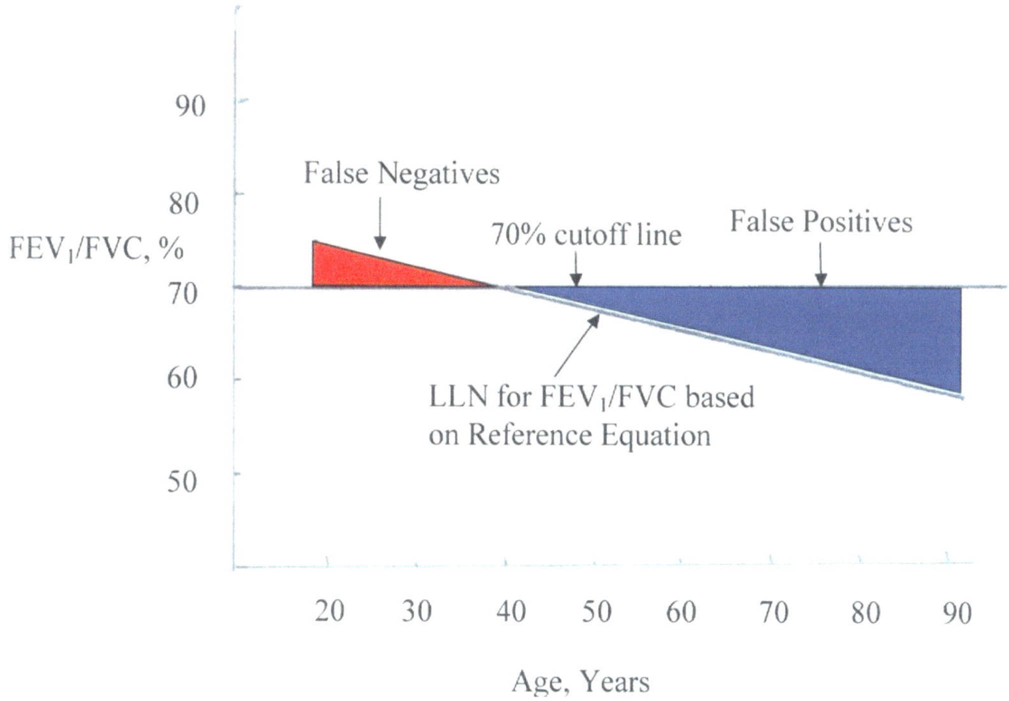

Figure 4. The difference for the interpretation of the presence of airflow obstruction by using an absolute cutoff of 70% or less for the ratio of FEV_1/FVC as the criteria for airflow obstruction compared to using values for this ratio that are lower than the lower limit of normal (LLN) based on the NHANES III reference equation [4]. The LLN line decreases with age as does the predicted ratio of FEV_1/FVC. As a result, the red area would include younger individuals who would be considered to be normal if a value of 70% is used for the interpretation of airflow obstruction but actually by use of the LLN would be considered to have airflow obstruction (false negative). On the other hand, those individuals in the blue area would be considered to have airflow obstruction by ratios of FEV_1/FVC below 70% but would be above the LLN (false positives).

Severe obstruction: FEV_1% predicted <49% but > 35%

Very Severe obstruction: FEV_1% predicted <34%

There may be patients whose results from spirometry testing or from complete pulmonary function testing (if available) may be equivocal for the presence of airflow limitation or COPD. In those cases, it is recommended that the patient be referred to the pulmonary specialists for further evaluation. This may also include the presence of emphysema as noted on imaging studies such as CT scans of the chest.

4.4. Problem with using spirometry to diagnose COPD

Although it has been recommended by those professional societies that a reduction in FEV_1/FVC using either a 70% cutoff or the LLN should be used to establish a diagnosis of COPD, there has been some controversy over this recommendation. The choice of either 70% or a LLN is an arbitrary value given that there are problems with an absolute cutoff of 70%

knowing the decline in FEV_1/FVC that occurs with aging and the LLN which was determined by a statistical analysis of the results of spirometry testing in a population of non-smoking, "normal" individuals [4]. Thus, the clinical significance of a value for FEV_1/FVC below either 70% or LLN is of questionable relevance given the pathological changes that can occur with COPD involving the airways and parenchyma [8]. It is known that there is not one physiological parameter that can completely describe all the changes that occur in the disease that is COPD. Unfortunately, until we develop better means to characterize this disease, we are left with using spirometry to diagnose and characterize the severity of the disease.

5. Summary

Airflow limitation as determined by spirometry testing is the hallmark of COPD. The spirometry testing criterion for airflow limitation is a reduced FEV_1/FVC ratio when compared to the lower limit of normal for that measurement from a reference population. It is critical that the test be done in an acceptable manner under the supervision of a trained technician. The results of spirometry testing can be useful in characterizing the presence and severity of the obstructive lung disease for that individual.

Author details

William L. Eschenbacher

Cincinnati VA Medical Center, Division of Pulmonary, Critical Care and Sleep, University of Cincinnati Medical Center, Cincinnati, USA

References

[1] Hogg JC. A Pathologist's View of Airway Obstruction in Chronic Obstructive Pulmonary Disease. Am J Respir Crit Care Med 2012; 186:v-vii.

[2] Miller MR, Hankinson J, Brusasco V, Burgos F, Casaburi R, et al. Standardization of Spirometry: Series "ATS/ERS Task Force: Standardization of Lung Function Testing". Eur Respir J 2005, 26:319-338.

[3] Pelligrino R, Viegi G, Brusasco V, Crapo RO, Burgos F, et al. Interpretative Strategies for Lung Function Tests: Series "ATS/ERS Task Force: Standardization of Lung Function Testing". Eur Respir J 2005, 26:948-968.

[4] Hankinson JL, Odencrantz JR, Fedan KB. Spirometric Reference Values from a Sample of the General U.S. Population. Am J Respir Crit Care Med 1999; 159:179-187.

http://dx.doi.org/10.5772/57549

[5] Global Strategy for the Diagnosis, Management, and Prevention of Chronic Obstructive Pulmonary Disease. Global Initiative for Chronic Obstructive Lung Disease. http://www.goldcopd.org/uploads/users/files/GOLD_Report_2013_Feb20.pdf

[6] VA/DoD Clinical Practice Guideline for Management of Outpatient Chronic Obstructive Pulmonary Disease. Department of Veteran Affairs/Department of Defense. Version 2.0 –2007. http://www.healthquality.va.gov/copd/copd_20.pdf

[7] Standards for the Diagnosis and Management of Patients with COPD. American Thoracic Society and European Respiratory Society. 2004. http://www.thoracic.org/clinical/copd-guidelines/resources/copddoc.pdf

[8] Rennard SI, Vestbo J, Agusti A. What is Chronic Obstructive Pulmonary Disease Anyway? Am J Respir Crit Care Med, 2013; 187:1036-1037.

Chapter 2

Asthma and COPD – Overlapping Disorders or Distinct Processes?

Peter H. Lenz and Ralph J. Panos

Additional information is available at the end of the chapter

http://dx.doi.org/10.5772/58234

1. Introduction

Historically, asthma and COPD (chronic obstructive pulmonary disease) have been considered separate and unique diseases with distinct characteristics. Classically, asthma has been characterized by reversible airways obstruction and COPD by fixed, less reversible, or irreversible airways obstruction. The definitions of asthma and COPD have undergone major revisions recently and COPD, like asthma, has now been recognized as an inflammatory disease of the airways [1, 2]. Even though asthma and COPD *can* be and are often *appropriately* separated as clinical entities, there are times when they are clinically and physiologically indistinguishable. As the American Thoracic Society guidelines for the diagnosis of COPD [3] state, "the obstruction in many patients with COPD may include a significant reversible component and that some patients with asthma may go on to develop irreversible airflow obstruction indistinguishable from COPD." This intersection of physiologic findings in asthma and COPD has led to the development of the concept of what is now known as the overlap syndrome of asthma and COPD [4]. As subcategories or phenotypes of asthma and COPD are identified, the distinction between these two disorders is less well defined. Some of the phenotypes exhibit very similar clinical, physiologic, and inflammatory profiles. The concept of asthma and COPD viewed as separate disease states has evolved as definitions and categorization of asthma and COPD change, and, as such, we are now encountering more overlap among these two disorders than was previously recognized. So we now pose the question: should asthma and COPD always be recognized and viewed as completely distinct diseases or is there enough similarity to view them equivalently at times? In essence, does an asthma-COPD overlap syndrome occur in some patients?

Multiple researchers have begun to view asthma as a diverse array of diseases distinguished by unique phenotypes. In other words, perhaps asthma is not one single disease entity, but a collection of multiple subgroupings. Similarly, recent evaluations of COPD suggest that it is also composed of multiple phenotypes [5, 6]. Furthermore, some of these COPD and asthma subgroupings or phenotypes share similar clinical presentations and characteristics [7]. So, from a clinical perspective, it may be appropriate to view these diseases as overlapping. Other authors have extended these observations to speculate that asthma and COPD are part of the same disease spectrum. Some offer the hypothesis that perhaps asthma turns into COPD or perhaps asthma and COPD have similar pathogenetic origins in individuals with similar host substrates and environmental exposures. Orie and coworkers [8] initiated a unified approach over five decades ago when they postulated common processes and evolution of asthma and COPD; they adopted the term chronic non-specific lung disease to include both disorders: "asthma, chronic bronchitis and emphysema should be considered as different expressions of one disease entity, in which both endogenous (host) and exogenous (environmental) factors play a role in the pathogenesis."

In addition, the new Global Initiative for Chronic Obstructive Lung Disease (GOLD) criteria that were established in 2011 [9] began to characterize patients with COPD based not just on their physiologic features, but also considered their clinical symptoms and risk for healthcare utilization. The GOLD guidelines proposed categorization of individuals with COPD into four distinct phenotypes based upon these characteristics (see Figure 1). Further, treatment guidelines are based upon the patient's categorization and phenotype.

New insights into asthma and COPD now recognize that there is much *heterogeneity* amongst individual patients with asthma and with COPD. However, when comparing asthma and COPD phenotypes, there appears to be cross-disease *homogeneity* amongst some of these specific asthma and COPD phenotypes. Therefore, as asthma and COPD research continues, the question remains: are asthma and COPD distinct and separate disease entities or are there enough similarities between them to allow us to view them equivalently at times? In other words, are asthma and COPD different disease states or is there significant overlap at the ends of the spectrum? Furthermore, are they two distinct phenotypes of a similar disease process?

In this chapter, we will investigate the historical definitions and perspectives of these two diseases and how they have been viewed and reported as distinct entities that are quite different from each other. While explaining the historical definitions of these diseases, we will highlight the differences and similarities in clinical manifestations, physiology, and airways inflammation between COPD and asthma. We also describe asthma and COPD phenotypes and discuss how separating asthma and COPD into multiple subcategories has paved the way to recognize the heterogeneity of these processes. These phenotypes can often overlap across disease states, especially those asthmatic patients that have a less-reversible form of airways obstruction that presents like that of COPD. We will review airway remodeling and how it can lead to chronic, more fixed obstruction in asthma. The concept of airways obstruction reversibility will be reviewed and the ambiguity and confusion of this nomenclature discussed. Finally, we will discuss the overlap of treatment and therapies now used to treat both asthma and COPD and where we are beginning to see success for the use of classical asthma treatments for COPD and vice-versa.

http://dx.doi.org/10.5772/58234

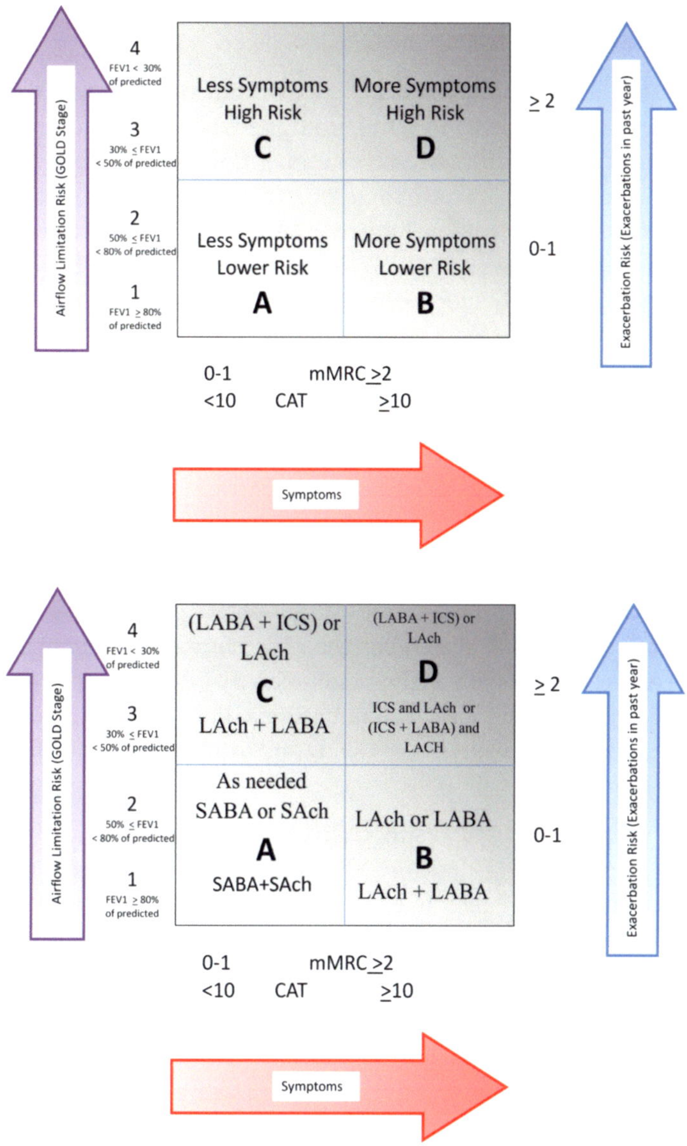

Abbreviations: *mMRC*-Modified Medical Research Council Dyspnea Scale, *CAT*-COPD Assessment Test questionnaire, *SABA*=short acting beta-agonist, *LABA*-long acting beta-agonist, *SAch*-short acting anti-cholinergic, *LAch*-long acting anti-cholinergic (also known as LAMA or long acting muscarinic antagonist), *ICS*-inhaled corticosteroid,

Figure 1. Adapted from [9]. A. Categorization of individuals according to the GOLD Guidelines [9] utilizes physiologic impairment based upon the reduction in the FEV1, symptoms measured by either the COPD Assessment Test (CAT) or the mMRC dyspnea scale, and risk measured by the number of exacerbations in the previous year. B. Use of the four GOLD categories to define management strategies. Note the risk assessments are now made on the vertical axes with airflow limitation and prior exacerbations taken into account, and the symptoms of the patient are also accounted for on the horizontal axis. The symptoms assessments are identified and scored by patient reported items such as the mMRC and CAT.

1.1. Ambiguous nomenclature and the bronchodilator response controversy: should we stop using the term reversible?

Although the historic definitions of asthma and COPD put an emphasis on the response to a bronchodilator, there are some instances and examples where this delineation may not be as useful. Although many asthmatics have normal lung function in between exacerbations or symptoms and require bronchoprovocation testing to induce airflow limitation, the majority of asthmatics experience relief of airflow limitation (AFL) when administered a bronchodilator (BD) in a laboratory setting. Between 39 and 73% of individuals with COPD also will experience significant improvement in AFL after receiving a BD [10]. In the Pulmonary Function Laboratory, an increase of 12% and at least 200 ml in either the FEV1 or FVC is usually defined as bronchodilator responsive airflow limitation [11] that many clinicians consider "reversible." Reversibility is also frequently used in the definitions of asthma and COPD: asthma is reversible and COPD is non-reversible airflow limitation; but in these definitions, reversible does not refer to the response to a bronchodilator but to the ability of airflow to return to normal or predicted levels in asthma and the inability to return to normal or predicted levels in COPD. Thus, *reversible* refers to *two very different concepts*: response to a bronchodilator (in the PFT lab) and normalization (in the definitions of COPD and asthma). This ambiguous use of the word reversible has led many clinicians to diagnose asthma when a patient has a measured response to bronchodilators in the PFT lab even when their lung function does not achieve predicted levels. Similarly, an individual with airflow limitation that does not improve with bronchodilators is often diagnosed with COPD and not asthma. Pulmonary physiology measured in the PFT lab can *assist* with the diagnosis of COPD and asthma but is insufficient to diagnosis either COPD or asthma.

Throughout this chapter, we will distinguish between bronchodilator responsivity and normalization of spirometric lung function and clarify use of the ambiguous term, reversibility. Bronchodilator responsivity will refer to improvement in either FEV1 or FVC by 12% and 200 cc after bronchodilator administration [12] and normalization will refer to a return to normal or predicted values for the FEV1 and FVC either during intercurrent periods of pulmonary disease activity or after bronchodilator use.

Thus, an individual with COPD will have non-normalizing lung function but could still have a bronchodilator response and most individuals with asthma will have normalizing lung function during periods of disease inactivity. Asthmatics with fixed airflow limitation have lost the ability to normalize their lung function and are inseparable physiologically from individuals with COPD.

In the December 2011 revision, the GOLD Guidelines [9] list several differences between asthma and COPD and stress the importance of the concept of "reversible" (normalizing) airflow obstruction. COPD is described as having onset in mid-life, slowly progressive symptoms, and a history of tobacco smoking or exposure to other types of smoke, whereas asthma begins early in life and symptoms vary widely from day to day. The definition of COPD in the GOLD guidelines clearly "excludes asthma ('reversible (normalizing) airflow limitation')" and also states that the presence of a post-bronchodilator FEV1/FVC < 0.70 confirms the presence of persistent (or non-normalizing) airflow limitation and thus of COPD. Once again, we see authors stress the importance of separating "reversible" from "non-reversible" airflow limitation as helping in defining and distinguishing asthma and COPD. However, as Pellegrino and colleagues [11] state, "The lack of a response to bronchodilator testing in a laboratory does not preclude a clinical response to bronchodilator therapy." Should we limit asthma therapy to only those patients who have normalizable AFL after BD? This decision could narrow a patient's therapeutic options and exclude potentially beneficial medications.

Certainly for the majority of patients a reasonable classification of asthma and COPD can be based on how airflow returns to predicted or normal levels after the administration of a bronchodilator. But many asthmatics can have fixed or non-normalizing airflow limitation after a bronchodilator is administered in a laboratory setting. Some asthma phenotypes have significant inflammation and airway remodeling that leads to non-normalizing AFL that does not respond to a bronchodilator. Therefore, it seems plausible that some asthma patients indeed have fixed airflow obstruction and approaching them as COPD patients may allow for more appropriate therapy. Using the normalization of AFL after BD may be useful for defining the majority of asthma and COPD patients but airway remodeling due to repetitive or persistent inflammation in asthmatics as they age and are chronically exposed to stimuli can account for the fact that some asthmatics show no significant spirometric change after BD administration in a laboratory. Patients with either asthma or COPD may respond to a BD so BD responsivity is neither sensitive nor specific in distinguishing asthma and COPD.

2. Why is overlap between asthma and COPD important?

In a 15 year longitudinal study of individuals with asthma, Lange and colleagues [13] concluded that some asthmatics progress to fixed airways obstruction suggesting that this asthmatic subgroup may exhibit non-normalizing lung function and be more similar to COPD. GOLD guidelines [9], NHLBI guidelines [14], and GINA [15] guidelines state that asthma and COPD are underdiagnosed and misdiagnosed. In addition, these guidelines attempt to distinguish asthma and COPD obviating recognition of potential overlap. Simply put, there are often times where guideline-driven therapy for COPD and asthma may preclude some patients from getting more tailored therapy. In the example of the asthma/COPD overlap patient, guideline driven care may not optimize or individualize treatment sufficiently. As listed in examples cited later in this chapter, many asthmatics with fixed or non-normalizing AFL may benefit from treatments that are traditionally only considered for patients with COPD. Thus, we feel it is imperative that a subgroup of patients with asthma and COPD may benefit by approaching them therapeutically as having an "overlap" syndrome of asthma and COPD. Furthermore, classic COPD and asthma medications may be used interchangeably and successfully for patients with overlapping phenotypes. Therefore, viewing asthma and COPD similarly for some patients can lead to more treatment options and possibly better outcomes.

3. Clinical perplexity emanating from overlapping definitions and ambiguous nomenclature

3.1. Defining these disorders has proven difficult

The recent movements to subcategorize asthma and COPD into distinctive phenotypes underscores the imprecise and evolving definitions of these disorders; neither asthma nor COPD are discrete diseases but rather syndromes that are defined or characterized by multifactorial listings of historical, physical examination, radiographic, cellular, biochemical, and physiologic features [9, 14, 15].

Historically, definitions have distinguished COPD with non-normalizing AFL in older adults from asthma with normalizing AFL in children with atopy or pulmonary inflammation. Figure 2 summarizes the features of asthma and COPD that have been used historically to distinguish these two disorders. Furthermore, as described in [4], "Asthma is recognized as an allergic disease that develops in childhood, characterised physiologically by "reversible" (normalizing) airflow obstruction, and has an episodic course with a generally favourable prognosis, responding well to anti-inflammatory treatment. In contrast, COPD is typically caused by tobacco smoking, develops in mid to later life and is characterised by incompletely"reversible" (non-normalizing) airflow limitation that results in a progressive decline in lung function leading to premature death."

Further, since these disorders are syndromes, there is not a single gold standard diagnostic test for either asthma or COPD. Bronchoprovocation testing has been advocated to complement spirometric measurement of FEV1 and FVC before and after bronchodilators for the diagnosis of asthma [14, 15]. For COPD, there is much debate over thresholds to define airflow obstruction – that is with a fixed FEV1/FVC ratio less than 0.70 or an FEV1/FVC ratio less than the lower limit of normal. Thus, it has been exceedingly difficult to define these disorders precisely based upon physiologic testing.

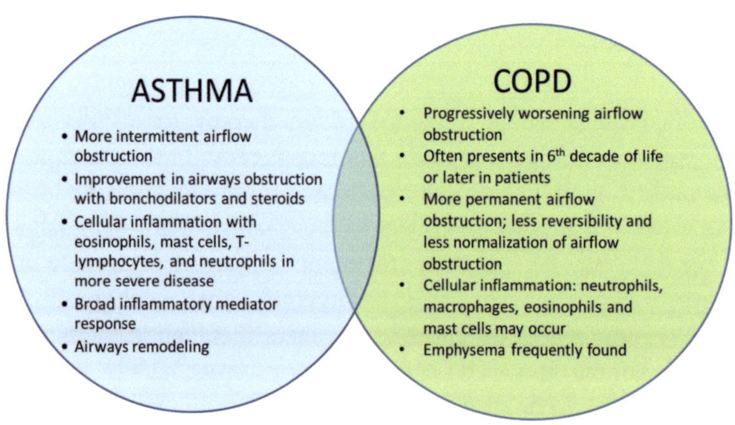

Figure 2. Historical characteristics of asthma and COPD, adapted from [16].

3.2. Revisiting the Dutch hypothesis and overlap syndrome proposals

Scientific and clinical evidence reinforces the overlap between COPD and asthma. The clinical manifestations of these disorders, cough, breathlessness, and wheezing, may be identical. AFL is present in both processes and BD responsiveness occurs frequently in either disorder. Cellular and biochemical assessments reveal inflammation and immunological derangements. The therapeutic pharmacologic armamentarium is very similar. Consequently, some investigators have surmised that asthma and COPD may share common pathophysiologic origins. As Bleecker suggests in [16], although the concepts of the Dutch hypothesis may be controversial, they have never been disproven and approaching these two diseases in a fashion that recognizes the possibility of similarities could pave the way for new approaches for both COPD and asthma.

Figure 3 illustrates the potential theoretical overlap among the obstructive lung diseases. The need to recognize overlap amongst asthma and COPD was highlighted by Gibson and Simpson [4] as the historical definitions of asthma and COPD are "limited because they do not fully depict the spectrum of obstructive airway disease that is seen in clinical practice. In particular, now that accelerated decline in lung function is recognized to occur in asthma, especially in those with asthma who smoke and COPD is increasingly considered to be a treatment-responsive disease, there is a need to re-evaluate the concept of asthma and COPD as separate conditions, and to consider situations when they may coexist, or when one condition may evolve into the other."

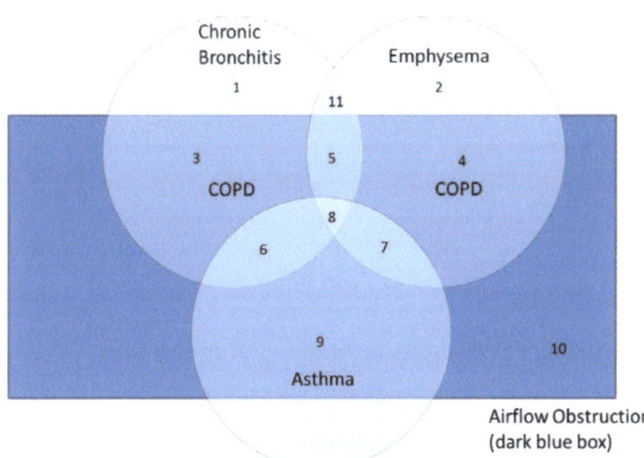

Figure 3. Overlapping of Obstructive Lung Diseases, reproduced from [3]. This non-proportional Venn diagram shows subsets of patients with chronic bronchitis, COPD, emphysema, and asthma and their intersection with airflow obstruction or airflow limitation (AFL) and each other. Patients with asthma whose airflow obstruction is reversible (normalizing) (subset 9), are not considered to have COPD. In many cases it is virtually impossible to differentiate patients with asthma whose airflow obstruction does not remit completely from persons with chronic bronchitis or COPD who have partially reversible (normalizing) airflow obstruction with airway hyperreactivity. Thus, some patients with unremitting asthma are classified as having COPD as shown by subsets 6, 7 and 8. Emphysema with AFL and chronic bronchitis with AFL comprise COPD patients, and are depicted in the darker circles labeled as subsets 3 and 4. Chronic bronchitis and emphysema with airflow obstruction often occur together as seen in subset 5, and some patients may have asthma associated with these two disorders as in subset 8. Individuals with asthma exposed to chronic irritation, as from cigarette smoke, may develop chronic productive cough, a feature of chronic bronchitis shown in subset 6. Such patients are often referred to in the United States as having asthmatic bronchitis or the asthmatic form of COPD. Persons with chronic bronchitis or emphysema without airflow obstruction, shown by subsets 1,2,11, are not classified as having COPD.

4. Phenotypic intersection – Clinical, physiologic, and inflammatory similarities and distinctions

4.1. Clinical – Asthma phenotypes and the 5th cluster

Moore and colleagues [7] categorized a large portion of the severe asthma research program (SARP) population into 5 distinct phenotypic groups based upon cluster analysis (see Table 1). The 5th cluster had more fixed airways obstruction (non-normalizing) with little bronchodilator responsivity, similar to the physiologic profile of a more classically defined COPD patient. This type of phenotypic approach to asthma may better suit some refractory asthma patients who require more tailored and individualized therapy [17-21].

Cluster 1 – 15% of participants	Atopic, mostly younger females with onset of asthma in childhood, with normal lung function and infrequent healthcare utilization or hospitalizations
Cluster 2 – 44% of participants	Atopic, mostly females, mostly older adults, with onset of asthma in childhood, with normal lung function and more asthma medication usage than cluster 1
Cluster 3 – 8% of participants	Non-Atopic, mostly females over the age of 50 with onset of asthma in adulthood and obese with body mass index >30, some decreased lung function, abundant asthma medication usage and corticosteroid usage with the most healthcare utilization and hospitalizations that appeared to be out of proportion to the degree of decreased lung function
Cluster 4 – 17% of participants	Atopic, equal males and females with onset of asthma in childhood and the most severe decline in lung function with most meeting a severe asthma definition and with only some bronchodilator responsivity on lung function testing
Cluster 5 – 16% of participants	Less Atopic, mostly females, with onset of asthma in childhood with most meeting a severe asthma definition and with worst lung function of all clusters and little bronchodilator responsivity

Table 1. Five Asthma Phenotypes Classified Using Cluster Analysis, adapted from [7].

4.2. Clinical – COPD phenotypes and the need for GOLD criteria revision in 2011

Not all COPD patients are alike. Some require oxygen and some do not. Some require one maintenance inhaler whereas others require three. Some have 2 or more exacerbations per year and some have few or no exacerbations. How can one account for these distinct differences in patient presentation or phenotype?

Prior to 2011, the GOLD guidelines [9] categorized COPD severity based solely upon physiologic criteria, especially the reduction in the FEV1. COPD patients are not always the same and carry different risk factors for worsening lung function and exacerbations. These concepts, that physiology does not adequately define groups of patients with similar therapeutic requirements and not all COPD patients are the same, were addressed by creating new GOLD classifications. In 2011, the use of level of lung dysfunction and airways obstruction continued, but further categorization based upon clinical symptoms as well as healthcare utilization or risk were added to the classification scheme, as seen in Figure 1. Patients are classified into four groups, A, B, C, and D based upon these three factors. Group A patients have better lung function, fewer symptoms, and lower risk for hospitalization. Group B patients have better lung function and lower risk for hospitalization but more symptoms; Group C patients have more impaired lung function and higher risk but are less symptomatic; and Group D patients have more impaired lung function, more symptoms, and greater risk for hospitalization. By restructuring the classification system, COPD patients can now be seen as a range of potentially diverse populations, with some patients not experiencing many symptoms or risk, whereas other COPD patients have greater risk of exacerbations and symptoms and will be treated more aggressively. In summary, the phenotypic differences between more symptomatic and/ or higher exacerbation risk coupled with physiologic function, are being used to not only categorize COPD patients but also guide therapeutic management.

The current GOLD classification scheme has progressed significantly beyond the historical labeling of patients with COPD as "pink puffers" or "blue bloaters." These descriptions may have addressed the physiologic differences between emphysema and chronic bronchitis patients, but these phenotypic descriptions did not translate into standardized approaches for medication usage or therapeutic management. The four phenotypes described in GOLD 2011 [9] now enable the patient's care team to choose therapeutic options based on level of pulmonary physiologic function, risk of exacerbation/healthcare utilization, and level of symptoms. Although still maintaining a stepped care approach, the use of phenotypic categories suggests therapies directed at reducing specific needs manifested by individuals within each category. The risk of exacerbations and significant lung function deterioration that can accompany them are now targeted and higher risk patients could have more access to novel therapies such as Phosphodiesterase-type 4 (PDE-4) inhibitors or chronic antibiotics like azithromycin as options to reduce their risk of COPD exacerbations [22, 23].

4.3. Airways inflammation: Often different but present in both, and sometimes similar amongst asthma & COPD

Both asthma and COPD are diseases of airway inflammation. In asthma, the inflammatory cells and cytokines include CD4+T-helper cell lymphocytes, eosinophils, and IL 4,5,10, and 13 along with GM-CSF and TNF-alpha whereas in COPD, the inflammatory profile usually consists of CD8+T-lymphocytes, neutrophils, and CD68+monocytes/macrophages [24]. Some investigators have divided asthma into eosinophilic and non-eosinophilic categories [25] emphasizing that non-eosinophilic asthma is a unique phenotype. Although there are significant differences in the inflammatory components encountered in asthma and COPD [24, 26], some asthmatics have a more neutrophil predominant inflammatory profile [27]. In contrast with these differences in the inflammatory components of asthma and COPD, there are some similar findings that occur in asthmatic and COPD patients who have fixed airways obstruction. Jeffrey [28] notes that remodeling and inflammation occur in both asthma and COPD and there are often major distinct differences in inflammation in the airways for COPD and asthma. However, these differences are most apparent when "nonsmoking patients with asthma and smokers with COPD from polar ends of the spectrum of "reversibility" (normalization) are compared" and as "disease becomes severe and the use of corticosteroids increases, the patterns of inflammation become more similar, mainly because of increases of neutrophils in both asthma and COPD"[28]. Further similarities in inflammatory patterns between asthma and COPD include:

- Distinct subpopulations of individuals with COPD and chronic bronchitis have a thickened reticular basement membrane (RBM) and bronchoalveolar lavage (BAL) eosinophilia that are similar to what is seen in the chronic inflammatory changes of asthma [29]. The RBM is thicker than normal in this subset of COPD patients who were smokers and showed significant airflow reversibility after 14 days of oral steroid therapy [29]. RBM thickening is usually considered a hallmark of severe asthma [30].

- The structural and inflammatory profiles observed in this subset of patients with COPD and a thickened RBM and BAL eosinophilia make the distinction between asthma and COPD less clear.

- Airway smooth muscle is increased both in COPD and asthma but the location of the smooth muscle hypertrophy and enlargement may differ [31]. Airway smooth muscle enlargement is also found in COPD but usually more in the smaller airways.

- The eosinophil has been a longstanding chronic inflammatory cell in asthma, whereas eosinophils in COPD appear to be more active during acute exacerbations of COPD [24, 28]. It has been postulated that the slight increase of eosinophils encountered in stable COPD perhaps do not degranulate [32].

As stated above there are stark contrasts in airway structure and inflammation in COPD and asthma yet the question remains: why do striking similarities exist between the two as well? As mentioned, the increase in airway smooth muscle mass that is observed ubiquitously in asthmatics can be seen in COPD patients, and the eosinophil appears to be a critical inflammatory cell in both diseases, albeit in COPD, its most significant role may be during acute exacerbations. Furthermore, it is interesting to see that there are some COPD patients who appear to have an inflammatory and airway structure profile that is more consistent with the classic findings of asthma. Perhaps these findings explain why we see benefits of inhaled steroids for some COPD patients. Compared with placebo, corticosteroids improve the outcomes of COPD patients hospitalized for acute exacerbations and decrease readmission rates [33]. In addition, the TORCH investigators [34] showed that inhaled corticosteroids reduced exacerbation rates and improved the health status of COPD patients. The similarities in airways inflammation and pathobiology seen in COPD and asthma may account for the clinical improvements associated with inhaled corticosteroids in COPD patients. We now see that the mainstay of therapy for asthma, inhaled corticosteroids, may improve outcomes in COPD patients. That is, a medication historically reserved for asthmatics is now widely used for COPD patients. Later in part 6 of this chapter, we will investigate this cross-treatment of COPD and asthma further.

5. How can an asthmatic evolve to chronic obstruction indistinguishable from COPD?

Airways remodeling in asthma can lead to more fixed, irreversible (non-normalizing) airways obstruction [13, 35]. Airways remodeling is a series of events that include structural and inflammatory changes that lead to fixed airways obstruction. Critical events in this pathway include reticular basement membrane (RBM) thickening, airway smooth muscle (ASM) hyperplasia and hyperreactivity, loss of ciliated epithelial cells, goblet cell (GC) hyperplasia and increased mucous production, as well as fibroblast and myofibroblast activation [35]. When extensive airway remodeling occurs, asthmatics can appear clinically and physiologically as if they had COPD with fixed, non-normalizing airways obstruction. Recent studies suggest that airway remodeling and airway smooth muscle (ASM) hyperplasia and hypertrophy occur at an early age, possibly even preceding the diagnosis of asthma and clinical symptoms [31, 36]. These studies suggest that reticular basement membrane thickening can occur even in childhood [37] and corroborate earlier investigations that showed that the lung function decline in some asthmatics occurred early in childhood, and not progressively throughout adulthood [38]. Thus, airway remodeling may precede both the clinical manifestations of asthma and the inflammation triggered by allergen exposure. The subsequent inflammation intensifies the remodeling process and leads to fixed airways obstruction in early adulthood. Thus, it seems plausible that the subset of asthma patients who have fixed obstruction may have defects in ASM regulatory mechanisms and that ASM hyperplasia may be an "early life event."For these individuals, the inflammation and ensuing asthma accentuates basement membrane dysregulation and ultimately leads to fixed airways obstruction in young asthma patients [31, 36-38].

6. Novel treatment paradigms: Asthma drugs treat COPD and vice-versa

According to current guidelines, inhaled corticosteroids (ICS) are the cornerstone and first line therapy of persistent asthma while long acting beta (LABA) agonists and long acting anti-muscarinic (LAMA) agents are first line therapy for COPD patients [9, 14, 15]. Despite this paradigm of "inhaled steroids first in asthma and long acting bronchodilators first in COPD", inhaled corticosteroids can be helpful for some COPD patients and long acting bronchodilators are commonly used as step up therapy in asthma when ICS therapy does not control symptoms alone. In addition, systemic corticosteroids are beneficial for the treatment of exacerbations of both diseases [9, 14, 15]. Recent investigations suggest that medications classically used for the treatment of asthma may be beneficial for COPD and pharmacologic treatments usually used for COPD may be advantageous in the management of some subpopulations of patients with asthma.

6.1. Asthma and anti-inflammatory medications used for COPD

Recent studies show that inhaled corticosteroids, the mainstay of asthma pharmacotherapy, improve multiple outcomes in individuals with COPD [9]. ICS can reduce the frequency of acute COPD exacerbations and improve respiratory health in patients with severe COPD [9, 34]. Although combined ICS and long acting beta agonist treatment slowed the reduction of lung function in individuals with COPD in the TORCH trial, these results have not been replicated in other trials [34, 39, 40]. However, as outlined in GOLD 2011 [9], inhaled corticosteroids have a significant role in the management of COPD, particularly for those at high risk for exacerbations and who are symptomatic despite long acting bronchodilator usage (GOLD class C,D). The summary of evidence [9, 34, 39-43] supporting the role of inhaled corticosteroids in the management of COPD includes the following:

- Long term treatment with inhaled steroids is recommended for patients with severe and very severe airflow limitation and for patients with frequent exacerbations not controlled by long acting bronchodilators.
- Inhaled steroids should be considered for GOLD class C and D patients.
- Long term monotherapy with inhaled steroids is not recommended in COPD as it is less effective than a combination of LABA and ICS together.

The inflammation present in COPD, for at least some COPD patients, appears to be helped by the addition of an inhaled steroid. Thus, historically labeled "asthma treatments" such as inhaled steroids may be beneficial for patients with COPD. Additionally, anti-leukotriene medications such as montelukast have shown some promise even in COPD patients as some authors propose that the inflammation in COPD can be a target of leukotriene receptor antagonist (LTRA) therapy. LTRA usage in elderly COPD patients appears to be safe and efficacious and may improve outcomes in respiratory health in this population [44, 45].

6.2. COPD and long-acting inhaler medications used for asthma

Alternatively, treatments that were relegated historically as mainstay therapy for COPD have also been used to treat asthma. Inhaled steroids are the principal treatment for persistent asthma, but for more severe asthmatics, LABA's are added to inhaled corticosteroids, similar to adding an inhaled corticosteroid to a LABA for a more severe COPD patient. LABAs are never used as monotherapy in asthma. However, combined LABA/ICS treatment is recommended for patients with severe asthma just as this combination is suggested therapy for patients with more severe COPD.

Based upon many trials, multiple guidelines identify inhaled corticosteroids as the recommended first line treatment for asthma [14, 15, 46]. LABA inhalers are effective as step up therapy, particularly in those asthmatics not controlled with inhaled corticosteroids alone [47, 48]. LABAs are indeed used in asthma; however, due to the risk of LABA monotherapy in asthma [49], these agents are recommended only for step up therapy in those asthmatics not controlled with an inhaled corticosteroid alone [14, 15]. Thus, LABAs can be used in both COPD and asthma, although for COPD they are first line therapeutic options and for asthma they are recommended only as add-on therapy choices in addition to inhaled corticosteroids. LABAs are not first line therapy for asthma. Inhaled corticosteroid and LABA combination therapy is recommended for both asthmatics and COPD patients with more severe disease [9, 14, 15].

http://dx.doi.org/10.5772/58234

What about long acting muscarinic antagonist usage (LAMA) or long acting anticholinergic (LAch) therapy in asthma? Recent studies show that treatment of severe asthmatics with a LAMA can reduce exacerbations and improve airflow obstruction [50]. In patients with asthma that is inadequately controlled with ICS, addition of a LAMA improves lung function and symptoms and is equivalent to the addition of a LABA [51]. Caution, however, has been advised by some authors including Bel [52], stating that the use of LAMAs and antimuscarinic agents may best be reserved for those asthma patients who have fixed airflow obstruction as evidenced by baseline FEV1/FVC ratios of <0.70.

Table 2 describes and summarizes some of these trials which have shown cross-therapy choices for asthma and COPD.

Trial & Reference	Medications Used/Disease	Summary of Meaningful Findings
TALC [51]	LAMA (tiotropium) use in asthma	Tiotopium as effective as long acting bronchodilator for uncontrolled asthmatics
Tiotropium added to asthmatics poorly controlled on LABA/ICS [50]	LAMA (tiotropium) use in asthma	LAMA use decreased exacerbations in severe asthmatics and showed minimal improvement in FEV1
Long-term montelukast in moderate to severe COPD [44, 45]	LTRA use in COPD	LTRA use appears safe and efficacious and may improve respiratory symptom control and exacerbations, particularly for elderly moderate to severe COPD patients
Meta-Analyses for ICS usage in more severe COPD or COPD with higher risk of exacerbations [41-43]	ICS for COPD	ICS reduce the risk of exacerbations, with an emphasis placed on more severe COPD patients
TORCH [34]	ICS for COPD	ICS therapy decreases exacerbations and modestly slows the progression of respiratory symptoms in COPD; possible or minimal impact found on lung function and mortality somewhat unique to TORCH trial.
UPLIFT [53]	Triple Therapy with LAMA, LABA and ICS for COPD patients	Suggests additive benefit to triple inhaler therapy for more advanced COPD patients

Abbreviations: *LTRA*-leukotriene receptor antagonist, *LAMA*-long acting muscarinic antagonist, *LABA*-long acting beta agonist, *ICS*-inhaled corticosteroid, *FEV1*-forced expiratory volume in 1 second, *COPD*-chronic obstructive pulmonary disease

Table 2. Summary of Novel Approaches Where Cross-Disease Therapeutic Options Have Shown Benefit.

7. Conclusion

We began this chapter with the question: are asthma and COPD completely distinct diseases or is there some degree of overlap? In response, we conclude that they are separate entities that are treated and approached in unique ways for the most part; however, for subpopulations of individuals with asthma or COPD, there is considerable clinical, physiologic, and inflammatory profile overlap. These disorders are syndromes defined by constellations of clinical, historical, physical examination, physiological, and inflammatory features. Recent investigations suggest that there are numerous subcategories of asthma and COPD and that some of these subcategories may have significant similarities.

Thus, COPD and asthma may coexist or overlap in individual patients or within specific phenotypic categories. Both diseases are characterized by airways inflammation and sometimes cannot be distinguished clinically. The physiologic differences between asthma and COPD are further confused by ambiguous use of reversibility to mean either responsiveness to bronchodilators or normalization of lung function. Historically, asthma has been associated with AFL that normalizes and returns to predicted levels with therapy whereas, in COPD, lung function progressively declines and no treatment has been shown to return it to predicted levels. However, there is a subpopulation of asthmatics that develop fixed AFL and despite treatment do not exhibit normalization of lung function.

Although the inflammatory profiles of asthma and COPD are traditionally considered to be distinct, more recent investigations and phenotypic categorizations suggest that there are populations of asthmatics with inflammatory profiles that are suggestive of COPD and some groups of patients with COPD may have inflammatory profiles that resemble those seen in asthma.

Although the principal guidelines for management of COPD and asthma are very different, considerable overlap in treatments does occur. Recent studies demonstrate that medications such as LAMAs that are traditionally used only for the treatment of COPD may be beneficial in patients with asthma and other drugs such as LTRAs that are usually only used for the treatment of asthma may be effective in patients with COPD. But, for most individuals with COPD or asthma, the initial treatment for COPD begins with maintenance long acting bronchodilators and for asthma with maintenance inhaled corticosteroids. Therefore, we feel that asthma and COPD can usually be addressed as separate entities but there are numerous times where the diseases and their treatments overlap.

In conclusion, it may be appropriate to approach some COPD patients as if they were more asthmatic, and some asthmatics as if they were more like COPD. The Dutch hypothesis suggesting that asthma and COPD may have common pathogenetic mechanisms is undergoing a resurgence as phenotypically distinct subpopulations of individuals with COPD and asthma are being identified. Although most of these subpopulations are distinct, some share similar clinical, physiologic, and inflammatory profiles. Finally, the therapeutic distinctions between asthma and COPD are blurring as medications traditionally used for one disorder are shown to be beneficial for the other. Ultimately, the goal is to develop therapeutic guidelines based upon a patient's phenotypic profile. As phenotypes become more descriptive, it may prove beneficial to categorize patients as "chronic obstructive asthma with fixed obstruction", or "COPD with asthmatic/more prominent eosinophilic airways inflammatory features", or "COPD with an allergic inflammatory component" to discern which COPD patients might benefit from inhaled corticosteroids or which asthmatics might improve with antimuscarinic bronchodilators.

Author details

Peter H. Lenz[1] and Ralph J. Panos[1,2]

1 Department of Pulmonary, Critical Care and Sleep Medicine, University of Cincinnati Medical Center, Cincinnati, Ohio, USA

2 Pulmonary, Critical Care, and Sleep Medicine, Cincinnati VAMC, Cincinnati, OH

References

[1] 2004 ATS/ERS Update on the standards for the diagnosis and treatment of patients with chronic obstructive pulmonary disease. Available from: http://thoracic.org/clinical/copd-guidelines/resources/copddoc.pdf.

[2] Barnes PJ, Shapiro SD, Pauwels RA. Chronic obstructive pulmonary disease: molecular and cellular mechanisms. The European respiratory journal. 2003;22(4):672-88.

[3] Standards for the diagnosis and care of patients with chronic obstructive pulmonary disease. American Thoracic Society 1995 [updated Nov; cited 152 5 Pt 2]. 1995/11/01: [S77-121].

[4] Gibson PG, Simpson JL. The overlap syndrome of asthma and COPD: what are its features and how important is it? Thorax. 2009;64(8):728-35.

[5] Carolan BJ, Sutherland ER. Clinical phenotypes of chronic obstructive pulmonary disease and asthma: recent advances. The Journal of allergy and clinical immunology. 2013;131(3):627-34; quiz 35.

[6] Barker BL, Brightling CE. Phenotyping the heterogeneity of chronic obstructive pulmonary disease. Clinical science (London, England : 1979). 2013;124(6):371-87.

[7] Moore WC, Meyers DA, Wenzel SE, Teague WG, Li H, Li X, et al. Identification of asthma phenotypes using cluster analysis in the Severe Asthma Research Program. American journal of respiratory and critical care medicine. 2010;181(4):315-23.

[8] Sluiter HJ, Koeter GH, de Monchy JG, Postma DS, de Vries K, Orie NG. The Dutch hypothesis (chronic non-specific lung disease) revisited. The European respiratory journal. 1991;4(4):479-89.

[9] Pocket Guide to COPD Diagnosis, Management, and Prevention 2011. Available from: http://www.goldcopd.org/uploads/users/files/GOLD_Pocket_May2512.pdf.

[10] Hanania NA, Celli BR, Donohue JF, Martin UJ. Bronchodilator reversibility in COPD. Chest. 2011;140(4):1055-63.

[11] Pellegrino R, Viegi G, Brusasco V, Crapo RO, Burgos F, Casaburi R, et al. Interpretative strategies for lung function tests. The European respiratory journal. 2005;26(5): 948-68.

[12] Lung function testing: selection of reference values and interpretative strategies. American Thoracic Society. The American review of respiratory disease. 1991;144(5): 1202-18.

[13] Lange P, Parner J, Vestbo J, Schnohr P, Jensen G. A 15-year follow-up study of ventilatory function in adults with asthma. The New England journal of medicine. 1998;339(17):1194-200.

[14] Guidelines for the Diagnosis and Management of Asthma, Summary Report 2007. Available from: http://www.nhlbi.nih.gov/guidelines/asthma/asthsumm.pdf.

[15] Global Strategy for Asthma Management and Prevention, Updated Summary 2012 2012. Available from: http://www.ginasthma.org/local/uploads/files/GINA_Report_March13.pdf.

[16] Bleecker ER. Similarities and differences in asthma and COPD. The Dutch hypothesis. Chest. 2004;126(2 Suppl):93S-5S; discussion 159S-61S.

[17] Miranda C, Busacker A, Balzar S, Trudeau J, Wenzel SE. Distinguishing severe asthma phenotypes: role of age at onset and eosinophilic inflammation. The Journal of allergy and clinical immunology. 2004;113(1):101-8.

[18] Wenzel SE, Schwartz LB, Langmack EL, Halliday JL, Trudeau JB, Gibbs RL, et al. Evidence that severe asthma can be divided pathologically into two inflammatory subtypes with distinct physiologic and clinical characteristics. American journal of respiratory and critical care medicine. 1999;160(3):1001-8.

[19] Green RH, Brightling CE, Bradding P. The reclassification of asthma based on subphenotypes. Current opinion in allergy and clinical immunology. 2007;7(1):43-50.

[20] Green RH, Brightling CE, Woltmann G, Parker D, Wardlaw AJ, Pavord ID. Analysis of induced sputum in adults with asthma: identification of subgroup with isolated sputum neutrophilia and poor response to inhaled corticosteroids. Thorax. 2002;57(10):875-9.

[21] The ENFUMOSA cross-sectional European multicentre study of the clinical phenotype of chronic severe asthma. European Network for Understanding Mechanisms of Severe Asthma. The European respiratory journal. 2003;22(3):470-7.

[22] Calverley PM, Rabe KF, Goehring UM, Kristiansen S, Fabbri LM, Martinez FJ. Roflumilast in symptomatic chronic obstructive pulmonary disease: two randomised clinical trials. Lancet. 2009;374(9691):685-94.

[23] Albert RK, Connett J, Bailey WC, Casaburi R, Cooper JA, Jr., Criner GJ, et al. Azithromycin for prevention of exacerbations of COPD. The New England journal of medicine. 2011;365(8):689-98.

[24] Jeffery PK. Comparison of the structural and inflammatory features of COPD and asthma. Giles F. Filley Lecture. Chest. 2000;117(5 Suppl 1):251s-60s.

[25] Berry M, Morgan A, Shaw DE, Parker D, Green R, Brightling C, et al. Pathological features and inhaled corticosteroid response of eosinophilic and non-eosinophilic asthma. Thorax. 2007;62(12):1043-9.

[26] Sutherland ER, Martin RJ. Airway inflammation in chronic obstructive pulmonary disease: comparisons with asthma. The Journal of allergy and clinical immunology. 2003;112(5):819-27; quiz 28.

[27] Simpson JL, Grissell TV, Douwes J, Scott RJ, Boyle MJ, Gibson PG. Innate immune activation in neutrophilic asthma and bronchiectasis. Thorax. 2007;62(3):211-8.

[28] Jeffery PK. Remodeling and inflammation of bronchi in asthma and chronic obstructive pulmonary disease. Proceedings of the American Thoracic Society. 2004;1(3):176-83.

[29] Chanez P, Vignola AM, O'Shaugnessy T, Enander I, Li D, Jeffery PK, et al. Corticosteroid reversibility in COPD is related to features of asthma. American journal of respiratory and critical care medicine. 1997;155(5):1529-34.

[30] Bourdin A, Neveu D, Vachier I, Paganin F, Godard P, Chanez P. Specificity of basement membrane thickening in severe asthma. The Journal of allergy and clinical immunology. 2007;119(6):1367-74.

[31] Stewart A. More muscle in asthma, but where did it come from? American journal of respiratory and critical care medicine. 2012;185(10):1035-7.

[32] Lacoste JY, Bousquet J, Chanez P, Van Vyve T, Simony-Lafontaine J, Lequeu N, et al. Eosinophilic and neutrophilic inflammation in asthma, chronic bronchitis, and chronic obstructive pulmonary disease. The Journal of allergy and clinical immunology. 1993;92(4):537-48.

[33] Niewoehner DE, Erbland ML, Deupree RH, Collins D, Gross NJ, Light RW, et al. Effect of systemic glucocorticoids on exacerbations of chronic obstructive pulmonary disease. Department of Veterans Affairs Cooperative Study Group. The New England journal of medicine. 1999;340(25):1941-7.

[34] Calverley PM, Anderson JA, Celli B, Ferguson GT, Jenkins C, Jones PW, et al. Salmeterol and fluticasone propionate and survival in chronic obstructive pulmonary disease. The New England journal of medicine. 2007;356(8):775-89.

[35] Limb SL, Brown KC, Wood RA, Wise RA, Eggleston PA, Tonascia J, et al. Irreversible lung function deficits in young adults with a history of childhood asthma. The Journal of allergy and clinical immunology. 2005;116(6):1213-9.

[36] James AL, Elliot JG, Jones RL, Carroll ML, Mauad T, Bai TR, et al. Airway smooth muscle hypertrophy and hyperplasia in asthma. American journal of respiratory and critical care medicine. 2012;185(10):1058-64.

[37] Barbato A, Turato G, Baraldo S, Bazzan E, Calabrese F, Panizzolo C, et al. Epithelial damage and angiogenesis in the airways of children with asthma. American journal of respiratory and critical care medicine. 2006;174(9):975-81.

[38] Phelan PD, Robertson CF, Olinsky A. The Melbourne Asthma Study: 1964-1999. The Journal of allergy and clinical immunology. 2002;109(2):189-94.

[39] Burge PS, Calverley PM, Jones PW, Spencer S, Anderson JA, Maslen TK. Randomised, double blind, placebo controlled study of fluticasone propionate in patients with moderate to severe chronic obstructive pulmonary disease: the ISOLDE trial. BMJ (Clinical research ed). 2000;320(7245):1297-303.

[40] Effect of inhaled triamcinolone on the decline in pulmonary function in chronic obstructive pulmonary disease. The New England journal of medicine. 2000;343(26): 1902-9.

[41] Alsaeedi A, Sin DD, McAlister FA. The effects of inhaled corticosteroids in chronic obstructive pulmonary disease: a systematic review of randomized placebo-controlled trials. The American journal of medicine. 2002;113(1):59-65.

[42] Gartlehner G, Hansen RA, Carson SS, Lohr KN. Efficacy and safety of inhaled corticosteroids in patients with COPD: a systematic review and meta-analysis of health outcomes. Annals of family medicine. 2006;4(3):253-62.

[43] Yang IA, Clarke MS, Sim EH, Fong KM. Inhaled corticosteroids for stable chronic obstructive pulmonary disease. The Cochrane database of systematic reviews. 2012;7:Cd002991.

[44] Celik P, Sakar A, Havlucu Y, Yuksel H, Turkdogan P, Yorgancioglu A. Short-term effects of montelukast in stable patients with moderate to severe COPD. Respiratory medicine. 2005;99(4):444-50.

[45] Rubinstein I, Kumar B, Schriever C. Long-term montelukast therapy in moderate to severe COPD--a preliminary observation. Respiratory medicine. 2004;98(2):134-8.

[46] Haahtela T, Jarvinen M, Kava T, Kiviranta K, Koskinen S, Lehtonen K, et al. Comparison of a beta 2-agonist, terbutaline, with an inhaled corticosteroid, budesonide, in newly detected asthma. The New England journal of medicine. 1991;325(6):388-92.

[47] Pauwels RA, Lofdahl CG, Postma DS, Tattersfield AE, O'Byrne P, Barnes PJ, et al. Effect of inhaled formoterol and budesonide on exacerbations of asthma. Formoterol

and Corticosteroids Establishing Therapy (FACET) International Study Group. The New England journal of medicine. 1997;337(20):1405-11.

[48] Faurschou P, Steffensen I, Jacques L. Effect of addition of inhaled salmeterol to the treatment of moderate-to-severe asthmatics uncontrolled on high-dose inhaled steroids. European Respiratory Study Group. The European respiratory journal. 1996;9(9):1885-90.

[49] Nelson HS, Weiss ST, Bleecker ER, Yancey SW, Dorinsky PM. The Salmeterol Multicenter Asthma Research Trial: a comparison of usual pharmacotherapy for asthma or usual pharmacotherapy plus salmeterol. Chest. 2006;129(1):15-26.

[50] Kerstjens HA, Engel M, Dahl R, Paggiaro P, Beck E, Vandewalker M, et al. Tiotropium in asthma poorly controlled with standard combination therapy. The New England journal of medicine. 2012;367(13):1198-207.

[51] Peters SP, Kunselman SJ, Icitovic N, Moore WC, Pascual R, Ameredes BT, et al. Tiotropium bromide step-up therapy for adults with uncontrolled asthma. The New England journal of medicine. 2010;363(18):1715-26.

[52] Bel EH. Tiotropium for asthma--promise and caution. The New England journal of medicine. 2012;367(13):1257-9.

[53] Tashkin DP, Celli B, Senn S, Burkhart D, Kesten S, Menjoge S, et al. A 4-year trial of tiotropium in chronic obstructive pulmonary disease. The New England journal of medicine. 2008;359(15):1543-54.

Chapter 3

Alpha-1 Antitrypsin Deficiency — A Missed Opportunity in COPD?

Tomás P. Carroll, M. Emmet O'Brien, Laura T. Fee,
Kevin Molloy, Blair Murray, Seshma Ramsawak,
Oisín McElvaney, Catherine O'Connor and
Noel G. McElvaney

Additional information is available at the end of the chapter

http://dx.doi.org/10.5772/58602

1. Introduction

The abundant serum protein alpha-1 antitrypsin (AAT) is the prototype chronic obstructive pulmonary disease (COPD) biomarker. AAT is an antiprotease which inhibits neutrophil-derived proteases and protects the fragile tissues of the lung. Absence of this key antiprotease renders the lung susceptible to proteolytic degradation. Alpha-1 antitrypsin deficiency (AATD) is a hereditary disorder characterised by low circulating levels of alpha-1 antitrypsin (AAT). The lung disease associated with the condition is characterized by neutrophil-dominated airway inflammation and elevated intra-pulmonary protease levels [1]. The SERPINA1 gene encodes for the AAT protein and the most common SERPINA1 mutation known to cause AATD is the Z mutation. The classic case of AATD is an individual homozygous for the Z mutation which causes a severe deficiency of circulating AAT. Intuitively, severe AATD is a proven genetic risk factor for the development of lung and less frequently, liver disease. The condition was previously estimated to play a causative role in approximately 1-2% of COPD cases [2]. However, when intermediate deficiency is included in any evaluation of the contribution of AATD to lung disease, we anticipate that this figure can rise to as high as 10%. Guidelines published by the World Health Organisation (WHO), the American Thoracic Society (ATS), and the European Respiratory Society (ERS) advocate a targeted screening approach for the detection of AATD. Together these organisations recommend testing for AATD in all individuals with COPD regardless of age or smoking history [3, 4]. Despite the clear and significant benefits of correct identification, AATD remains an under-diagnosed condition with the majority of cases undetected or misdiagnosed as COPD. Less than 10% of ZZ individuals have been correctly identified in Ireland and the same is true in many other countries [5]. In addition, long delays between the presentation of first symptoms and correct diagnosis are commonplace [6]. A diagnosis of AATD can present the doctor and the affected individual with a unique opportunity for early medical intervention and the prevention or postponement of COPD. This is an opportunity that, if seized, has enormous benefits for the affected individual and extended family relatives. This chapter aims to provide healthcare professionals with an overview of AATD and with clinically relevant information to assist them in the recognition, diagnosis, and management of this rarely diagnosed hereditary condition. It is our hope that this information can help counteract the nihilism related to AATD and the reluctance to test that can sometimes exist.

2. What is alpha-1 antitrypsin?

2.1. Clinical manifestations & presentation of AATD

To understand the deficiency, one must first understand the protein. Alpha-1 antitrypsin (AAT) is a 52 kDa glycosylated plasma protein. It belongs to a group of serine protease inhibitors and is encoded by the SERPINA1 gene on chromosome 14q32.1-32.3 [7]. Production of circulating AAT is predominantly the liver and the normal plasma concentration of AAT is 1.5 g/L (1.0-2.0 g/L) with a half-life of 4–5 days [8]. Production of AAT protein has also been shown in other cells such as monocytes, macrophages, pulmonary alveolar cells and intestinal epithelial cells [9-12], hinting at an important role in the local response to tissue inflammation. AAT is an acute phase protein and plasma levels can rise two to five fold in response to cytokine release (e.g. TNF-α, IL-1 and IL-6) during infection or inflammation [13, 14] with local concentrations at sites of inflammation reaching even higher levels [15].

The association of an absent alpha-globulin band on serum plasma electrophoresis with a possible hereditary form of pulmonary emphysema was first reported by Laurell and Eriksson in 1963 [16]. The observation that these individuals were susceptible to a severe form of hereditary emphysema led to a major breakthrough in our understanding of the role of protease-antiprotease imbalance in the pathogenesis of COPD [17]. Subsequently it was also discovered that people with AATD were also at risk of liver cirrhosis [18]. In the absence of familial or population screening for AATD the majority of people present with clinical symptoms, often at a stage where significant morbidity from the condition has already developed.

2.2. Pulmonary manifestations

Adults with AATD are susceptible to the premature development of lung diseases such as emphysema, chronic bronchitis, bronchiectasis, and asthma. Patients with AATD usually present with exertional breathlessness, wheeze, cough, and frequent pulmonary exacerbations often, but not exclusively with a background history of smoking [19]. Symptoms usually begin from the age of 30 and the clinical suspicion for underlying asthma or chronic obstructive pulmonary disease (COPD) prompts referral for spirometric assessment. The finding of reversibility on spirometry is common (approximately 50%) and often belies concomitant asthma and emphysema. Reversibility can be associated with a worse prognosis, possibly due to ongoing airway inflammation [19, 20]. The diagnosis of fixed airway obstruction in AATD, indicative of COPD, is often made at a much younger age (<40 years) than the general population. However, screening for AATD is recommended for all adults with COPD or incompletely reversible asthma [4]. Analysis of the Danish AATD registry data of index and non-index cases indicates that the median life expectancy in ZZ homozygotes is reduced dramatically from 69 years to 49 years in smokers compared to non-smokers, and baseline forced expiratory volume in 1 second (FEV1) was the single most important predictor of survival [21, 22]. Cigarette smoke exposure in AATD results in severe impairment of lung function and an accelerated decline in lung function, and affected individuals should be counselled to stop smoking immediately. Occupational exposure to chemicals and pollutants is also independently associated with a decline in lung function in AATD and patients should be advised of using personal protective respiratory equipment where necessary [23, 24].

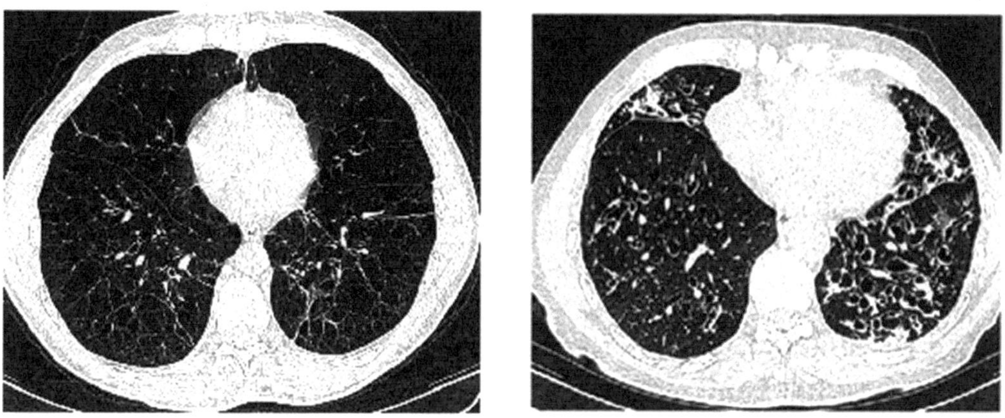

Figure 1. HRCT findings in ZZ individuals with emphysema (left) and bronchiectasis (right).

The classic pathological finding of bibasal panacinar emphysema can be now readily visualised with the widespread availability of high resolution computed tomography (HRCT) imaging, and the unexpected detection of these changes should prompt the clinician to screen for AATD. CT imaging with lung densitometry measurement facilitates monitoring of disease progression in AATD [25] and may be a superior outcome measure to change in FEV1 in clinical trials examining the effect of augmentation therapy in AATD [26]. CT imaging also permits the identification of bronchiectasis, which may or may not be clinically significant. The reported prevalence of bronchiectasis varies considerably but may occur independently of emphysema and can be severe [27, 28]. Symptoms of bronchiectasis are often difficult to distinguish from COPD and the prevalence and impact of this airway disease in AATD may be underestimated.

2.3. Liver manifestations

A small proportion of ZZ homozygotes present with a neonatal hepatitis syndrome, usually within the first 3-4 months of life. AATD is one of the commonest causes for neonatal hepatitis and can account for up to 29% of cases in some paediatric centres [29]. A large infant screening study of 200,000 newborns identified 120 with the ZZ phenotype, 22 (18.3%) had evidence of a hepatic abnormality. Of this cohort, 14 (11.7%) had prolonged obstructive jaundice and 9 (7.5%) had severe clinical liver disease [30]. The SZ phenotype is also associated with biochemical liver abnormalities, and can lead to end-stage liver disease requiring transplantation, although this is observed less frequently than in ZZ cohorts [31]. A number of risk factors for AATD associated liver disease in childhood have been identified including male gender, renal or pulmonary complications [29], and a first degree relative with AATD-related liver disease [32]. The reported outcomes of childhood liver disease are variable, with one study reporting mortality of 20/74 (27%) and persistent cirrhosis in a similar number [32], although most studies report complete clinical and biochemical recovery of liver function in the majority of cases [29].

Data from the Irish National AATD Registry allowed an investigation of the prevalence of liver abnormalities in a cohort of 115 ZZ individuals (Table 1). A total of 36% had liver function test (LFT) abnormalities on the first assessment, most commonly alanine aminotransferase (ALT), and this did not correlate with increasing age. A further 24% (30/115) were found to have abnormal liver findings by radiology. Fatty infiltration was the most common radiological finding (17%) after examination of abdominal ultrasound results, followed by cirrhosis, liver cysts, and haemangioma. No differences in body mass index (BMI) or alcohol consumption were observed in those with or without liver abnormalities which suggests the frequency of fatty liver was not due to increased obesity or alcohol but more likely to be attributable to the accumulation of Z AAT protein in the liver.

	Total ZZ	**Abnormal Ultrasound**
No. of subjects	115	30
Gender (M/F)	62/53	20/10
Age, years (mean +/- SD)	52+/- 12	44 +/- 11
Mean FEV1 (% predicted)	65 +/- 33	50 +/- 28
Mean BMI	26.5	27.4
Alcohol (total respondents)	80	21
Active	61	17
Past	4	1
Never	15	3

Table 1. Liver abnormality findings in ZZ cohort on Irish National AATD Registry.

In adulthood, a strong relation between AATD and cirrhosis has been reported (OR=7.8; CI 2.4 to 24.7) and primary liver cancer (OR=20; CI 3.5 to 114.3), particularly affecting men [33]. Cirrhosis is usually complicated by portal hypertension, ascites, gastrointestinal bleeding, spontaneous bacterial peritonitis, hepatic encephalopathy, and hepatocellular carcinoma. The prevalence of liver cirrhosis increases with age and usually occurs in those who have never smoked, perhaps as a consequence of the prolonged survival in this group [4, 34]. Both genetic and environmental modifiers play a role in the pathogenesis of liver disease in AATD. Reports of putative candidate modifier genes for AATD-related liver disease have emerged [35-37], however, no specific gene or polymorphism has been conclusively demonstrated to have clinical utility and prognostic value. In addition, the high prevalence of MZ phenotypes in liver disease cohorts and the role of heterozygous AATD in worsening liver disease has been highlighted by several studies [38-40]. Thankfully, the natural history of those with fulminant AATD related liver disease has been dramatically altered by liver transplantation [41] and excellent survival rates have been achieved in adult and paediatric transplant recipients [31, 42].

2.4. Extra-pulmonary manifestations

The rare occurrence of recurrent panniculitis has been noted in individuals with AATD and is thought to relate to persistent neutrophilic inflammation at the affected sites [43]. A number of case reports have reported the panniculitis to be responsive to intravenous augmentation therapy [44-46]. AATD has been associated with a variety of other medical conditions, the best described being ANCA-associated vasculitis and in particular granulomatosis with polyangiitis (GPA). A recent genome wide association study identified the Z allele of SERPINA1 to be associated with Proteinase 3 (PR3)-ANCA positivity [47]. PR3 is inhibited by AAT and some case reports of PR3-ANCA vasculitis in ZZ homozygotes report a severe disease phenotype [48, 49]. The role of AAT in diseases of the circulatory system is incompletely understood. Oxidised AAT can bind to the Apolipoprotein B100 component of LDL in the circulation and may contribute to atherogenesis [50], additionally the cleaved C36 peptide fragment of AAT has been found complexed within atherosclerotic plaques indicating a role in monocyte recruitment within the intima of arterial walls [51]. AAT complexes with IgA were found in the joints and sera of patients with rheumatoid arthritis [52, 53] though there appears to be no strong link between the two conditions [54]. A recent development is the association of diabetes mellitus with low AAT levels [55] and the emerging scientific data demonstrating improved islet cell graft survival in mice transfected with human AAT [56]. However, it is too soon to determine if any sustained benefit can be achieved. Clinical trials are planned to investigate the efficacy of AAT augmentation therapy in diabetes (NCT01183455, NCT02093221).

2.5. AATD heterozygosity: A risk factor for COPD?

An accurate determination of the risk of COPD in AATD heterozygotes is vitally important given the large number of individuals who are potentially affected. We know MZ individuals have moderately reduced levels of AAT but clarifying the risk of COPD in this group has been controversial. The Irish National AATD Targeted Detection Programme has identified over

1,600 MZ individuals in the 12,000 individuals tested to date. While this heterozygote group does include cases identified through family screening, this means that approximately 1 in 8 individuals tested are MZ. Anecdotally, a significant number of MZ individuals from our AATD clinic, both smokers and non-smokers, develop COPD at a relatively young age. Approximately 250,000 individuals on the island of Ireland [5] and 6 million individuals in the United States possess the MZ genotype [57]. A deeper appreciation of the risk of COPD in heterozygotes could lead to the prevention or postponement of lung disease in this group, lessening the growing global healthcare burden of COPD.

During the past 40 years, over 100 studies have attempted to assess the risk of lung disease in MZ individuals. A meta-analysis by Hersh *et al* estimated that the combined odds ratio for COPD in MZ compared to MM individuals was 2.31. This risk was attenuated in studies which adjusted for cigarette smoke exposure [58]. An accurate determination of the risk of COPD has been fraught with difficulty. Many previous attempts to ascertain the contribution of MZ heterozygosity to the development of COPD have been met with various methodological and design flaws; most notably selection bias and inadequate control for cigarette smoke exposure. A recent study which aimed to clarify the risk of COPD in MZ heterozygotes has addressed many of the concerns which hampered an accurate risk estimate from previous attempts to answer this vitally important question. The issue of selection bias was addressed in the study design by using a family based approach. Index cases or probands were MZ individuals who had a confirmed diagnosis of COPD based on the following spirometric criteria: a post-bronchodilator FEV1/FVC ratio < 0.7 and an FEV1 (% predicted) < 80%. All first degree family members of the index case (probands) underwent AAT phenotyping, pre-and post-bronchodilator spirometry as well as completing the ATS-DLD Epidemiology Questionnaire. For the final analysis, the probands were excluded and the risk of COPD in the MM and MZ first degree relatives was determined. While the main strength of this study was elimination of ascertainment bias, additional strengths included the use of a genetically homogenous population, a standardised criterion for the diagnosis of COPD and adequate control for covariates including age, sex and cigarette smoke exposure. The adjusted odds ratio (OR) for COPD in MZ compared with MM group was 5.18 and this was higher (OR, 10.65) in ever-smoking individuals [59].

A significant gene-by-environment interaction exists to influence the development of COPD in MZ individuals. MZ individuals who have a low exposure to cigarette smoke (< 20 pack-years) have more airflow obstruction compared to MM individuals [59] in addition to more emphysema on quantitative analysis of chest CT scans [60]. This indicates that MZ heterozygosity and cigarette smoke exposure are a potent combination of risk factors in the pathogenesis of COPD. While these studies focused on direct exposure to cigarette smoke, the effect of passive cigarette smoke exposure and occupational exposure are less well defined. The MZ genotype in conjunction with cigarette smoke exposure modifies a MZ heterozygote's longitudinal decline in lung function following occupational exposure to vapours, dusts, fumes and gases [61]. An accurate estimate of the effect of passive cigarette smoke exposure on MZ individuals has yet to be determined but the harmful effect of environmental tobacco smoke was found to be greater in MZ schoolchildren [62].

http://dx.doi.org/10.5772/58602

The recent advances in our understanding of COPD risk in MZ individuals make it more important than ever to test individuals for AATD. Knowledge that the MZ genotype can significantly interact with environment to influence susceptibility to COPD is a powerful message and this should help deter heterozygotes from exposing themselves to potentially harmful environmental risk factors. The timely detection of at risk MZ individuals underpins the importance of diagnosing this condition early in order to reduce smoking initiation rates [63] and also increase smoking cessation [64].

2.6. AATD heterozygosity: A biological perspective

Analysis of sputum from non-smoking asymptomatic MZ individuals without evidence of airflow obstruction demonstrates increased neutrophil counts and IL-8 levels compared with MM individuals [65]. This indicates that the co-expression of the Z allele could have pro-inflammatory consequences. Harbouring the Z mutation may confer a survival advantage as the formation of polymers at sites of inflammation could potentially focus and amplify the immune response to aid the eradication of invading pathogens [66]. However, this advantage is abolished by environmental exposure to cigarette smoke via enhanced polymerization of the Z protein which potentiates a deleterious pro-inflammatory milieu in the AAT deficient lung, culminating in an increased risk of developing COPD [67].

The observed increased risk of COPD in MZ smokers challenges some of the underlying tenets of the protease-antiprotease theory. Given that MZ individuals have intermediate levels of circulating AAT, it is biologically plausible that an imbalance in pulmonary neutrophil elastase and a suboptimal protective level of AAT may be responsible for the observed increased risk of airflow obstruction and COPD in MZ heterozygotes. Reactive oxygen species in cigarette smoke can inactivate pulmonary AAT on the one hand and also promote a pro-inflammatory environment by increasing neutrophilic influx into the lung by the promotion of polymerisation of Z AAT on the other [68]. The biological mechanism by which cigarette smoke is presumed to enhance the risk of COPD in MZ heterozygotes is summarised in Figure 2.

The increased risk of COPD in MZ heterozygotes should lead to a reconsideration of what is the true protective threshold. This has implications not only for our understanding of the pathogenesis of COPD but also for AAT replacement therapy. Plasma purified AAT has been administered for almost 30 years by intravenous infusion to severe AATD individuals [69] with the aim of maintaining the plasma levels of AAT above the 11 μM level (approximately 0.56 g/l) throughout the duration of therapy [70]. The conflicting results and the paucity of clinical evidence for AAT replacement therapy [71] in severe AAT deficiency (ZZ) may be the result of targeting a sub-therapeutic threshold and augmenting the threshold to a higher MZ level may lead to improved treatment efficacy. The original threshold was based on mean AAT plasma concentration in the SZ phenotype as these individuals were thought to rarely develop COPD [72]. The SZ phenotype is more common than ZZ but studies in this area have been relatively few [73, 74]. However, an accurate determination of this risk would be very difficult as it would require a similar family based approach to that employed to determine the risk in MZ individuals including rigorous control for cigarette smoke exposure and a number of different patient groups encompassing the Z, S and M alleles. Until such information is

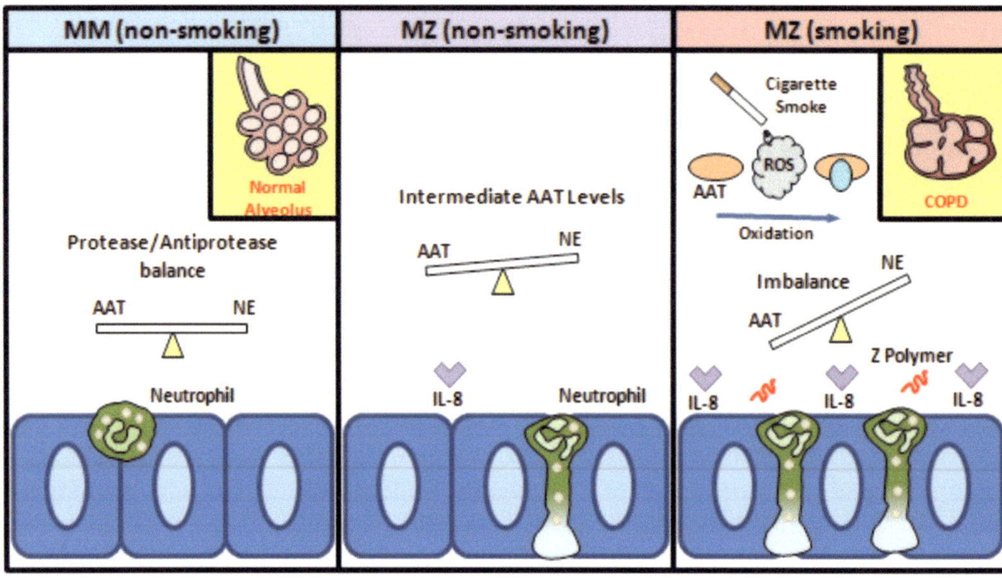

Figure 2. Pathogenesis of COPD in MZ heterozygotes. A normal protease/antiprotease balance exists in MM individuals (left panel). Non-smoking MZ individuals have intermediate levels of AAT and increased sputum IL-8 levels and neutrophil counts (middle panel). Reactive oxygen species in cigarette smoke inactivate AAT resulting in a protease/antiprotease imbalance with increased amounts of neutrophil elastase. Polymerisation of Z AAT protein and increased amounts of IL-8 increase neutrophil influx into the MZ lung. An overwhelmed anti-protease defence contributes to the development of COPD (right panel).

available it may be prudent to consider a new protective threshold as MZ individuals are not likely to develop lung disease in the absence of cigarette smoke exposure.

The emerging weight of evidence regarding the risk of COPD in MZ heterozygotes raises several important questions for further research. Firstly, what are the biological mechanisms by which cigarette smoking confers MZ heterozygotes with an increased risk of COPD? Secondly, in a longitudinal family based study, does the slope of lung function decline differ significantly between MZ and MM first degree relatives? What is the true protective threshold level of AAT and would increasing this threshold level result in greater therapeutic efficacy of AAT augmentation therapy?

2.7. When does AATD present – An Irish perspective

Trends in diagnosis and clinical presentation of severe AATD individuals in Ireland were recently investigated in a study of ZZ individuals enrolled in the Irish National AATD Registry. A total of 120 ZZ AATD individuals attending the national AATD centre completed a detailed questionnaire. For the entire group, the mean age of reported symptom onset was 37.8+/-1.6 years (range 0.03-80) while the mean age at diagnosis was 44.1+/-1.6 years (range 0.03-80). This leaves a mean interval between reported onset of first symptoms and diagnosis of AATD of 6.5+/-1.0 years (range 0 – 46). However, when subjects identified through family screening were excluded, the diagnostic delay increased to 8.5+/-1.2 years (range 1 – 46). In

http://dx.doi.org/10.5772/58602

addition, the average number of physicians seen by the entire group prior to a diagnosis of AATD was 3 (range 1 – 13). The findings are similar to data from other registries and reflect the diagnostic odyssey that individuals are often subjected to before a correct diagnosis is reached [6, 28, 75]. This further highlights the under-recognition of AATD that persists.

2.8. Who should be tested?

Guidelines published by the World Health Organisation (WHO) and the American Thoracic Society/European Respiratory Society (ATS/ERS) recommend the establishment of targeted screening programmes for the detection of individuals with AATD [3, 4]. In comparison to general population screening which can be more difficult and expensive to perform, targeted detection programmes offer a much higher rate of detection and are significantly more cost effective. The Irish National AATD Targeted Detection Programme began in 2004 and follows the ATS/ERS and WHO guidelines for the diagnosis of AATD. The ATS/ERS guidelines recommend targeted screening of patients with COPD, non-responsive asthma, cryptogenic liver disease and also first-degree relatives of known AATD individuals, termed type A recommendations (Table 2).

ATS/ERS Recommendations for Diagnostic Testing (Type A)
Adults with symptomatic emphysema or COPD (regardless of age or smoking history)
Adults with asthma with airflow obstruction that is incompletely reversible after aggressive treatment with bronchodilators
Asymptomatic individuals with persistent obstruction on pulmonary function tests with identifiable risk factors (e.g. cigarette smoking, occupational exposure)
Adults with necrotising panniculitis
Siblings of individuals with AATD
Individuals with unexplained liver disease, including neonates, children, and adults, particularly the elderly

Table 2. ATS/ERS recommendations for diagnostic testing for AATD (type A recommendations).

In addition to these groups, ATS/ERS guidelines also recommend testing should be considered in a number of other scenarios as outlined in table 3 (type B recommendations).

ATS/ERS Recommendations for Diagnostic Testing (Type B)
Adults with bronchiectasis without evident etiology
Adolescents with persistent airflow obstruction
Asymptomatic individuals with persistent airflow obstruction and no risk factors
Adults with C-ANCA-positive (anti-proteinase 3-positive) vasculitis

Table 3. ATS/ERS recommendations for diagnostic testing for AATD (type B recommendations).

3. How do we test for AATD?

The laboratory diagnosis of AATD is usually performed by following two steps; determination of AAT concentration in serum or plasma (quantitative) and identification of allelic variants by phenotyping or genotyping (qualitative) [76-78]. Quantification of AAT is generally the first investigation and has the advantages of being quick and relatively inexpensive. Clinically, a simple rule of thumb is the lower the level of AAT, the higher the risk of COPD. AAT quantification is routinely performed in most clinical chemistry, biochemistry, and immunology hospital laboratories. If quantification of AAT reveals a level below a pre-determined cut-off point or threshold (for example 1.0 g/l or 100 mg/dl) the sample should be automatically reflexed to phenotyping [79, 80]. This is the most cost-efficient and prudent algorithm. If necessary, genotyping using allele-specific PCR (usually to Z and S) and/or direct sequencing of the AAT gene can be performed either as a further investigation or on a complementary basis. The choice of using phenotyping or genotyping depends on resources available and the type of sample being referred, and there are advantages and disadvantages associated with both qualitative methods.

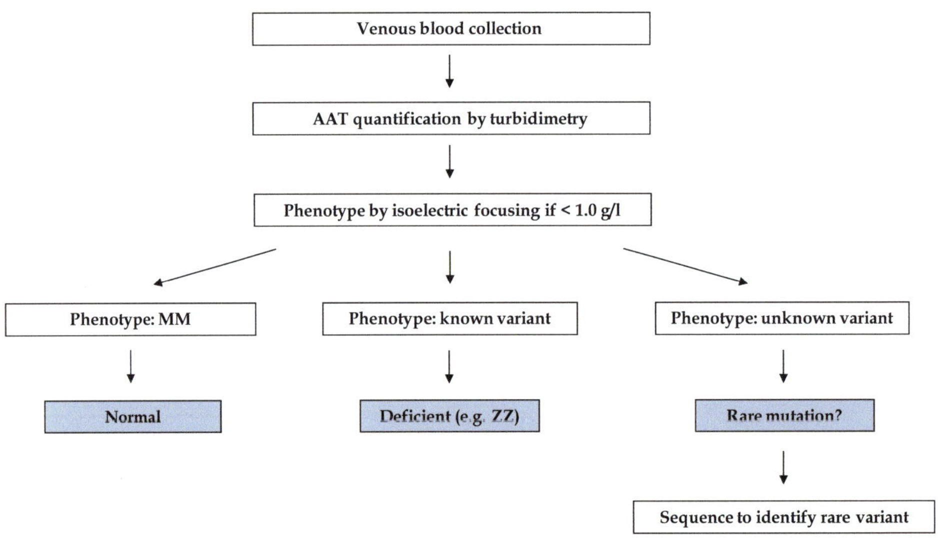

Figure 3. AATD diagnostic algorithm for whole blood, serum, and plasma in the Irish National AATD Targeted Detection Programme.

3.1. AAT quantification

AAT levels are measured routinely by immunoassay techniques such as nephelometry and turbidimetry, or less commonly by radial immunodiffusion [81, 82]. AAT levels measured in our centre are determined using immune turbidimetry on an Olympus AU540 analyser. The WHO and ATS/ERS guidelines recommend that AAT levels should be measured at least once in COPD patients. Although a substantial correlation between AAT phenotype and circulating

AAT concentrations has been established by several groups [70, 80, 83], confounding factors include normal intra-individual variation, depression of AAT production in liver disease, malnutrition, and the fact that AAT is an acute phase protein [84, 85]. Potential analytical variation may also occur; however, this variation is generally not significant. The increasing availability of external quality assurance schemes and accreditation programmes has led to improvements in testing accuracy, sensitivity, and reproducibility. In terms of which type of blood sample to use for AATD testing, a study by Miles *et al* in 2004 [86] which compared results from serum and heparinised plasma samples for 45 different chemistry tests addressed this concern. No statistically significant difference was observed in AAT concentrations measured in serum compared to plasma.

As an acute phase reactant, AAT levels are increased during the acute phase response, for example during infection or surgery [13]. Therefore, markers of inflammation such as CRP should be considered when assessing the concentration of AAT, and this has been discussed comprehensively elsewhere [87]. If CRP is indeed elevated, the quantification of AAT should be repeated once the acute phase response has subsided. The acute phase response will however, not result in a significant increase in AAT level in severe AATD (e.g. ZZ, Z/null). In contrast, AAT levels in heterozygotes (e.g. MZ, SZ) can be falsely elevated to levels similar to those observed in MM individuals, masking the underlying deficiency. For this reason, quantification of AAT levels alone is not a definitive test, and is no substitute for phenotype or genotype analysis, neither of which is affected by the acute phase.

Phenotype	Cases	Mean AAT (g/l +/- SEM)	Range AAT (g/l)
MS	1209	1.23 +/- 0.01	0.40 – 3.82
MZ	1657	0.91 +/- 0.01	0.44 – 4.08
SS	60	0.91 +/- 0.01	0.56 – 1.54
SZ	165	0.65 +/- 0.01	0.35 – 1.17
ZZ	219	0.25 +/- 0.001	0.11 – 0.61

Table 4. Mean AAT in deficient phenotypes identified in the Irish National AATD Targeted Detection Programme.

In the formulation of diagnostic algorithms for AATD the cut-off or threshold AAT value is critical to effective screening efforts and the identification of at risk individuals. A study by Donato *et al* in 2012 found a cut-off of 1.0 g/L was sufficient for the detection of severe (ZZ, Z/null) and intermediate AATD (e.g. MZ and SZ heterozygotes) [79]. Intermediate AATD has been an area of some controversy, with previous guidelines adopting stringently low cut-off values (for example 0.6 g/l) which would fail to detect large at risk populations of intermediate AATD. We know now that SZ and MZ individuals are also at risk of lung disease, particularly if they smoke [59, 74], and this knowledge has led to a change in diagnostic algorithms and increased the heterozygote detection rate. In light of the Donato study and our own data from screening 12,000 individuals we employ a cutoff point of 1.0 g/l at our centre as this is optimal for the detection of severe and intermediate AATD. Using this cut off value reduces laboratory costs and unnecessary testing, while maximising the detection of at risk individuals. An exception where a cut off value may not apply is when screening individuals due to a family history of AATD, as in this case it should be recommended the phenotype is checked regardless of AAT level.

3.2. AAT phenotyping

The ATS/ERS guidelines identify serum phenotyping as the 'gold standard' for the diagnosis of AATD. The qualitative detection and characterisation of AAT variants is carried out in our centre by isoelectric focusing followed by immunofixation using a kit which is the only FDA-approved method for AAT phenotype determination [88]. The isoelectric focusing (IEF) method on agarose gel has an added immunofixation step which utilises a specific antibody to AAT. This renders it superior to traditional IEF techniques due to its high resolution and reproducibility. IEF is also advantageous due to the fact it can easily detect rare and novel phenotypes. IEF identifies the various isoglycoforms and highlights the microheterogeneity of AAT in terms of carbohydrate side chains, but more importantly highlights the macroheterogeneity of AAT in terms of genetic variation. AAT phenotype is determined by comparison to three reference standards (e.g. MM, MS, and ZZ) and by visual inspection by a minimum of two independent observers. All IEF results are checked and correlated with the corresponding AAT levels. The recent publication of a reference compendium of known AAT phenotypes is a helpful resource for interpreting IEF migration patterns of AAT variants [89].

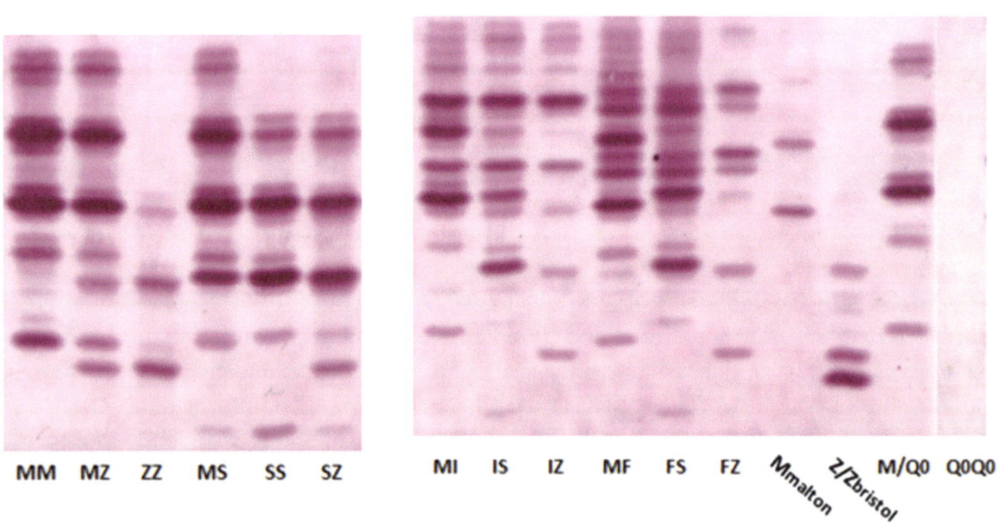

Figure 4. IEF migration pattern of common (left) and rare (right) AAT phenotypes identified in Ireland.

There are some cases in which analytical errors may occur using the IEF technique. Patients who are on augmentation therapy receive intravenous administration of purified AAT (isolated from MM donor individuals). The M variant will be detected in samples obtained from individuals receiving therapy and could result in discordant or unidentifiable migration patterns (e.g. a ZZ individual on therapy may appear MZ). Another error is possible with the presence of null mutations, which are a class of mutations characterised by a total absence of AAT secretion. Therefore, heterozygote null cases such as M/null, Z/null, S/null will appear as homozygous MM, ZZ, SS respectively [90, 91]. M/null and S/null phenotypes can be identified by the lower than expected AAT level. More difficult to identify are the Z/null phenotypes as the AAT level in ZZ compared to Z/null phenotypes is so low as to be practically indistinguishable. Similarly, caution must be taken with samples from individuals following a blood transfusion; this may also result in an incorrect diagnosis due to the possibility of the phenotype of the donor being present. If necessary genotyping using PCR and/or direct sequencing of the SERPINA1 gene can be achieved either in a complementary investigation to investigate discordant results or to identify rare and novel phenotypic variants.

3.3. AAT genotyping and sequencing

The adoption of dried blood spot (DBS) samples in an attempt to increase testing rates by making sampling easier, coupled with advances in molecular diagnostics, has resulted in the development of genotyping assays for AATD. Genotyping assays are commonly performed by melt curve analysis on real-time PCR instruments with primers and probes designed for specific mutations or less frequently by PCR-based restriction fragment length polymorphism (RFLP) analysis [92, 93], although RFLP methods have been replaced by the faster and more efficient melt curve methods. Allowing for the fact the DBS method has the convenience of allowing home testing and easier transportation of samples [94], in our centre we encourage the collection of serum or plasma samples for phenotyping by isoelectric focusing. This is primarily due to the nature of the sample referral centres which are large hospitals with specialist respiratory clinics, and also due to cost and logistical reasons.

Genotyping has the advantage of facilitating the rapid screening of both dried blood spots and DNA isolated from blood and is arguably less prone to interpretation errors which may occur with phenotyping. A downside to the method is that many laboratories, generally for cost and logistical reasons, employ primers for selected mutations, often the most common Z and S. In some cases, this can lead to rare mutations such as I, F, and M_{malton} not being detected and misclassified as normal [90]. For this reason, in certain laboratories the genotyping method is used on a complementary or a clarification basis, unless specific M primers are being used.

For the precise identification of rare and unusual phenotypes observed in our centre we reflex to sequencing the gene for AAT (SERPINA1, RefSeq: NG_008290). This involves the isolation of DNA and sequencing the coding exons (II-V) of the SERPINA1 gene [95]. The detailed genetic analysis has led to the identification and characterisation of many rare and novel SERPINA1 alleles (Table 5).

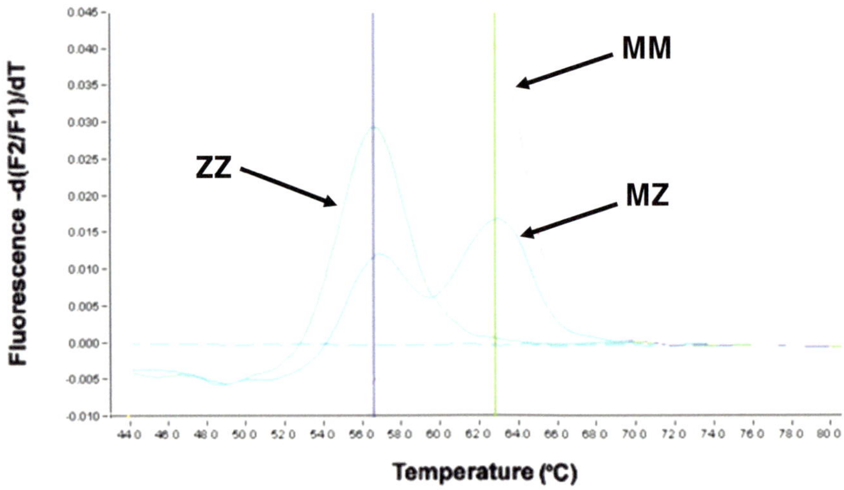

Figure 5. Genotyping assay for the Z allele by melting curve analysis on a real-time PCR system [93].

Variant	Mechanism	Effect	Disease Risk
Z	GAG – AAG, Glu342Lys	Polymerisation, impaired secretion and severe deficiency	Lung & liver
S	GAA – GTA, Glu264Val	Impaired secretion and mild deficiency	Lung & liver (in compound heterozygotes e.g. SZ)
I	CGC – TGC, Arg39Cys	Impaired secretion and mild deficiency	Lung & liver (case reports in compound heterozygotes e.g. IZ)
F	CGT – TGT, Arg223Cys	Defective protease inhibition	Lung (case reports in compound heterozygotes e.g. FZ)
Null (Q0)	Mutations causing gene deletion, premature stop codon or mRNA degradation	No AAT produced	Lung
M_{malton}	ΔTTC, ΔPhe52	Polymerisation, impaired secretion and severe deficiency	Lung & liver
$Z_{bristol}$	ACG – ATG Thr85Met	Intracellular accumulation & defective glycosylation	Lung
$M_{wurzburg}$	CCC – TCC Pro369Ser	Block in secretion	Lung & liver

Table 5. Common and rare pathological AATD variants detected in Ireland.

http://dx.doi.org/10.5772/58602

4. Why should we test?

There are clear benefits to a diagnosis of AATD for the clinician and the individual. Unfortunately, these benefits are often ignored to the detriment of the affected individual and the extended family.

4.1. Smoking cessation and occupational exposure considerations

The deleterious consequences of smoking on lung health in general and on the lungs of individuals with AATD in particular are well known and the origins of this can be traced back to the late 1960s. The twin discoveries of AATD and its association with COPD [16], and the induction of emphysema by the protease neutrophil elastase (NE) [96] led to an explosion in research surrounding proteolysis and lung disease. Importantly, NE was found to be exquisitely sensitive to inhibition by AAT by Aaron Janoff in 1968 [97]. The pathological effects of smoking were further elucidated when it was found products of cigarette smoke were able to destroy the anti-NE activity of AAT [98]. Despite being an excellent inhibitor of NE, the active site methionine residue at position 358 of the AAT molecule is easily oxidised by cigarette smoke and oxidants released by immune cells [99-101]. These studies provided the clear and irrefutable evidence that smoking causes a functional deficiency in the antiprotease screen. Therefore, in those individuals who develop COPD solely due to smoking, this functional deficiency contributes to the pathogenesis of disease. In individuals with AATD who develop COPD, the deficiency which contributes to the pathogenesis of disease is genetic.

So, we know that the small and precious quantity of AAT that does eventually reach the lung in ZZ individuals is knocked out by cigarette smoke. This is the reason why AAT deficient individuals who smoke develop early onset lung disease [102]. Cigarette smoke is by far the single most important risk factor for the development of COPD in AATD individuals [103-105]. In fact, smoking can reduce the life expectancy of a ZZ patient by up to 25 years [102]. Carpenter *et al* in a 2007 study revealed higher smoking cessation rates in individuals with a diagnosis of AATD compared to COPD individuals [64]. In this study severely deficient individuals (ZZ and SZ) had a 59% quit attempt rate, compared to a 26% quit attempt rate in unaffected MM individuals. This information is vital in the clinic as it shows that knowledge of AATD motivates the affected individual toward smoking cessation. Every ZZ, SZ, and MZ AATD individual should be educated about the incredibly harmful effects of cigarette smoke in AATD. Smoking cessation and the avoidance of occupational and environmental exposures (for example particulate matter, chemical vapours, and agricultural dusts) is paramount. AATD individuals without apparent lung disease should also be encouraged to quit smoking as this cohort offers the most realistic chance of delaying or possibly preventing the development of COPD. A decision to quit smoking is the most important decision a person with AATD can make. The decision to modify this behaviour is strongly influenced by the quality of the information provided and how this is communicated to at risk individuals.

Ireland is a leader in Europe in terms of anti-smoking measures with the introduction of the first ban on smoking in the workplace [106]. However, a 2007 Irish Government study (Slán 2007 Survey of Lifestyle, Attitudes and Nutrition in Ireland) found that 34% of Irish 30 – 44 year olds currently smoke and this is the age bracket that AATD individuals first begin to report deterioration in lung health. To assess the effect of smoking on lung health in AATD we analysed lung function data from 120 ZZ individuals enrolled in the Irish National AATD Registry and correlated this to smoking history. While the relative contribution of occupational exposures was not taken into account, the mean FEV1 (% predicted) and diffusion capacity of carbon monoxide (DLCO, % predicted) was significantly higher in ZZ subjects who never smoked compared to ZZ subjects who were past or active smokers (Figure 6). This clearly demonstrates the destructive consequences of smoking for ZZ individuals.

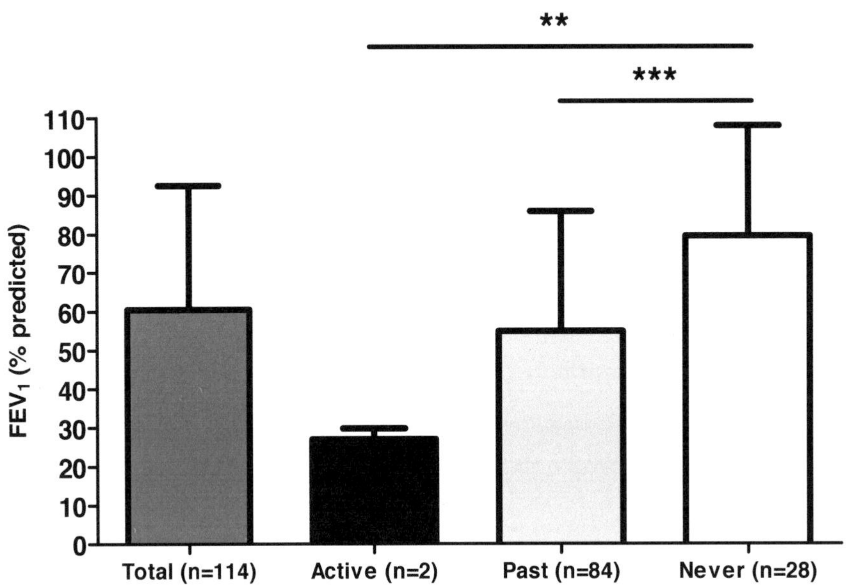

Figure 6. FEV1 (% predicted) stratified by smoking in ZZ individuals enrolled in Irish National AATD Registry (***$p < 0.0001$, **$p < 0.001$, t-test).

Interestingly, smoking cessation rates were also analysed as part of this study. In the past smokers cohort 36% stopped smoking within the first 12 months after AATD diagnosis; 24% stopped smoking after the first 12 months post-AATD diagnosis and 40% had already stopped smoking prior to AATD diagnosis. This supports the findings of the earlier Carpenter study and demonstrates the positive effect of AATD diagnosis on smoking cessation rates.

4.2. Family screening

The area of family screening offers the greatest possibility for the prevention or at least postponement of COPD [107]. An early diagnosis of AATD provides tantalising opportunities for behaviour modification and lifestyle changes, the single most important of which is smoking cessation. Interim data from the Irish National AATD Registry demonstrates that ZZ

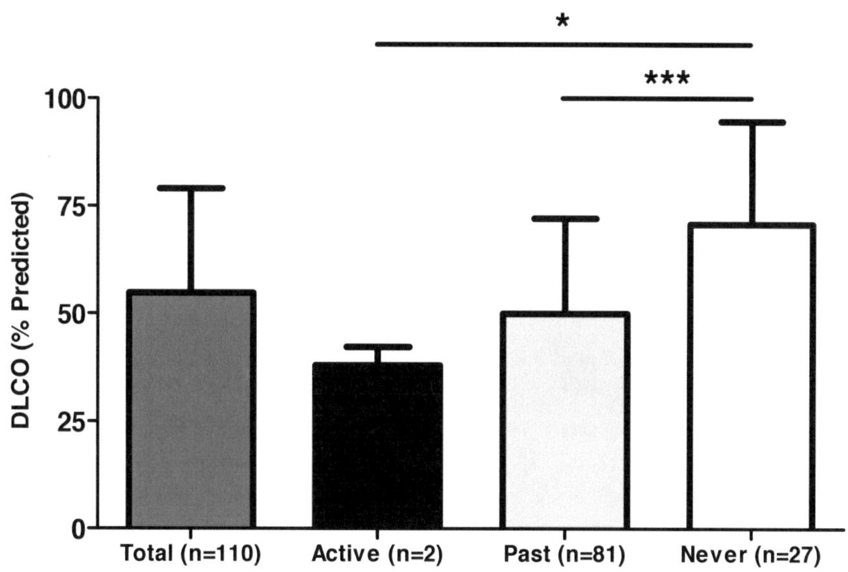

Figure 7. DLCO (% predicted) stratified by smoking in ZZ individuals enrolled in Irish National AATD Registry (***$p < 0.0001$, *$p < 0.05$, t-test).

individuals detected by family screening tend to have preserved lung function compared to those identified by symptomatic screening (Figure 8).

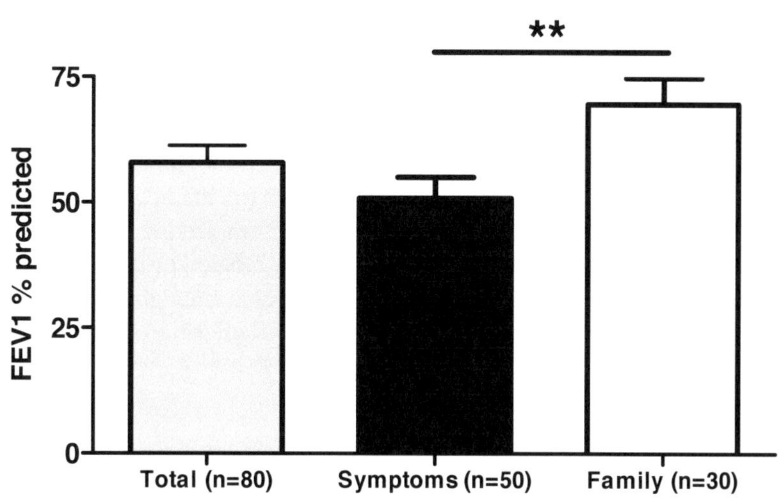

Figure 8. FEV1 (% predicted) in ZZ individuals diagnosed by symptomatic screening versus those diagnosed by family screening enrolled in Irish National AATD Registry (**$p < 0.001$, t-test).

An excellent example of the family screening possibilities opened up by a diagnosis of AATD is presented in a large family study from the Irish AATD Registry (Figure 9). In this example, the index case was diagnosed with AATD because of lung disease. Six of the nine siblings were subsequently tested revealing 3 ZZ individuals, 2 MZ individuals, and 1 MM individual.

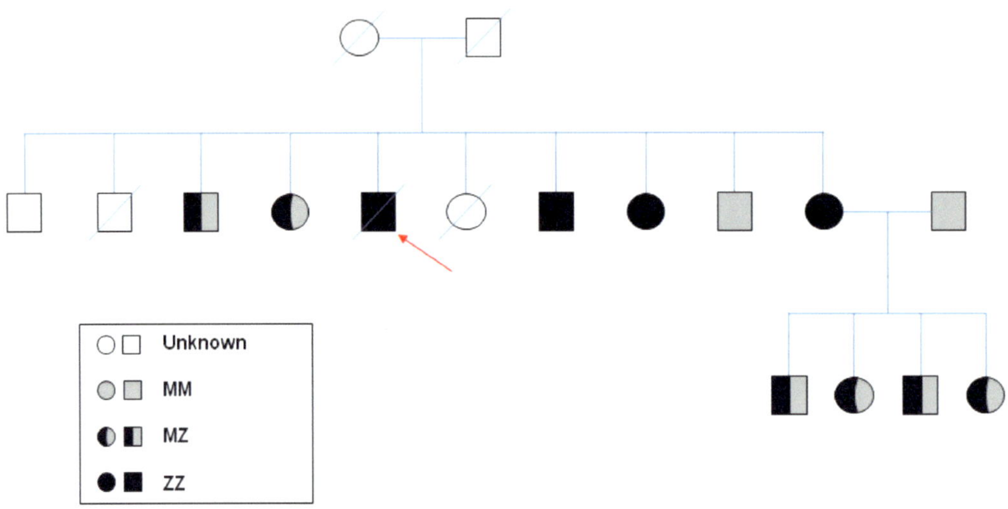

Figure 9. Identification of ZZ proband (red arrow) and subsequent identification of at risk relatives by family screening.

4.3. Liver assessment

A baseline liver assessment should be performed in a newly-diagnosed AATD individual to investigate the presence of liver abnormalities. The primary tools for assessment are liver function tests and abdominal ultrasound. This is a practise not routine in the specialist respiratory clinic and ignorance of AATD and the potential for liver disease can be fatal. Early recognition is important for two reasons. The first reason is to prevent, recognize, and treat early the complications of AATD-related liver disease, which can include portal hypertension, encephalopathy, and tumours [108]. The second reason is to advise the patient to avoid injurious habits, such as alcohol consumption, which can accelerate disease. Interestingly, patients who undergo liver transplantation for other causes have a higher incidence of being heterozygous for AATD than the general population [40].

4.4. Vaccination

Influenza and pneumococcal vaccinations are recommended for all individuals with AATD [4]. A 2007 study investigated the practice of vaccinations and respiratory outcomes in AATD individuals in the USA and found over 80% of AATD individuals had received adequate influenza and pneumococcal vaccinations during the influenza season [109]. However, there was no significant difference in severity or rate of exacerbations between vaccinated and unvaccinated individuals but the authors concluded that the vaccinated group may represent 'sicker' AATD individuals. Influenza and pneumococcal vaccinations in COPD patients are recommended in several guidelines for COPD [110, 111] and the unique susceptibility of AATD individuals provides additional motivation for vaccination, especially during influenza season.

4.5. Exacerbation management

Exposure to bacterial and viral infections can result in a respiratory exacerbation. Symptoms include increased dyspnoea, cough, and production of sputum [112]. The aggressive treatment of infections is recommended in AATD individuals as per ATS/ERS guidelines [4]. This is particularly important as frequent exacerbations have been shown to be related to worsening health-related quality of life (HRQoL). An English study investigated health status in AATD individuals over 12 months and recorded exacerbations, lung function and HRQoL. The authors concluded exacerbations occur commonly in AATD individuals and correlate to worse health status. Exacerbations were associated with a decline in the gas transfer of the lung for carbon monoxide over time (DLCO), but not FEV1 [113]. Interestingly, a study investigated exacerbation frequency in AATD individuals with COPD who were receiving augmentation therapy and found subjects with frequent exacerbations had the worst baseline HRQoL scores, as well as more physician visits and hospitalizations. Unfortunately, AATD individuals not receiving augmentation therapy were not included for comparison [114]. A recent longitudinal study undertaken in the USA, evaluated the effectiveness of a disease management and prevention programme for AATD individuals and involved 905 individuals over a 2 year period. The programme included written educational material for self-study and individualised treatment plans for exacerbations. Improved compliance was observed in the use of bronchodilators, oxygen therapy, and steroids during exacerbations. The management programme significantly reduced medical visits and showed a slower deterioration of HRQoL during exacerbations [115]. A follow-up study providing additional evidence to evaluate the long-term benefits of an AATD disease management programme would be beneficial.

4.6. Augmentation therapy

Augmentation therapy is the only specific therapy available for severe AATD, and comprises of intravenous administration of AAT derived from human plasma [116]. This treatment is available in several European countries and the USA [117]. The therapy comprises of weekly or fortnightly intravenous infusions of AAT preparations that augment the low levels of circulating AAT in severe AATD. However, its efficacy remains to be definitively proven and uncertainty persists concerning the therapy's cost effectiveness [118]. Ongoing randomised clinical trials are being performed to definitively assess the efficacy of the treatment. Previous trials have been under-powered and have mostly demonstrated only biochemical efficacy with AAT levels restored to above the putative threshold in the blood and lung, with a failure to show clear clinical efficacy in randomised controlled trials [71, 119]. Nevertheless, there is evidence that augmentation therapy can slow lung function decline in AATD individuals, and moderately obstructed cohorts are most likely to benefit [120].

4.7. Pulmonary rehabilitation

Pulmonary rehabilitation is a tailored exercise programme aimed at restoring the best possible quality of life in patients with lung disease, particularly focused on reducing breathlessness, as well as improving independence and the physical ability to tolerate stress [121]. It is defined as a complex, multimodal treatment regimen for patients with pulmonary diseases [122]. The goal is to help patients become more physically active, to learn more about their disease, treatment options, and how to cope. Patients are encouraged to become actively involved in providing their own health care, more independent in daily activities, and less dependent on health professionals and expensive medical resources. Rather than focusing solely on reversing the disease process, rehabilitation attempts to reduce symptoms and reduce disability from the disease. In general, patients with COPD secondary to AATD tend to be younger compared to patients with usual COPD, and less comorbidity is observed. This suggests the potential for greater improvement in AATD individuals participating in rehabilitation programmes.

5. Why is testing not taking place?

The reasons for the continuing under-diagnosis of AATD are diverse and can include low medical and public awareness, the misconception that it is a rare disease, the belief that testing is complicated and expensive, and testing fatigue [123]. Current data suggests that less than 10% of individuals with severe AATD have been recognised globally [124], and increasing detection rates is the most pressing, and vexing issue for leaders in the AATD community. Unfortunately, some clinicians adopt the attitude of "what difference does a diagnosis of AATD actually make". This is a challenge for all stakeholders and the benefits of AATD testing must be clearly stated in a simple powerful message to lung health professionals and policy-makers. In particular, the potential economic benefits are not being stressed enough [125]. Early diagnosis of AATD is an example of preventative medicine. The newly-diagnosed individual and healthcare provider have the power to arrest or prevent the development of COPD through lifestyle choices, close medical observation, and focused treatment. This in turn means that the long term financial burden on the health system is reduced and by remaining healthy the individual continues to contribute to society and the exchequer. There is also the consideration of the large direct medical cost to the symptomatic AATD individual [125]. So why does testing in COPD cohorts not occur if the ATS/ERS and WHO guidelines are so clear and the benefits so convincing?

Many early guidelines for AATD advocated testing early-onset COPD patients and this fallacy was to the detriment of screening efforts. The age at which manifestations of airway obstruction, pulmonary emphysema, or chronic bronchitis appear in ZZ individuals is highly variable [102]. While a common feature of AATD is indeed early-onset COPD, a significant AATD cohort do not develop symptoms until much later in life, particularly if non-smokers [126, 127]. In fact, among never-smokers the risk of liver disease increases with age in ZZ individuals [127, 128]. Numerous case reports have described AATD in elderly individuals with COPD who were lifelong never smokers [129]. Taken together, it is clear that screening for AATD

http://dx.doi.org/10.5772/58602

Belief that AATD is a rare disorder
Perception that only early-onset non-smokers are affected
Therapeutic nihilism due to lack of specific treatments
Fear of genetic discrimination
Lack of education and awareness (in healthcare professionals & public)
Testing fatigue
Failure to admit lack of knowledge
Reluctance to lose patients to specialist centres
Lack of communication between clinicians and laboratory scientists
Absence of effective national guidelines
No access to testing methods
Privacy concerns
Perceived stigma

Table 6. Reasons why testing for AATD is not taking place.

should be automatically performed in all COPD regardless of age or smoking history, especially as failure to do so has serious clinical repercussions for undiagnosed family members.

The fear of genetic discrimination, financial concerns, and privacy concerns are real barriers to testing for AATD in the COPD population [130]. Fears of genetic discrimination have been allayed in recent years with preventative legislation enacted in several countries, including Ireland and the US. Genetic discrimination was made illegal in Ireland from December 31st 2005 when the Irish government enacted new legislation. It became illegal to use or process the results of genetic testing for insurance, life assurance or mortgage purposes. This also applies in the case of employment, health insurance and occupational pension. What is assessed when a person is being considered for a financial product or insurance policy are the usual criteria including health history (symptom-related questions), lifestyle choices (smoking, alcohol, etc.), and the regular questions surrounding family history of particular illnesses. There are still reasons to be wary in this area. Following the advent of the Genetic Information Non-Discrimination Act (GINA) in the US in 2008, discrimination can be implicit, indirect and subtle, rather than explicit, direct and overt; and as a result can be harder to prove [131].

6. How can we increase detection of AATD?

Initiatives to increase detection rates might include automatic physician alerts suggesting AATD testing on pulmonary function test reports of patients with fixed airflow obstruction [132], better medical and patient education in the area of AATD [133], changes to national COPD guidelines, and a red flag to recommend testing for AATD on laboratory reports of patient with low AAT levels. The advent of finger-prick tests using dried blood spots (DBS) as a source of DNA has allowed home testing for AATD, with easier transportation of samples to the laboratory [94]. This method of testing eliminates the fear of needles for the individual, and is also cheaper as the test does not require a visit to a general practitioner.

Improve education in undergraduate and postgraduate medical and scientific training
Include primary care physicians and hepatologists in awareness efforts
Educate and empower respiratory nurse specialists
Public awareness campaigns
Patient empowerment
Update WHO and ATS/ERS guidelines for AATD
Refine COPD guidelines to include automatic testing for AATD
Laboratory red-flags
Pulmonary function test red-flags
Electronic health record prompts
Embed as routine test by creating COPD care templates and physician order reminders
Joint seminars between pulmonologist and laboratory scientists
Presentations at national conferences
Provision of free testing kits

Table 7. Strategies to improve the detection of AATD.

An attractive strategy is the use of electronic red-flags on low AAT laboratory reports. This prompts the clinician to investigate low AAT results and reflex to phenotyping and/or genotyping. During our efforts to increase awareness at a national level in Ireland, we have advocated that hospital laboratories should include the following recommendation on AAT reports; "*Serum AAT < 1.0 g/L may indicate alpha-1 antitrypsin deficiency and further investigation is recommended. Information is available from the Alpha One Foundation on www.alpha1.ie. AAT is an acute phase reactant and serum concentrations can increase significantly during trauma, acute infection or surgery.*" This cost-neutral approach has been successfully implemented at 9 large hospitals in Ireland and has directly led to increased diagnosis of AATD in these centres and surrounding hinterlands. Implementation was achieved by presenting to lung specialists and laboratory scientists on site, and in the same room. This twin track approach is most effective and it is often the first time for each party to meet – those requesting the test and those performing the quantitative AAT assay. The aim is to eliminate missed diagnosis of AATD when a low AAT is reported but not acted upon. A particularly striking aspect of this strategy is that incidental findings of AATD are common, and hitherto asymptomatic cases can be detected. As AAT is an acute phase protein and a robust marker of inflammation, the test can

http://dx.doi.org/10.5772/58602

be requested during routine blood work with the expectation that it will be dramatically increased. However, the opposite is sometimes the case. The inadvertent low finding is highlighted by the electronic red-flag and the ensuing diagnosis of AATD is the positive outcome. We are hopeful that this system will eventually be adopted on a nationwide basis and are in consultation with the government and various stakeholders to effect this change.

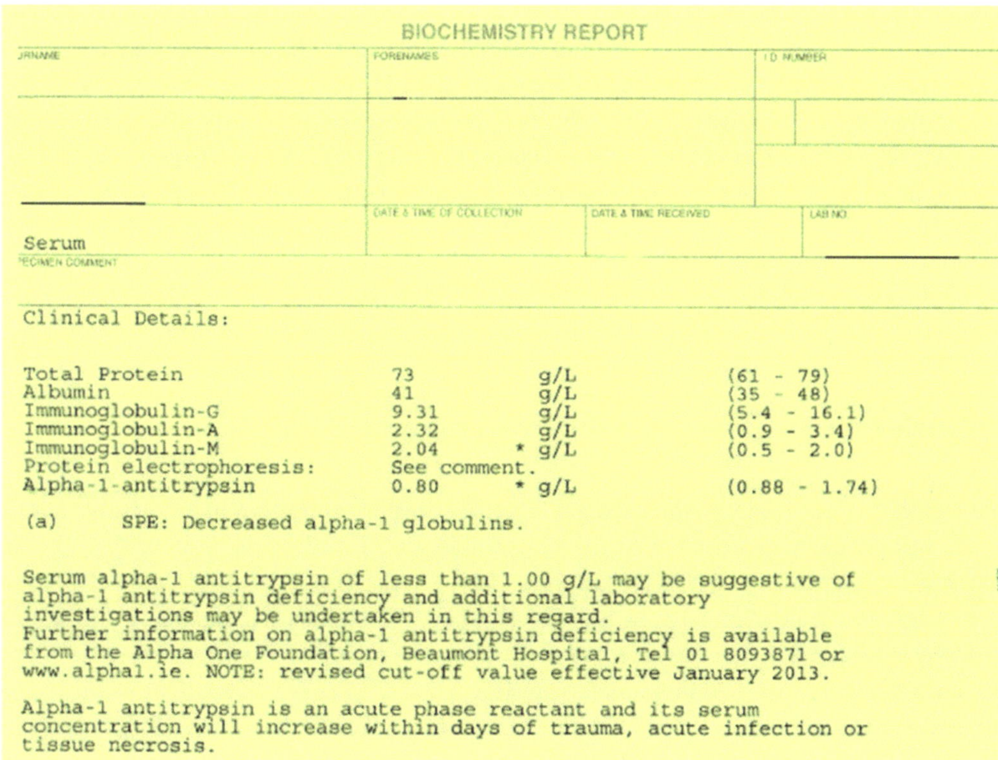

BIOCHEMISTRY REPORT

SURNAME | FORENAMES | I D NUMBER

DATE & TIME OF COLLECTION | DATE & TIME RECEIVED | LAB NO

Serum

SPECIMEN COMMENT

Clinical Details:

Total Protein	73	g/L	(61 - 79)
Albumin	41	g/L	(35 - 48)
Immunoglobulin-G	9.31	g/L	(5.4 - 16.1)
Immunoglobulin-A	2.32	g/L	(0.9 - 3.4)
Immunoglobulin-M	2.04	* g/L	(0.5 - 2.0)
Protein electrophoresis:	See comment.		
Alpha-1-antitrypsin	0.80	* g/L	(0.88 - 1.74)

(a) SPE: Decreased alpha-1 globulins.

Serum alpha-1 antitrypsin of less than 1.00 g/L may be suggestive of alpha-1 antitrypsin deficiency and additional laboratory investigations may be undertaken in this regard.
Further information on alpha-1 antitrypsin deficiency is available from the Alpha One Foundation, Beaumont Hospital, Tel 01 8093871 or www.alpha1.ie. NOTE: revised cut-off value effective January 2013.

Alpha-1 antitrypsin is an acute phase reactant and its serum concentration will increase within days of trauma, acute infection or tissue necrosis.

Figure 10. Example of a laboratory red-flag on low AAT results from a biochemistry laboratory at a large Irish hospital.

In the era of the electronic medical record, technology can help deliver or enhance specific clinical practices, such as testing for AATD. For example, if physicians were prompted to consider this condition when they received the results of pulmonary function tests (PFT) showing fixed airflow obstruction, testing for AATD should increase. Also, if eliciting a family history of COPD or chronic liver disease prompted a physician alert on the electronic medical record to test the serum AAT level, testing could increase. For example, a small pilot study found that the frequency of AATD testing increased when a prompt to test for AATD was included on the PFT reports of patients with airflow obstruction [132]. Another similar study looked at the impact of a clinical decision support system within an electronic health record which facilitated testing for AATD [134]. The alert within the electronic health record resulted in a four-fold increase in testing for AATD.

7. Other strategies

There are a host of other strategies which could lead to increased detection of AATD. These include continuing medical education lectures, AATD teaching in medical school and clinical chemistry curricula, public awareness campaigns, lobbying of public health officials, and making available free testing kits. Moreover, the WHO and ATS/ERS guidelines need urgent updating. AATD is often relegated to a footnote in many clinical guidelines for COPD. A summary of the ATS and ERS document outlining standards for the diagnosis and treatment of patients with COPD published in 2004 mentions AATD once, stating that "patients presenting with airflow limitation at a relatively early age (4th or 5th decade) and particularly those with a family history of COPD should be tested for alpha-1 antitrypsin deficiency" [135]. Narrow definitions such as these are damaging to efforts to increase AATD detection. Another strategy to promote testing is to empower patients by providing free, high-quality, easy to understand information available, such as the information material prepared by the Alpha-1 Foundation (www.alpha-1foundation.org).

8. Conclusion

The fact that cigarette smoking is often a coincident historical finding in the assessment of COPD has probably contributed to the remarkable global under-diagnosis of AATD. For example, of the estimated 3,000 ZZ individuals on the island of Ireland, less than 10% have been diagnosed. Unfortunately for the clinician and the patient, testing for AATD is not routinely considered in the assessment of COPD. Any model for COPD diagnosis, assessment and management must include automatic testing for AATD as one of the first steps. Large variability exists in the clinical course of lung disease in AATD and therefore all COPD patients should be tested for AATD, regardless of age or smoking history. The under-diagnosis of AATD in COPD is a situation that must not be allowed to continue.

Acknowledgements

We thank all the AATD individuals attending our centre for their continued collaboration in research, awareness and detection efforts. The Irish National AATD Targeted Detection Programme is supported by funding from the Irish Government. We thank Dr. Ilaria Ferrarotti, Dr. Stefania Ottaviani, and Prof. Maurizio Luisetti from the University of Pavia for their continued assistance with rare and novel variant identification. We would like to thank John Walsh and Angela McBride of the Alpha-1 Foundation (USA) for their continued support and encouragement. Finally, we wish to thank Pat O'Brien and Emma Pentony in the Department of Chemical Pathology in Beaumont Hospital for help with sampling and turbidimetry.

http://dx.doi.org/10.5772/58602

Author details

Tomás P. Carroll[1*], M. Emmet O'Brien[2], Laura T. Fee[1], Kevin Molloy[2], Blair Murray[2], Seshma Ramsawak[2], Oisín McElvaney[2], Catherine O'Connor[1] and Noel G. McElvaney[2]

*Address all correspondence to: tcarroll@rcsi.ie

1 Alpha One Foundation, RCSI Education and Research Centre, Beaumont Hospital, Dublin, Ireland

2 Department of Medicine, RCSI Education and Research Centre, Beaumont Hospital, Dublin, Ireland

References

[1] Greene CM, Miller SD, Carroll T, McLean C, O'Mahony M, Lawless MW, O'Neill SJ, Taggart CC, McElvaney NG: Alpha-1 antitrypsin deficiency: a conformational disease associated with lung and liver manifestations. *J Inherit Metab Dis* 2008, 31:21-34.

[2] Lieberman J, Winter B, Sastre A: Alpha 1-antitrypsin Pi-types in 965 COPD patients. *Chest* 1986, 89:370-373.

[3] Alpha 1-antitrypsin deficiency: memorandum from a WHO meeting. *Bull World Health Organ* 1997, 75:397-415.

[4] American Thoracic Society/European Respiratory Society statement: standards for the diagnosis and management of individuals with alpha-1 antitrypsin deficiency. *Am J Respir Crit Care Med* 2003, 168:818-900.

[5] Carroll TP, O'Connor CA, Floyd O, McPartlin J, Kelleher DP, O'Brien G, Dimitrov BD, Morris VB, Taggart CC, McElvaney NG: The prevalence of alpha-1 antitrypsin deficiency in Ireland. *Respir Res* 2011, 12:91.

[6] Stoller JK, Sandhaus RA, Turino G, Dickson R, Rodgers K, Strange C: Delay in diagnosis of alpha1-antitrypsin deficiency: a continuing problem. *Chest* 2005, 128:1989-1994.

[7] Carrell RW, Jeppsson JO, Laurell CB, Brennan SO, Owen MC, Vaughan L, Boswell DR: Structure and variation of human alpha 1-antitrypsin. *Nature* 1982, 298:329-334.

[8] Jones EA, Vergalla J, Steer CJ, Bradley-Moore PR, Vierling JM: Metabolism of intact and desialylated alpha 1-antitrypsin. *Clin Sci Mol Med* 1978, 55:139-148.

[9] Perlmutter DH, Kay RM, Cole FS, Rossing TH, Van Thiel D, Colten HR: The cellular defect in alpha 1-proteinase inhibitor (alpha 1-PI) deficiency is expressed in human

monocytes and in Xenopus oocytes injected with human liver mRNA. *Proc Natl Acad Sci U S A* 1985, 82:6918-6921.

[10] Molmenti EP, Perlmutter DH, Rubin DC: Cell-specific expression of alpha 1-antitrypsin in human intestinal epithelium. *J Clin Invest* 1993, 92:2022-2034.

[11] Carroll TP, Greene CM, O'Connor CA, Nolan AM, O'Neill SJ, McElvaney NG: Evidence for unfolded protein response activation in monocytes from individuals with alpha-1 antitrypsin deficiency. *J Immunol* 2010, 184:4538-4546.

[12] Cichy J, Potempa J, Travis J: Biosynthesis of alpha1-proteinase inhibitor by human lung-derived epithelial cells. *J Biol Chem* 1997, 272:8250-8255.

[13] Voulgari F, Cummins P, Gardecki TI, Beeching NJ, Stone PC, Stuart J: Serum levels of acute phase and cardiac proteins after myocardial infarction, surgery, and infection. *Br Heart J* 1982, 48:352-356.

[14] Kossmann T, Hans VH, Imhof HG, Stocker R, Grob P, Trentz O, Morganti-Kossmann C: Intrathecal and serum interleukin-6 and the acute-phase response in patients with severe traumatic brain injuries. *Shock* 1995, 4:311-317.

[15] Perlmutter DH, May LT, Sehgal PB: Interferon beta 2/interleukin 6 modulates synthesis of alpha 1-antitrypsin in human mononuclear phagocytes and in human hepatoma cells. *J Clin Invest* 1989, 84:138-144.

[16] Laurell CB, Eriksson SE: The electrophoretic alpha-globulin pattern of serum in alpha1-antitrypsin deficiency. *Scand J Clin Lab Invest* 1963, 15:132-140.

[17] Gadek JE, Fells GA, Crystal RG: Cigarette smoking induces functional antiprotease deficiency in the lower respiratory tract of humans. *Science* 1979, 206:1315-1316.

[18] Sharp HL, Bridges RA, Krivit W, Freier EF: Cirrhosis associated with alpha-1-antitrypsin deficiency: a previously unrecognized inherited disorder. *J Lab Clin Med* 1969, 73:934-939.

[19] McElvaney NG, Stoller JK, Buist AS, Prakash UB, Brantly ML, Schluchter MD, Crystal RD: Baseline characteristics of enrollees in the National Heart, Lung and Blood Institute Registry of alpha 1-antitrypsin deficiency. Alpha 1-Antitrypsin Deficiency Registry Study Group. *Chest* 1997, 111:394-403.

[20] Eden E, Mitchell D, Mehlman B, Khouli H, Nejat M, Grieco MH, Turino GM: Atopy, asthma, and emphysema in patients with severe alpha-1-antitrypysin deficiency. *Am J Respir Crit Care Med* 1997, 156:68-74.

[21] Seersholm N, Kok-Jensen A, Dirksen A: Decline in FEV1 among patients with severe hereditary alpha 1-antitrypsin deficiency type PiZ. *Am J Respir Crit Care Med* 1995, 152:1922-1925.

[22] Seersholm N, Kok-Jensen A, Dirksen A: Survival of patients with severe alpha 1-antitrypsin deficiency with special reference to non-index cases. *Thorax* 1994, 49:695-698.

[23] Piitulainen E, Tornling G, Eriksson S: Effect of age and occupational exposure to airway irritants on lung function in non-smoking individuals with alpha 1-antitrypsin deficiency (PiZZ). *Thorax* 1997, 52:244-248.

[24] Mayer AS, Stoller JK, Bucher Bartelson B, James Ruttenber A, Sandhaus RA, Newman LS: Occupational exposure risks in individuals with PI*Z alpha(1)-antitrypsin deficiency. *Am J Respir Crit Care Med* 2000, 162:553-558.

[25] Stolk J, Ng WH, Bakker ME, Reiber JH, Rabe KF, Putter H, Stoel BC: Correlation between annual change in health status and computer tomography derived lung density in subjects with alpha1-antitrypsin deficiency. *Thorax* 2003, 58:1027-1030.

[26] Parr DG, Dirksen A, Piitulainen E, Deng C, Wencker M, Stockley RA: Exploring the optimum approach to the use of CT densitometry in a randomised placebo-controlled study of augmentation therapy in alpha 1-antitrypsin deficiency. *Respir Res* 2009, 10:75.

[27] Parr DG, Guest PG, Reynolds JH, Dowson LJ, Stockley RA: Prevalence and impact of bronchiectasis in alpha1-antitrypsin deficiency. *Am J Respir Crit Care Med* 2007, 176:1215-1221.

[28] Piras B, Ferrarotti I, Lara B, Martinez MT, Bustamante A, Ottaviani S, Pirina P, Luisetti M, Miravitlles M: Clinical phenotypes of Italian and Spanish patients with alpha1-antitrypsin deficiency. *Eur Respir J* 2013, 42:54-64.

[29] Moroz SP, Cutz E, Cox DW, Sass-Kortsak A: Liver disease associated with alpha1-antitrypsin deficiency in childhood. *J Pediatr* 1976, 88:19-25.

[30] Sveger T: Liver disease in alpha1-antitrypsin deficiency detected by screening of 200,000 infants. *N Engl J Med* 1976, 294:1316-1321.

[31] Carey EJ, Iyer VN, Nelson DR, Nguyen JH, Krowka MJ: Outcomes for recipients of liver transplantation for alpha-1-antitrypsin deficiency-related cirrhosis. *Liver Transpl* 2013, 19:1370-1376.

[32] Psacharopoulos HT, Mowat AP, Cook PJ, Carlile PA, Portmann B, Rodeck CH: Outcome of liver disease associated with alpha 1 antitrypsin deficiency (PiZ). Implications for genetic counselling and antenatal diagnosis. *Arch Dis Child* 1983, 58:882-887.

[33] Eriksson S, Carlson J, Velez R: Risk of cirrhosis and primary liver cancer in alpha 1-antitrypsin deficiency. *N Engl J Med* 1986, 314:736-739.

[34] Voide N, Ardigo S, Morris M, Rubbia-Brandt L, Rougemont AL, Morard I, Vischer UM: Alpha-1-antitrypsin deficiency in a 78-year-old woman with isolated liver cirrhosis. *J Am Geriatr Soc* 2010, 58:415-416.

[35] Pan S, Huang L, McPherson J, Muzny D, Rouhani F, Brantly M, Gibbs R, Sifers RN: Single nucleotide polymorphism-mediated translational suppression of endoplasmic

reticulum mannosidase I modifies the onset of end-stage liver disease in alpha1-antitrypsin deficiency. *Hepatology* 2009, 50:275-281.

[36] Scott CM, Kruse KB, Schmidt BZ, Perlmutter DH, McCracken AA, Brodsky JL: ADD66, a gene involved in the endoplasmic reticulum-associated degradation of alpha-1-antitrypsin-Z in yeast, facilitates proteasome activity and assembly. *Mol Biol Cell* 2007, 18:3776-3787.

[37] Zhang B, Zheng C, Zhu M, Tao J, Vasievich MP, Baines A, Kim J, Schekman R, Kaufman RJ, Ginsburg D: Mice deficient in LMAN1 exhibit FV and FVIII deficiencies and liver accumulation of alpha1-antitrypsin. *Blood* 2011, 118:3384-3391.

[38] Regev A, Guaqueta C, Molina EG, Conrad A, Mishra V, Brantly ML, Torres M, De Medina M, Tzakis AG, Schiff ER: Does the heterozygous state of alpha-1 antitrypsin deficiency have a role in chronic liver diseases? Interim results of a large case-control study. *J Pediatr Gastroenterol Nutr* 2006, 43 Suppl 1:S30-35.

[39] Cacciottolo TM, Gelson WT, Maguire G, Davies SE, Griffiths WJ: Pi*Z heterozygous alpha-1 antitrypsin states accelerate parenchymal but not biliary cirrhosis. *Eur J Gastroenterol Hepatol* 2014, 26:412-417.

[40] Kok KF, Wahab PJ, Houwen RH, Drenth JP, de Man RA, van Hoek B, Meijer JW, Willekens FL, de Vries RA: Heterozygous alpha-I antitrypsin deficiency as a co-factor in the development of chronic liver disease: a review. *Neth J Med* 2007, 65:160-166.

[41] Hood JM, Koep LJ, Peters RL, Schroter GP, Weil R, 3rd, Redeker AG, Starzl TE: Liver transplantation for advanced liver disease with alpha-1-antitrypsin deficiency. *N Engl J Med* 1980, 302:272-275.

[42] Francavilla R, Castellaneta SP, Hadzic N, Chambers SM, Portmann B, Tung J, Cheeseman P, Rela M, Heaton ND, Mieli-Vergani G: Prognosis of alpha-1-antitrypsin deficiency-related liver disease in the era of paediatric liver transplantation. *J Hepatol* 2000, 32:986-992.

[43] Irvine C, Neild V, Stephens C, Black M: Alpha-1-antitrypsin deficiency panniculitis. *J R Soc Med* 1990, 83:743-744.

[44] Dowd SK, Rodgers GC, Callen JP: Effective treatment with alpha 1-protease inhibitor of chronic cutaneous vasculitis associated with alpha 1-antitrypsin deficiency. *J Am Acad Dermatol* 1995, 33:913-916.

[45] Gross B, Grebe M, Wencker M, Stoller JK, Bjursten LM, Janciauskiene S: New Findings in PiZZ alpha1-antitrypsin deficiency-related panniculitis. Demonstration of skin polymers and high dosing requirements of intravenous augmentation therapy. *Dermatology* 2009, 218:370-375.

[46] Blanco I, Lara B, de Serres F: Efficacy of alpha1-antitrypsin augmentation therapy in conditions other than pulmonary emphysema. *Orphanet J Rare Dis* 2011, 6:14.

[47] Lyons PA, Rayner TF, Trivedi S, Holle JU, Watts RA, Jayne DR, Baslund B, Brenchley P, Bruchfeld A, Chaudhry AN, et al: Genetically distinct subsets within ANCA-associated vasculitis. *N Engl J Med* 2012, 367:214-223.

[48] Segelmark M, Elzouki AN, Wieslander J, Eriksson S: The PiZ gene of alpha 1-antitrypsin as a determinant of outcome in PR3-ANCA-positive vasculitis. *Kidney Int* 1995, 48:844-850.

[49] Fortin PR, Fraser RS, Watts CS, Esdaile JM: Alpha-1 antitrypsin deficiency and systemic necrotizing vasculitis. *J Rheumatol* 1991, 18:1613-1616.

[50] Mashiba S, Wada Y, Takeya M, Sugiyama A, Hamakubo T, Nakamura A, Noguchi N, Niki E, Izumi A, Kobayashi M, et al: In vivo complex formation of oxidized alpha(1)-antitrypsin and LDL. *Arterioscler Thromb Vasc Biol* 2001, 21:1801-1808.

[51] Dichtl W, Moraga F, Ares MP, Crisby M, Nilsson J, Lindgren S, Janciauskiene S: The carboxyl-terminal fragment of alpha1-antitrypsin is present in atherosclerotic plaques and regulates inflammatory transcription factors in primary human monocytes. *Mol Cell Biol Res Commun* 2000, 4:50-61.

[52] Swedlund HA, Hunder GG, Gleich GJ: Alpha 1-antitrypsin in serum and synovial fluid in rheumatoid arthritis. *Ann Rheum Dis* 1974, 33:162-164.

[53] Scott LJ, Evans EL, Dawes PT, Russell GI, Mattey DL: Comparison of IgA-alpha1-antitrypsin levels in rheumatoid arthritis and seronegative oligoarthritis: complex formation is not associated with inflammation per se. *Br J Rheumatol* 1998, 37:398-404.

[54] Cox DW, Huber O: Rheumatoid arthritis and alpha-1-antitrypsin. *Lancet* 1976, 1:1216-1217.

[55] Sandstrom CS, Ohlsson B, Melander O, Westin U, Mahadeva R, Janciauskiene S: An association between Type 2 diabetes and alpha-antitrypsin deficiency. *Diabet Med* 2008, 25:1370-1373.

[56] Ye J, Liao YT, Jian YQ, Zhang XD, Wei P, Qi H, Deng CY, Li FR: Alpha-1-antitrypsin for the improvement of autoimmunity and allograft rejection in beta cell transplantation. *Immunol Lett* 2013, 150:61-68.

[57] de Serres FJ, Blanco I: Prevalence of alpha1-antitrypsin deficiency alleles PI*S and PI*Z worldwide and effective screening for each of the five phenotypic classes PI*MS, PI*MZ, PI*SS, PI*SZ, and PI*ZZ: a comprehensive review. *Ther Adv Respir Dis* 2012, 6:277-295.

[58] Hersh CP, Dahl M, Ly NP, Berkey CS, Nordestgaard BG, Silverman EK: Chronic obstructive pulmonary disease in alpha1-antitrypsin PI MZ heterozygotes: a meta-analysis. *Thorax* 2004, 59:843-849.

[59] Molloy K, Hersh CP, Morris VB, Carroll TP, O'Connor CA, Lasky-Su JA, Greene CM, O'Neill SJ, Silverman EK, McElvaney NG: Clarification of the risk of chronic obstruc-

tive pulmonary disease in alpha1-antitrypsin deficiency PiMZ heterozygotes. *Am J Respir Crit Care Med* 2014, 189:419-427.

[60] Sorheim IC, Bakke P, Gulsvik A, Pillai SG, Johannessen A, Gaarder PI, Campbell EJ, Agusti A, Calverley PM, Donner CF, et al: alpha(1)-Antitrypsin protease inhibitor MZ heterozygosity is associated with airflow obstruction in two large cohorts. *Chest* 2010, 138:1125-1132.

[61] Mehta AJ, Thun GA, Imboden M, Ferrarotti I, Keidel D, Kunzli N, Kromhout H, Miedinger D, Phuleria H, Rochat T, et al: Interactions between SERPINA1 PiMZ genotype, occupational exposure and lung function decline. *Occup Environ Med* 2014, 71:234-240.

[62] Corbo GM, Forastiere F, Agabiti N, Dell'Orco V, Pistelli R, Massi G, Perucci CA, Valente S: Passive smoking and lung function in alpha(1)-antitrypsin heterozygote schoolchildren. *Thorax* 2003, 58:237-241.

[63] Wall M, Moe E, Eisenberg J, Powers M, Buist N, Buist AS: Long-term follow-up of a cohort of children with alpha-1-antitrypsin deficiency. *J Pediatr* 1990, 116:248-251.

[64] Carpenter MJ, Strange C, Jones Y, Dickson MR, Carter C, Moseley MA, Gilbert GE: Does genetic testing result in behavioral health change? Changes in smoking behavior following testing for alpha-1 antitrypsin deficiency. *Ann Behav Med* 2007, 33:22-28.

[65] Malerba M, Ricciardolo F, Radaeli A, Torregiani C, Ceriani L, Mori E, Bontempelli M, Tantucci C, Grassi V: Neutrophilic inflammation and IL-8 levels in induced sputum of alpha-1-antitrypsin PiMZ subjects. *Thorax* 2006, 61:129-133.

[66] Lomas DA: The selective advantage of alpha1-antitrypsin deficiency. *Am J Respir Crit Care Med* 2006, 173:1072-1077.

[67] Alam S, Li Z, Atkinson C, Jonigk D, Janciauskiene S, Mahadeva R: Z alpha-1 antitrypsin confers a pro-inflammatory phenotype that contributes to COPD. *Am J Respir Crit Care Med* 2014.

[68] Alam S, Li Z, Janciauskiene S, Mahadeva R: Oxidation of Z alpha1-antitrypsin by cigarette smoke induces polymerization: a novel mechanism of early-onset emphysema. *Am J Respir Cell Mol Biol* 2011, 45:261-269.

[69] Wewers MD, Casolaro MA, Sellers SE, Swayze SC, McPhaul KM, Wittes JT, Crystal RG: Replacement therapy for alpha 1-antitrypsin deficiency associated with emphysema. *N Engl J Med* 1987, 316:1055-1062.

[70] Brantly ML, Wittes JT, Vogelmeier CF, Hubbard RC, Fells GA, Crystal RG: Use of a highly purified alpha 1-antitrypsin standard to establish ranges for the common normal and deficient alpha 1-antitrypsin phenotypes. *Chest* 1991, 100:703-708.

[71] Dickens JA, Lomas DA: Why has it been so difficult to prove the efficacy of alpha-1-antitrypsin replacement therapy? Insights from the study of disease pathogenesis. *Drug Des Devel Ther* 2011, 5:391-405.

[72] Current status of alpha-1-antitrypsin replacement therapy: recommendations for the management of patients with severe hereditary deficiency. Ad Hoc Committee on Alpha-1-Antitrypsin Replacement Therapy of the Standards Committee, Canadian Thoracic Society. *CMAJ* 1992, 146:841-844.

[73] Turino GM, Barker AF, Brantly ML, Cohen AB, Connelly RP, Crystal RG, Eden E, Schluchter MD, Stoller JK: Clinical features of individuals with PI*SZ phenotype of alpha 1-antitrypsin deficiency. alpha 1-Antitrypsin Deficiency Registry Study Group. *Am J Respir Crit Care Med* 1996, 154:1718-1725.

[74] Dahl M, Hersh CP, Ly NP, Berkey CS, Silverman EK, Nordestgaard BG: The protease inhibitor PI*S allele and COPD: a meta-analysis. *Eur Respir J* 2005, 26:67-76.

[75] Kohnlein T, Janciauskiene S, Welte T: Diagnostic delay and clinical modifiers in alpha-1 antitrypsin deficiency. *Ther Adv Respir Dis* 2010, 4:279-287.

[76] Snyder MR, Katzmann JA, Butz ML, Wiley C, Yang P, Dawson DB, Halling KC, Highsmith WE, Thibodeau SN: Diagnosis of alpha-1-antitrypsin deficiency: An algorithm of quantification, genotyping, and phenotyping. *Clin Chem* 2006, 52:2236-2242.

[77] Miravitlles M, Herr C, Ferrarotti I, Jardi R, Rodriguez-Frias F, Luisetti M, Bals R: Laboratory testing of individuals with severe alpha1-antitrypsin deficiency in three European centres. *Eur Respir J* 2010, 35:960-968.

[78] Bornhorst JA, Procter M, Meadows C, Ashwood ER, Mao R: Evaluation of an integrative diagnostic algorithm for the identification of people at risk for alpha1-antitrypsin deficiency. *Am J Clin Pathol* 2007, 128:482-490.

[79] Donato LJ, Jenkins SM, Smith C, Katzmann JA, Snyder MR: Reference and interpretive ranges for alpha(1)-antitrypsin quantitation by phenotype in adult and pediatric populations. *Am J Clin Pathol* 2012, 138:398-405.

[80] Ferrarotti I, Thun GA, Zorzetto M, Ottaviani S, Imboden M, Schindler C, von Eckardstein A, Rohrer L, Rochat T, Russi EW, et al: Serum levels and genotype distribution of alpha1-antitrypsin in the general population. *Thorax* 2012, 67:669-674.

[81] Gaidulis L, Muensch HA, Maslow WC, Borer WZ: Optimizing reference values for the measurement of alpha 1-antitrypsin in serum: comparison of three methods. *Clin Chem* 1983, 29:1838-1840.

[82] Viedma JA, de la Iglesia A, Parera M, Lopez MT: A new automated turbidimetric immunoassay for quantifying alpha 1-antitrypsin in serum. *Clin Chem* 1986, 32:1020-1022.

[83] Bornhorst JA, Greene DN, Ashwood ER, Grenache DG: alpha1-Antitrypsin phenotypes and associated serum protein concentrations in a large clinical population. *Chest* 2013, 143:1000-1008.

[84] Lisowska-Myjak B: AAT as a diagnostic tool. *Clin Chim Acta* 2005, 352:1-13.

[85] Ritchie RF, Palomaki GE, Neveux LM, Navolotskaia O: Reference distributions for the positive acute phase proteins, alpha1-acid glycoprotein (orosomucoid), alpha1-antitrypsin, and haptoglobin: a comparison of a large cohort to the world's literature. *J Clin Lab Anal* 2000, 14:265-270.

[86] Miles RR, Roberts RF, Putnam AR, Roberts WL: Comparison of serum and heparinized plasma samples for measurement of chemistry analytes. *Clin Chem* 2004, 50:1704-1706.

[87] Ottaviani S, Gorrini M, Scabini R, Kadija Z, Paracchini E, Mariani F, Ferrarotti I, Luisetti M: C reactive protein and alpha1-antitrypsin: relationship between levels and gene variants. *Transl Res* 2011, 157:332-338.

[88] Zerimech F, Hennache G, Bellon F, Barouh G, Jacques Lafitte J, Porchet N, Balduyck M: Evaluation of a new Sebia isoelectrofocusing kit for alpha 1-antitrypsin phenotyping with the Hydrasys System. *Clin Chem Lab Med* 2008, 46:260-263.

[89] Greene DN, Elliott-Jelf MC, Straseski JA, Grenache DG: Facilitating the laboratory diagnosis of alpha1-antitrypsin deficiency. *Am J Clin Pathol* 2013, 139:184-191.

[90] Rodriguez-Frias F, Vila-Auli B, Homs-Riba M, Vidal-Pla R, Calpe-Calpe JL, Jardi-Margalef R: Diagnosis of Alpha-1 Antitrypsin Deficiency: Limitations of Rapid Diagnostic Laboratory Tests. *Arch Bronconeumol* 2011, 47:415-417.

[91] Lieberman J, Gaidults L, Schleissner LA: Intermediate alpha1-antitrypsin deficiency resulting from a null gene (M-phenotype). *Chest* 1976, 70:532-535.

[92] Ferrarotti I, Zorzetto M, Scabini R, Mazzola P, Campo I, Luisetti M: A novel method for rapid genotypic identification of alpha 1-antitrypsin variants. *Diagn Mol Pathol* 2004, 13:160-163.

[93] Rodriguez F, Jardi R, Costa X, Cotrina M, Galimany R, Vidal R, Miravitlles M: Rapid screening for alpha1-antitrypsin deficiency in patients with chronic obstructive pulmonary disease using dried blood specimens. *Am J Respir Crit Care Med* 2002, 166:814-817.

[94] Costa X, Jardi R, Rodriguez F, Miravitlles M, Cotrina M, Gonzalez C, Pascual C, Vidal R: Simple method for alpha1-antitrypsin deficiency screening by use of dried blood spot specimens. *Eur Respir J* 2000, 15:1111-1115.

[95] Zorzetto M, Russi E, Senn O, Imboden M, Ferrarotti I, Tinelli C, Campo I, Ottaviani S, Scabini R, von Eckardstein A, et al: SERPINA1 gene variants in individuals from

the general population with reduced alpha1-antitrypsin concentrations. *Clin Chem* 2008, 54:1331-1338.

[96] Gross P, Pfitzer EA, Tolker E, Babyak MA, Kaschak M: Experimental Emphysema: Its Production with Papain in Normal and Silicotic Rats. *Arch Environ Health* 1965, 11:50-58.

[97] Janoff A, Scherer J: Mediators of inflammation in leukocyte lysosomes. IX. Elastinolytic activity in granules of human polymorphonuclear leukocytes. *J Exp Med* 1968, 128:1137-1155.

[98] Johnson D, Travis J: The oxidative inactivation of human alpha-1-proteinase inhibitor. Further evidence for methionine at the reactive center. *J Biol Chem* 1979, 254:4022-4026.

[99] Carp H, Miller F, Hoidal JR, Janoff A: Potential mechanism of emphysema: alpha 1-proteinase inhibitor recovered from lungs of cigarette smokers contains oxidized methionine and has decreased elastase inhibitory capacity. *Proc Natl Acad Sci U S A* 1982, 79:2041-2045.

[100] Hubbard RC, Ogushi F, Fells GA, Cantin AM, Jallat S, Courtney M, Crystal RG: Oxidants spontaneously released by alveolar macrophages of cigarette smokers can inactivate the active site of alpha 1-antitrypsin, rendering it ineffective as an inhibitor of neutrophil elastase. *J Clin Invest* 1987, 80:1289-1295.

[101] Taggart C, Cervantes-Laurean D, Kim G, McElvaney NG, Wehr N, Moss J, Levine RL: Oxidation of either methionine 351 or methionine 358 in alpha 1-antitrypsin causes loss of anti-neutrophil elastase activity. *J Biol Chem* 2000, 275:27258-27265.

[102] Survival and FEV1 decline in individuals with severe deficiency of alpha1-antitrypsin. The Alpha-1-Antitrypsin Deficiency Registry Study Group. *Am J Respir Crit Care Med* 1998, 158:49-59.

[103] Janoff A, Carp H: Possible mechanisms of emphysema in smokers: cigarette smoke condensate suppresses protease inhibition in vitro. *Am Rev Respir Dis* 1977, 116:65-72.

[104] Seersholm N, Kok-Jensen A: Survival in relation to lung function and smoking cessation in patients with severe hereditary alpha 1-antitrypsin deficiency. *Am J Respir Crit Care Med* 1995, 151:369-373.

[105] Mayer AS, Stoller JK, Vedal S, Ruttenber AJ, Strand M, Sandhaus RA, Newman LS: Risk factors for symptom onset in PI*Z alpha-1 antitrypsin deficiency. *Int J Chron Obstruct Pulmon Dis* 2006, 1:485-492.

[106] McElvaney NG: Smoking ban--made in Ireland, for home use and for export. *N Engl J Med* 2004, 350:2231-2233.

[107] Hogarth DK, Rachelefsky G: Screening and familial testing of patients for alpha 1-antitrypsin deficiency. *Chest* 2008, 133:981-988.

[108] Tzakis A: Early recognition of alpha-1 antitrypsin deficiency and considerations for liver transplantation. *Gastroenterol Hepatol (N Y)* 2013, 9:110-112.

[109] Campos MA, Alazemi S, Zhang G, Sandhaus RA, Wanner A: Influenza vaccination in subjects with alpha1-antitrypsin deficiency. *Chest* 2008, 133:49-55.

[110] Halpin D: NICE guidance for COPD. *Thorax* 2004, 59:181-182.

[111] Fromer L, Cooper CB: A review of the GOLD guidelines for the diagnosis and treatment of patients with COPD. *Int J Clin Pract* 2008, 62:1219-1236.

[112] Hoogendoorn M, Feenstra TL, Hoogenveen RT, Al M, Molken MR: Association between lung function and exacerbation frequency in patients with COPD. *Int J Chron Obstruct Pulmon Dis* 2010, 5:435-444.

[113] Needham M, Stockley RA: Exacerbations in {alpha}1-antitrypsin deficiency. *Eur Respir J* 2005, 25:992-1000.

[114] Campos MA, Alazemi S, Zhang G, Wanner A, Salathe M, Baier H, Sandhaus RA: Exacerbations in subjects with alpha-1 antitrypsin deficiency receiving augmentation therapy. *Respir Med* 2009, 103:1532-1539.

[115] Campos MA, Alazemi S, Zhang G, Wanner A, Sandhaus RA: Effects of a disease management program in individuals with alpha-1 antitrypsin deficiency. *COPD* 2009, 6:31-40.

[116] Stoller JK, Aboussouan LS: alpha1-Antitrypsin deficiency. 5: intravenous augmentation therapy: current understanding. *Thorax* 2004, 59:708-712.

[117] Chapman KR, Stockley RA, Dawkins C, Wilkes MM, Navickis RJ: Augmentation therapy for alpha1 antitrypsin deficiency: a meta-analysis. *COPD* 2009, 6:177-184.

[118] McCarthy C, Dimitrov BD: Augmentation therapy for alpha-1 antitrypsin deficiency--not enough evidence to support its use yet! *COPD* 2010, 7:234; author reply 235-236.

[119] Mohanka M, Khemasuwan D, Stoller JK: A review of augmentation therapy for alpha-1 antitrypsin deficiency. *Expert Opin Biol Ther* 2012, 12:685-700.

[120] Modrykamien A, Stoller JK: Alpha-1 antitrypsin (AAT) deficiency-what are the treatment options? *Expert Opin Pharmacother* 2009, 10:2653-2661.

[121] Celli BR: Pulmonary rehabilitation for patients with advanced lung disease. *Clin Chest Med* 1997, 18:521-534.

[122] Ries AL, Bauldoff GS, Carlin BW, Casaburi R, Emery CF, Mahler DA, Make B, Rochester CL, Zuwallack R, Herrerias C: Pulmonary Rehabilitation: Joint ACCP/AACVPR Evidence-Based Clinical Practice Guidelines. *Chest* 2007, 131:4S-42S.

http://dx.doi.org/10.5772/58602

[123] Stoller JK, Fromer L, Brantly M, Stocks J, Strange C: Primary care diagnosis of alpha-1 antitrypsin deficiency: issues and opportunities. *Cleve Clin J Med* 2007, 74:869-874.

[124] Aboussouan LS, Stoller JK: Detection of alpha-1 antitrypsin deficiency: a review. *Respir Med* 2009, 103:335-341.

[125] Mullins CD, Huang X, Merchant S, Stoller JK, Alpha One Foundation Research Network Registry I: The direct medical costs of alpha(1)-antitrypsin deficiency. *Chest* 2001, 119:745-752.

[126] Campos MA, Alazemi S, Zhang G, Salathe M, Wanner A, Sandhaus RA, Baier H: Clinical characteristics of subjects with symptoms of alpha1-antitrypsin deficiency older than 60 years. *Chest* 2009, 135:600-608.

[127] Tanash HA, Nilsson PM, Nilsson JA, Piitulainen E: Clinical course and prognosis of never-smokers with severe alpha-1-antitrypsin deficiency (PiZZ). *Thorax* 2008, 63:1091-1095.

[128] Willson AB, Seow C, Zimmerman M: Severe alpha-1 antitrypsin deficiency diagnosed in an 86-year-old man. *Intern Med J* 2004, 34:653-654.

[129] Jack CI, Evans CC: Three cases of alpha-1-antitrypsin deficiency in the elderly. *Postgrad Med J* 1991, 67:840-842.

[130] Fanos JH, Strange C: "The lion, the witch and the wardrobe": impact on sibs of individuals with AAT deficiency. *Am J Med Genet A* 2004, 130A:251-257.

[131] Klitzman R: Views of discrimination among individuals confronting genetic disease. *J Genet Couns* 2010, 19:68-83.

[132] Rahaghi F, Ortega I, Rahaghi N, Oliveira E, Ramirez J, Smolley L, Stoller JK: Physician alert suggesting alpha-1 antitrypsin deficiency testing in pulmonary function test (PFT) results. *COPD* 2009, 6:26-30.

[133] Fromer L: Improving diagnosis and management of alpha-1 antitrypsin deficiency in primary care: translating knowledge into action. *COPD* 2010, 7:192-198.

[134] Jain A, McCarthy K, Xu M, Stoller JK: Impact of a clinical decision support system in an electronic health record to enhance detection of alpha(1)-antitrypsin deficiency. Chest 2011, 140:198-204.

[135] Celli BR, MacNee W, Force AET: Standards for the diagnosis and treatment of patients with COPD: a summary of the ATS/ERS position paper. Eur Respir J 2004, 23:932-946.

Chapter 4

Antiproteases as Therapeutics to Target Inflammation in Chronic Obstructive Pulmonary Disease

Cormac McCarthy, Ciara A. O'Dwyer,
David A. Bergin, Noel G. McElvaney and
Emer P. Reeves

Additional information is available at the end of the chapter

http://dx.doi.org/10.5772/57455

1. Introduction

Chronic obstructive pulmonary disease (COPD) is characterized by progressive inflammation of the airways and is one of the major causes of death in the elderly. COPD leads to development of airflow limitation as evident by decreased forced expiratory volume in one second (FEV_1) and reduction in the percentage of FEV_1/ vital capacity. Standardised spirometric tests showing the presence of airflow obstruction are used in clinical diagnosis and more recently the use of high resolution CT scanning has been employed to detect early emphysematous changes which may be present prior to severe airflow obstruction (Figure 1).

In the lungs of patients with COPD elevated levels of pro-inflammatory cytokines such as interleukin (IL)-8, leukotriene-B_4 (LTB_4) and tumour necrosis factor-α (TNFα) have been recorded which can act as neutrophil chemoattractants. Once recruited to the airways, neutrophils are activated and release various compounds including reactive oxygen species, proteases and cationic proteins in order to clear infections. When released in excessive amounts however, these molecules can cause extensive damage to the respiratory epithelium resulting in yet more pro-inflammatory cytokine release and further neutrophil influx, thereby creating a cycle of inflammation.

It is now clear that neutrophil serine proteases, including neutrophil elastase (NE), proteinase 3 (PR3) and cathepsin G (CathG) are major pathogenic determinants in chronic airway inflammatory disorders. Moreover, accumulating evidence indicates that the expression of matrix metalloproteases (MMPs) is dysregulated in COPD and these proteins are involved in small airway remodelling. Increased levels of both MMPs and serine proteases can participate in proteolytic attack on the alveolar wall matrix and, as a consequence the lung extracellular matrix is damaged, resulting in obstruction of small airways and development of emphysema.

Due to their implication in the pathology of COPD airways disease both MMPs and serine proteases have been in focus for drug-development efforts over the last two decades. Such concepts are further reinforced by scientific findings indicating that a variety of broad spectrum serine protease and MMP inhibitors significantly ameliorate emphysema in experimental animal models of COPD. To this end, in recent years continued efforts to identify and optimize novel mechanism-based inhibitors have led to a number of new inhibitors being reported. For example three natural protease inhibitors, secretory leucocyte protease inhibitor (SLPI), elafin and alpha-1 antitrypsin (AAT), have therapeutic potential for reducing the protease-induced inflammatory response and show promising potency and selectivity profiles. Other therapy options for the modulation of inflammation associated with excessive protease activity is the use of recombinant, synthetic or semi synthetic protease inhibitors. In this chapter we aim to describe the clinical and scientific evidence for the involvement of proteases and their proposed mode of action in COPD development and progression. Potential intervention with natural or synthetic inhibitors in the management of emphysematous symptoms associated with COPD will be reviewed in this chapter.

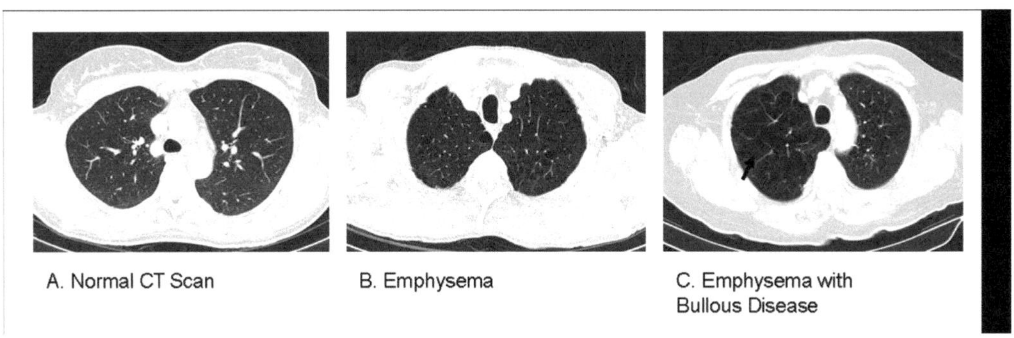

Figure 1. Chest high resolution CT scan of COPD. A) A single slice from a high resolution CT (HRCT) scan of thorax demonstrating normal healthy lung parenchyma. B) A single HRCT thorax image of the upper lobes demonstrating loss of lung density in keeping with emphysematous change. C) Severe emphysema of the upper lobes showing markedly reduced lung density and bullous disease present (indicated by the arrow).

2. The role of proteases in COPD

There are several classes of proteases and these include serine-, cysteine-, aspartate-, threonine-proteases and metalloproteases. For the purpose of this chapter we will focus on proteases which have been implicated in the pathogenesis of COPD and discuss particularly serine proteases and metalloproteases including NE, PR3, cathepsins and matrix metalloproteases.

2.1. Serine proteases

Serine proteases are a class of proteases which are involved in various physiological and pathological processes throughout the body and universally contain a serine as the amino acid at the active site of the enzyme [1]. Serine proteases include NE, CathG and PR3. They are primarily inactivated by serine protease inhibitors, the archetypal member of this family being AAT [2]. The main model for the protease-antiprotease imbalance is AAT deficiency, thus providing us with an insight into the importance of proteases in the development of emphysema [3, 4].

NE, PR3 and CathG are produced during neutrophil development in the bone marrow and are stored in the azurophilic (primary) granules of neutrophils [5]. These serine proteases are found in high concentrations in airway secretions of patients with inflammatory lung conditions [6, 7] and are seen in the circulating plasma of patients with severe sepsis and acute respiratory distress syndrome [8]. They have effects upon a broad range of extracellular matrix proteins including elastin, collagens, fibronectin, proteoglycans and laminin [9, 10]. Apart from AAT deficiency a large number of experimental animal studies also support the role of the protease/antiprotease imbalance in the pathogenesis of COPD, including the involvement of NE and PR3 in the development of emphysema [11, 12].

2.1.1. The serine protease neutrophil elastase

NE is a single polypeptide glycoprotein comprising 218 amino acids and is quite homologous with other serine proteases including PR3 and CathG [13]. NE is stored in the primary granules of neutrophils and when neutrophils are activated or primed by cytokines, it is released from the cell to the extracellular environment and may also rebind and become expressed on the cell surface [14]. The activity of NE is primarily inhibited and regulated by AAT [2, 15] but other inhibitors of NE have been reported including monocyte neutrophil elastase inhibitor (MNEI/Serpin B1) [16], elafin [17, 18] and SLPI [19, 20]. Of interest, the converse has also been shown whereby NE has been shown to inactivate and cleave SLPI. [21]

Smoking may lead to an imbalance between proteases and antiproteases through the reduction of the functional activity of AAT in the lung and also as described earlier by increasing the number of proteases produced hence increasing the proportion of elastolysis in the lung. Moreover, cigarette smoke has been reported to inhibit the anti-NE activity of AAT in bronchoalveolar lavage (BAL) fluid of smokers compared to healthy non-smoking control subjects [22, 23], however some studies have argued against this point [24, 25]. Cigarette smoke has also been shown to induce the release of NE in BAL fluid [26] and also to increase the circulating NE levels seen in plasma [27]. This implicates NE in the pathogenesis of emphysema and studies in BAL from COPD patients demonstrated a direct correlation between the NE burden in BAL and the degree of emphysema seen on CT scans. Further to this, results showed an inverse relationship between the anti-elastase activity in the BAL of COPD patients and the degree of emphysema and diffusing capacity, supporting the protease-antiprotease imbalance theory of emphysema [28].

Further studies on the presence of NE in the airways have shown that NE can cleave a number of epithelial cell surface receptors [29], cell activators and signalling cytokines [30] thereby potentially orchestrating the airway inflammatory milieu. Moreover, data have shown that alveolar macrophages may bind and internalise NE [31] and a later study has reported increased levels of NE in alveolar macrophages of patients with emphysema, providing further evidence of the increased protease burden [32]. NE has also been demonstrated using immunohistochemistry to be localised to the elastin fibres in the lung parenchyma of patients with emphysema [33]. The theory of NE induced emphysema has been supported not only from human studies but excellent animal models. Indeed, tracheal instillation of NE has been shown to induce the infiltration of neutrophils into the lung and cause emphysema in experimental models [11, 34].

Apart from the well-known role of NE as a protease in the protease/antiprotease imbalance in emphysema it exerts additional effects which contribute to the pathogenesis of COPD. For example NE exposure has been shown to significantly increase macrophage production of cathepsin B and latent and active MMP-2 [35], whilst the addition of AAT to BAL fluid greatly reduced NE-induced cathepsin B and MMP-2 expression in macrophages *in vitro* [36]. Additionally, NE is involved in the hypersecretion of mucus seen in COPD and is also a secretagogue, inducing the submucosal gland cells and goblet cells to secrete mucus [37-39]. NE has been shown to induce the expression of MUC5AC at the gene level in epithelial cells and hence increase the production of mucin in the airway. This mechanism has been shown to be dependent on the presence of reaction oxygen species, linking the role of NE inducing mucus hypersecretion to smoking [40, 41]. Moreover, not only does NE increase the amount of mucus produced in the lung but it also interrupts the mucociliary clearance mechanism by decreasing the ciliary beat frequency of bronchial epithelial cells [42].

The importance of the immune system and the inflammatory process in the pathogenesis of COPD is becoming more apparent and NE is involved in several of these immune mechanisms. NE can induce the expression of IL-8 in bronchial epithelial cells via TLR-4, subsequently leading to neutrophil chemotaxis and increasing the inflammatory burden in the lung [43, 44]. NE also plays an important role in neutrophil migration both through the cleavage of fibrin [45] and through the chemo-attractant properties of NE complexed with AAT [46]. The immune function can be further affected by NE through the cleavage of CD4 and CD8 glycoproteins from the surface of T-cells, thus impairing the function of T-cells and contributing to the inflammation seen in COPD [47]. Moreover, NE up-regulates the expression of TGF-β1 in smooth airway muscle via the NFκB pathway and this may further contribute to the airflow limitation seen in COPD [48]. Additionally, NE plays a role in the apoptosis seen in the pathogenesis of emphysematous lesions. Accordingly NE has been demonstrated to induce endothelial cell apoptosis [49], cytolysis of epithelial cells [42, 50] and cleaves the hydrophobic phospholipid substrate phophatidylserine receptor on macrophages, which subsequently impairs the ability of macrophages to clear apoptotic cells [51]. Collectively, these documented reports demonstrate that NE is an integral enzyme involved in the pathogenesis of COPD and emphysema and is a key target for therapeutic intervention.

2.1.2. *Neutrophil derived proteinase 3*

PR3 is the most abundant serine protease found in the neutrophil [52] and consequently more PR3 than NE is released by the neutrophil during the phagocytosis process [53]. Similar to NE, following activation of neutrophils by inflammatory cytokines, PR3 can be expressed on the surface of neutrophils [52] and AAT potently inhibits PR3 in the circulation [2, 54]. In contrast to AAT, SLPI has no effect upon PR3 and in fact PR3 is capable of degrading SLPI, thereby enhancing the activities of NE and other serine proteases [55].

Animal studies have demonstrated that PR3 plays a role in the development of emphysema, with studies showing that instillation of PR3 intra-tracheally leads to emphysematous lung disease in hamsters [12]. PR3 is found in the sputum of both stable COPD patients and AAT deficient individuals and increases at times of pulmonary exacerbations. Elevated PR3 levels correlate with an increase in neutrophilic burden [56]. However, its elastolytic rate is relatively low compared to NE, suggesting possibly a more minor role in the pathogenesis of emphysema [57]. Studies have also shown that PR3 maintains pro-inflammatory properties, possessing the ability to activate TNFα and IL-1β [58]. PR3 also has a strong effect on promoting the secretion of mucus in the airways [59] and can lead to cell apoptosis in the lung [49, 60].

2.1.3. *Cathepsin G and other cathepsins*

Not all cathepsins are serine proteases and in fact include aspartate and cysteine proteases. In this section we will discuss CathG, a serine protease related to NE and PR3 and briefly discuss other cathepsins and their role in COPD. Of major importance, increased levels of cathepsins have been demonstrated in BAL fluid of emphysema patients and therefore may play a role in the pathogenesis of the condition [61].

CathG is a serine protease and is stored in the primary granules of neutrophils. Upon release, activity of this protease is under the regulation of AAT and SLPI [19]. Increased levels of cathepsins can be seen in the BAL fluid of patients with emphysema [61] but unlike NE and PR3, *in vivo* animal studies have not demonstrated the same effect of CathG in inducing emphysema [62]. Similar to the other serine proteases however, CathG can induce secretion of mucus, hence adding to the airflow limitation and symptoms found in COPD [37]. Moreover, CathG can impair T-cell function by cleaving trans-membrane glycoprotein co-receptors on the cell surface in a similar fashion to NE [47].

Increased levels and activity of cathepsin L and cathepsin S have been shown in alveolar macrophages of smokers [63, 64]. The expression of cathepsin S is induced by INF-γ and this occurs in multiple cell types including smooth muscle cells. Subsequently, it has been shown that over-expression of IFN-γ can increase the expression of cathepsin B, D, L and S [65]. Moreover, in murine investigational studies cysteine-protease inhibitors markedly reduced the amount of airway inflammation and emphysema associated with over expression of cathepsins B, H, K, L and S [66]. In addition, bacterial killing by the antimicrobial peptide LL-37 and by human beta-defensins is inhibited due to proteolytic degradation by cathepsin D [67] and inactivation by the cysteine proteases cathepsins B, L, and S, respectively [68]. Although there is far less evidence and reported studies on cathepsins they most likely play a contributory role to the pathogenesis of emphysema and should also be considered as possible therapeutic targets in the future.

3. Matrix metalloproteases in COPD

MMPs are proteolytic enzymes which degrade components of the lung matrix, including collagens and elastins. This occurs both under normal physiological conditions and during abnormal pathological processes. MMPs are secreted as pro-enzymes and are activated by proteolytic conversion and have a close relationship with cytokines and growth factors [69, 70]. MMPs have both collagenase and elastase activity and account for 50% of the elastolytic activity of BAL fluid in smokers [71]. Indeed, MMPs account for the majority of the elastolytic activity of macrophages in COPD patients [72] and are counteracted by tissue inhibitors of matrix metalloproteases known as TIMPs. Additionally, MMPs do not only demonstrate degrading properties but also are pro-inflammatory in nature, with liberated matrix fragments possessing pro-inflammatory and monocytic chemotactic properties [73, 74].

3.1. Macrophage derived matrix metalloprotease-12

MMP-12, also known as macrophage-metalloelastase, is perhaps the most studied and best understood MMP in emphysema and COPD and numerous animal models have demonstrated its role in lung disease. It is involved directly in matrix degradation and is also a pro-inflammatory peptide. A recombinant form of human MMP-12 has been used to demonstrate the direct role that MMP-12 plays in the inflammatory process in the airways of mice [75]. This recombinant form of MMP-12 caused an increase in neutrophils and in macrophages accompanied by increased levels of pro-inflammatory cytokines and MMPs. Human studies have reported that the number of alveolar macrophages in BAL fluid expressing MMP-12 was higher in COPD patients than in controls [76]. MMP-12 can also be produced by bronchial epithelial cells [77] and is expressed by airway smooth muscle [78]. Cigarette smoke has been repeatedly shown to up-regulate both the release and production of MMP-12 [79]. How this occurs is complex in nature and likely through several mechanisms. For example, upon exposure to smoke, proteins including plasminogen and prothrombin are released into the alveolar space where they are converted to plasmin and thrombin, both of which are serine proteases. Their action upon proteinase activated receptor-1 (PAR-1) subsequently leads to the secretion and activation of MMP-12 [80, 81]. A second mechanism by which smoke may activate MMP-12 has been shown in mice where it was shown to up-regulate GM-CSF production which in turn controls MMP-12 release [82]. Moreover, the gene expression of MMP-12 in epithelial cells is affected by reactive oxygen species [83] and in murine studies a direct link between MMP-12 and cigarette smoke induced airway inflammation has been demonstrated [84-86]. Moreover, in MMP-12 knockout mice a marked reduction in monocyte recruitment and in IL-13 and IFN-γ induced emphysema has been demonstrated, implicating the importance of MMP-12 in the inflammatory response seen in COPD [65, 66]. How MMP-12 exerts this inflammatory effect is multifactorial. One reported mechanism involves the pro-inflammatory action of MMP-12 through the release and activation of TNFα [87]. Secondly, MMP-12 has also been shown to possess the ability to induce the production and release of IL-8 via the EGFR pathway in epithelial cells [88]. The importance of MMP-12 in inducing airway inflammation is further supported by the use of MMP-12 inhibitors which were shown to ameliorate emphysema in experimental animals [89] and to lower both the concentration of immune cells in BAL fluid, and to affect inflammation [90]. MMP-12 also impacts upon the activity of other proteases, especially neutrophil derived enzymes including NE, PR3 and cathepsins, and can degrade AAT hence up-regulating the activity of these serine proteases [91].

Despite convincing evidence provided by experimental models and compelling data showing an association between MMP-12 and emphysema, the data from human studies is conflicting and not as clear cut. A number of studies have suggested increased expression of MMP-12 in alveolar macrophages and increased MMP-12 protein in sputum of COPD individuals compared to healthy controls [76, 92, 93] while others have shown no difference [94-96]. Thus further studies on MMP-12 are essential to confirm the role of this matrix metalloprotease in inflammation and tissues destruction associated with COPD.

3.2. Neutrophil released matrix metalloprotease-9

The next most studied and understood MMP in COPD is MMP-9. Also known as gelatinase-B and similarly to other matrix metalloproteases MMP-9 has multiple substrates including collagens IV, V, VII, X and XI as well as elastin, gelatin, pro-MMP9 and pro-MMP13. MMP-9 is secreted by bronchial epithelial cells, mast cells, neutrophils, eosinophils and alveolar macrophages in response to TGFβ, IL-13 and IL-8 [79].

Increased levels of MMP-9 have been demonstrated in smokers with and without airflow obstruction [97, 98] and a correlation between the levels of MMP-9 in sputum and the extent of airflow obstruction and symptoms in COPD has been reported [99]. There are also increased levels of MMP-9 in AAT deficient individuals, where levels correlated with clinical parameters including FEV1, DLCO, lung density and exacerbation frequency [98, 100]. Elevated levels of MMP-9 in COPD individuals have been demonstrated to correlate to the number of neutrophils, implicating MMP-9 in the inflammatory burden in COPD [98, 101]. Moreover, polymorphism in the promoter region of the human MMP-9 gene has been shown associated with emphysema in 2 separate Japanese cohorts [102, 103] and with COPD in a Chinese population [104].

In support of a role for the involvement of MMP-9 in COPD, *ex vivo* studies have shown that alveolar macrophages from BAL fluid in emphysema patients demonstrate increased expression of MMP-9 and MMP-1 compared to control subjects [95]. This is also true for smokers with and without COPD where there is increased expression of MMP-9 on alveolar macrophages compared to healthy controls [105, 106]. In a study comparing COPD patients to smokers with no evidence of airflow obstruction, alveolar macrophages from COPD individuals released increased levels of MMP-9 and *in vitro* the stimulation of these cells by IL-1β, lipopolysaccharides (LPS) and cigarette smoke increased the secretion of MMP-9 [106].

Consequently, emphysematous lung tissue has been shown to contain higher levels of MMP-9 compared to disease free tissue [107, 108].

Other studies of interest that provide evidence for the involvement of MMP-9 in the inflammatory process associated with COPD include data that demonstrate that MMP-9 possesses levels of TACE (TNFα converting enzyme) like activity and mediates acute cigarette smoke-induced inflammation via TNFα release [87]. MMP-9 may also be involved in the link between destruction of alveolar tissue and fibrotic proliferation observed in emphysema, potentially mediated by proteolytic cleavage of latent TGF-binding-protein-1 with subsequent release of TGFβ-1, possibly linking elastolysis and fibrosis [109, 110]. Interestingly, MMP-9 may be activated by NE via cleavage of pro-MMP-9 to active MMP-9 [111]. Moreover, NE has been shown to degrade TIMP-1 thereby leading to enhanced MMP-9 activity [112], implicating both NE and MMP-9 in the pathogenesis of COPD. Finally, a role for MMP-9 in mucus hypersecretion in COPD patients has been suggested, as MMP-9 activates epidermal growth factor which in turn increases the expression of MUC5AC production hence leading to increased mucus secretion [113, 114].

3.3. Matrix metalloprotease-1 and other matrix-metalloproteases

MMP-1, also known as interstitial collagenase-1, is active against multiple collagens including collagen I, II, III and VII, gelatin and pro-MMP9 and over-expression in mice has been associated with development of emphysema [115]. Loss of collagen type II leads to an increase in lung compliance and hence the development of emphysema [116]. In humans, BAL fluid from emphysema patients has increased MMP-1 expression compared to healthy controls [117] and increased expression of MMP1 was reported in the lungs of patients with emphysema [94]. This expression was localised to type II epithelial cells but not alveolar macrophages. MMP-1 is also expressed by airway smooth muscle [118] and the production of MMP-1 is driven by the MAPK pathway and also by hydrogen peroxide, an important pathogenic component of cigarette smoke [119]. In mouse models, MMP-1 has been shown to contribute to alveolar destruction leading to emphysema development [120, 121]. Similar to MMP-9, MMP-1 also possesses levels of TACE like activity which may contribute to the inflammation seen in COPD [87].

MMP-2 which is also known as gelatinase-A has activity against collagens I-V, VII, X, XI and XIV as well as elastin, fibronectin and gelatin. Increased levels of MMP-2 have been demonstrated in COPD lungs [107, 108] and also in experimental mice exposed to cigarette smoke [122]. Interestingly, in guinea pigs exposed to wood-smoke increased expression of MMP2 was recorded, possibly providing an insight into the pathogenesis of emphysema in individuals not exposed to cigarette smoke [123]. Moreover, increased levels of both MMP-8 and MMP-10 are seen in sputum of COPD patients and have been shown to correlate with airflow obstruction [97, 124], with increased levels of MMP-8 recorded at the time of acute pulmonary exacerbation [125]. Finally, MMP-12 is up-regulated in mice exposed to cigarette smoke [126] and elevated levels of MMP-13 are seen in individuals with emphysema [127].

Collectively, this information on MMPs contributes to the protease/antiprotease theory in COPD pathogenesis and provides targets that may be investigated when developing future therapeutic strategies. MMPs play a mixed role in COPD and are involved in the proteolytic destruction of lung tissue and possess a close relationship to neutrophil derived serine proteases. These latter processes are intertwined and hence targeting certain elements of protease induced inflammatory processes may provide encouraging and exciting therapeutic options.

4. Approaches to treatment

Current therapies for the treatment of COPD are similar between the non-genetically inherited form of the lung disease and COPD as a result of AAT deficiency, and are in line with the American Thoracic Society/European Respiratory Society published guidelines [128]. Of particular importance is the cessation of smoking for individuals diagnosed with the disorder, as smoking aggravates the condition and is a predominant prognostic factor for the outcome of COPD patients. Therapeutic strategies aimed at the protease-antiprotease imbalance can be expected to have the greatest effect on lung disease associated with COPD and AAT deficiency. Ensuing sections will focus on AAT augmentation therapy in both intravenous and aerosolized forms, transgenic and recombinant forms of AAT and administration of either natural (elafin and SLPI) or synthetic (Sivelestat) antiproteases for treatment of COPD.

4.1. AAT replacement therapy

The importance of the protease: antiprotease balance is evident by the development of emphysema in AAT deficient individuals due to unopposed NE activity, of which AAT is the major inhibitor. Indeed the most logical approach to treatment is the reestablishment of physiological levels of AAT. The minimum level of AAT required to protect the lung from protease mediated damage was set as 11μmol/L (or 80mg/dL), and this has been referred to as the "protective" threshold level [129]. This value is based on the levels of AAT recorded in non-smoking individuals with the PiSZ phenotype, which is not thought to confer an increased risk of developing lung disease. Intravenous infusion of human plasma derived AAT, also referred to as AAT augmentation therapy, provides a method of maintaining this protective threshold and thus delays the progression of emphysema (Table 1). In 1981, researchers developed a method for partially purifying AAT from pooled human plasma and with the knowledge that the serum half-life of AAT is 5.4 days [130], devised an infusion schedule that allowed once weekly administration of purified AAT to AAT deficient individuals. Following such infusions the results of this study demonstrated that significant amounts of AAT, with full anti-NE capacity, diffused to the lower respiratory tract. Consequently, infusion of purified human plasma AAT at a dose of 60mg per kilogram of body weight per week, a dose that was sufficient to maintain serum levels ≥ 11μmol/ L, was FDA-approved and is now widely used in Europe and North America in treatment of AAT deficient individuals [131]. The first available preparations of AAT included pooled human plasma AAT prepared by pasteurisation (Prolastin, Bayer, West Haven, CT, USA). In turn, more recent studies examined the biochemical effectiveness of AAT purified by solvent detergent and nano-filtration methodology (Aralast, Baxter, Westlake Village, CA, USA) [132] and a third preparation (Zemaira,

CSL Behring, PA USA) has received US FDA approval [133]. Currently there are six FDA approved AAT preparations available in the USA. The clinical effects of infused AAT therapy documented to date consist of patient outcome measures including the rate of FEV_1 decline [134, 135], the level of desmosine as a biomarker of elastin degradation [136, 137], the incidence of acute exacerbations [138], frequency of lung infections [139] and the change in lung density [140] calculated by CT scanning [141]. Nevertheless, though studies have demonstrated that infusion of AAT is safe and well tolerated [142], there remains considerable debate over the clinical benefits and the cost-effectiveness of the treatment [134, 143, 144].

Study Type	AAT Infusion	Reference	Patient outcome
Observational	Weekly	(Ma et al. 2013)	Reduced elastin degradation in treated group
Observational	Weekly	(Tonelli et al. 2009)	Slower rate of decline in FEV1% predicted in augmentation group
Randomized	Weekly	(Dirksen et al. 2009)	Attenuated loss of lung tissue in treated cohort measured by CT lung density
Observational	Weekly	(Wencker et al. 2001)	Reduced rate of FEV1 decline post augmentation therapy
Descriptive	Weekly	(Gottlieb et al. 2000)	Elastin degradation was not reduced
Observational	56% weekly & 26% biweekly	(Lieberman 2000)	Decline in number of infections per year
Randomized controlled	4-weekly	(Dirksen et al. 2009)	Reduced loss of lung tissue by CT densitometry with augmentation
Observational parallel controls	51% weekly & 25% biweekly	(group 1998)	Slowed decline in FEV1 of 27ml/year in treated group
Observational parallel controls	Weekly	(Seersholm et al. 1997)	Reduced rate of decline of FEV1 in treated group of 21ml/year.

Table 1. Treatment of patients with AAT deficiency with augmentation therapy

The biochemical efficacy of AAT augmentation therapy has been examined in a number of studies and in 1987 Wewers and colleagues demonstrated that a weekly dosage of 60mg/kg not only restored AAT levels in serum and BAL fluid but also increased anti-NE capacity from a baseline value of 5.4 ± 0.1μM in the serum to 13.3 ± 0.1μM [142]. Indeed, additional studies have focused on the impact of augmentation therapy on the inflammatory environment of the lung. For example, AAT deficiency is characterised by increased neutrophil numbers and thus increased sputum and BAL fluid levels of NE [145]. This burden of neutrophils in the lung as a result of excessive trafficking is attributed to chemotactic agents such as IL-8 and LTB_4 and significantly higher levels of these chemo-attractants have been recorded in sputum from individuals with AAT deficiency compared to COPD patients. To understand this further, an *in vitro* study discovered increased release of LTB_4 from AAT deficient alveolar macrophages as a result of unopposed NE activity. Of relevance, the addition of exogenous AAT reduced the amount of LTB_4 being released by macrophages in response to NE [146]. In confirmation of this latter study, Stockley *et al* demonstrated that sputum samples from AAT deficient individuals on day one post infusion of AAT augmentation therapy possessed reduced NE activity and a dramatic attenuation of LTB_4 concentration from a level of 13.46nM to 8.62nM [147]. Moreover, the anti-inflammatory effects of AAT augmentation therapy were confirmed as decreased concentrations of IL-8, and the chemotactic activity mediated by this chemokine, were reduced to normal levels in AAT deficient individuals post treatment. [148, 149]

One of the first studies to examine the effect of AAT augmentation therapy compared the ΔFEV_1 of 97 ex-smokers from a Danish AAT deficient registry to a German group of 198 patients treated with weekly infusions of AAT (60mg/kg) for at least one year. Overall, the ΔFEV_1 in the treated group was significantly lower than in the untreated group, with annual declines of 53 mL yr^{-1} and 75 mL yr^{-1}, respectively (p=0.02). However, there was no beneficial effect of augmentation therapy in 103 patients with an initial $FEV_1 \leq 30$ or in the 25 patients with an $FEV_1 > 65\%$ [134]. In 1998, one of the largest observational studies (n=1129) centred on the NHLBI Registry for individuals with severe AAT deficiency [150] was carried out. Although no overall difference in FEV_1 decline was recorded between the augmentation-therapy treated and untreated groups, in a subgroup with FEV_1 between 39-45% predicted there was a significant difference of -27ml/year between treated and untreated. This study also suggested that survival was enhanced in individuals receiving augmentation therapy. The risk ratio for death in augmentation therapy recipients was 0.64, significantly lower than non-recipients (P=0.02) and the risk ratio for individuals receiving augmentation therapy with stage II COPD was 0.21 (P<0.001). The possibility that these differences may have been due to other factors, such as the socioeconomic status of enrolled patients could not be ruled out and this latter point is a potential limitation of this study. In a subsequent randomised study of 164 AAT deficient individuals enrolled in the Alpha-1 foundation DNA and tissue bank, when adjusted by age at baseline, sex, smoking status, baseline FEV_1 % of predicted, a slower rate of decline in FEV_1% predicted was observed in the augmentation group (10.6±21.4 ml/year) in comparison to the non-augmented group (36.96±12.1ml/year). The authors of this study concluded that augmentation therapy was effective in subjects with AAT deficiency, favouring ex-smoker subjects with an FEV_1 below 50% of predicted [151].

Results from studies measuring changes in urine desmosine levels, a marker of elastin breakdown, in response to AAT augmentation therapy have been mixed. One study of two AAT deficient patients observed a 35% reduction in urine desmosine levels after monthly doses of 260mg/kg AAT [152]. In contrast, a larger study by Gottelieb *et al* showed no change in the level of elastin breakdown after eight weeks of augmentation therapy (P=0.85). Although this latter study recruited only twelve AAT deficient individuals, the authors suggested that elastin degradation at this point in the disease was possibly NE independent [137]. In a recent study desmosine levels were assessed in plasma, BAL fluid and urine in a cohort of AAT deficient patients receiving AAT augmentation therapy. A 13.9% reduction in plasma and 37% reduction in BAL fluid desmosine levels were observed 12 weeks after receiving IV augmentation therapy compared to baseline levels prior to treatment [153]. The study showed that augmentation therapy maintained the ability to inhibit NE and to reduce degradation of elastin both systemically and in the lungs, however the findings suggested that the dose of AAT was not sufficient to reduce elastin degradation to that of control levels of healthy individuals. There is a relatively limited body of clinical evidence supporting the benefits of 60mg/kg dosage, with some even questioning the recommendation of this dose of AAT to AAT deficient patients [154]. The concentration of 60mg/kg aims to increase AAT levels to values above that of the protective threshold (11μM) yet levels are still below that of serum AAT concentration observed in non-AAT deficient individuals (20-53μM) [155]. To address this issue Campos *et al* assessed the safety and efficacy of an increased 120mg/kg weekly dose of AAT in 30 adults with AAT deficiency in a multicentre, randomised, double-blind crossover study. A weekly dose of 120mg/kg resulted in a serum concentration of 27.7μM four weeks after treatment, well within the healthy control range, compared to 17.3μM at the same time period for the group receiving 60mg/kg. Concurrently, this increased dosage was considered to be safe and well-tolerated, however further investigation is warranted due to the relatively small cohort size and the lack of analysis of clinical parameters such as FEV_1 and CT densitometry [156].

Currently desmosine is the only clinical biomarker for assessment of lung tissue destruction, however it is limited by lack of specificity and may be influenced by diet and renal function which may in part provide an explanation for the lack of association between desmosine levels in the urine and FEV_1 [157-159]. Current research is aimed at identifying cost effective yet stable novel biomarkers that are central to the pathophysiological process, which can act as a predictor of disease progression and are sensitive to therapeutic intervention [160, 161]. In this regard, a novel potential biomarker has been recently reported specific to cleavage of fibrinogen and related to NE in the lungs [136]. The fibrinogen cleavage product $A\alpha\text{-}Val^{360}$ was measured in plasma from subjects recruited in the EXACTLE trial and the levels of this product were decreased in subjects receiving AAT replacement therapy while remaining unchanged in the placebo group.

Determining exacerbation rates in patients receiving therapy is an additional parameter that is employed to determine the efficacy of AAT replacement therapy. In a web based questionnaire prepared by Lieberman and colleagues, key questions addressed issues such as frequency of respiratory infections pre- and post-AAT augmentation therapy [139]. Out of eighty nine individuals who had received augmentation therapy for more than one year, seventy four felt that the treatment was of benefit, with almost half accrediting the benefits to a reduction in the number of infectious exacerbations from approximately five down to one per year ($P<0.001$). CT lung density measurements are currently considered to be a more sensitive outcome to measure the impact of AAT replacement therapy. The first of these studies was a double blind trial with 26 Danish and 30 Dutch ex-smokers, randomized to either AAT (250 mg/kg) or albumin (625 mg/kg) infusions at 4 week intervals for at least 3 years [140]. Using self-administered spirometry, no difference was found in FEV_1 decline between treatment and placebo. Conversely, upon analysis of CT scans (slices 5 cm below carina), a trend towards a slower rate in loss of lung density was observed in augmentation receiving patients with measurements of 2.6 ± 0.41 g/L/yr for placebo as compared with 1.5 ± 0.41 g/L/yr for AAT infusion, however the reported differences were shown to be non-significant (P=0.07), possibly due to the inadequate study size. Following this, in 2009, Dirksen *et al*. carried out a randomised, double-blind, placebo-controlled, parallel-group study conducted at three European centres (Copenhagen (Denmark), Birmingham (UK), and Malmö (Sweden)) known as the EXACTLE trial. CT scans were performed at baseline and at 12 and 24 months and the difference in the decline of lung density between treated and placebo groups suggested a trend towards a beneficial treatment effect, with P values for treatment difference ranging from 0.049 to a non-significant value of 0.084 depending on the outcome algorithm chosen. In 2010, Stockley and colleagues analysed the combined outcome measures of the EXACTLE and Danish-Dutch trial and concluded that augmentation therapy conferred a significant decline in the rate of CT densitometric loss but not in FEV_1 decline [162].

A number of studies have addressed the potential clinical use of AAT augmentation therapy in treatment of disorders outside the context of AAT deficiency, including transplant rejection, type1 diabetes mellitus, inflammatory bowel disease, rheumatoid arthritis, viral infection and cystic fibrosis [163]. In light of this, there is a need that goes beyond that afforded by purified human plasma and thus transgenic and recombinant AAT have been considered.

4.2. Recombinant and transgenic AAT

Despite the accumulation of encouraging data supporting the use of AAT augmentation therapy, significant questions remain regarding the cost-effectiveness of this intravenous strategy for treatment of AAT deficient related COPD, which is estimated to cost the US $100,000 per patient per year worldwide [143]. Such deliberation has prompted the development of new strategies, including the use of recombinant and transgenic protein to boost the natural antiprotease screen. A variety of systems have been employed to produce humanized recombinant AAT including plants, yeast fungi, animals, insect cells, bacteria and mammalian cells. One of the approaches involved expression of recombinant AAT in *E. coli,* but AAT produced via this system lacked glycosylation and consequently exhibited a short half-life within the circulation. To address this issue the presence of a single thiol residue at the surface of AAT was exploited by researchers, who conjugated maleimido-polyethylene glycol to the thiol group. Results revealed that site-specific conjugation with polyethylene glycol at Cys^{232} of nonglycosylated recombinant human AAT gave rise to active inhibitor with prolonged *in vivo* stability [164]. An alternative approach included production of a secreted fully functional AAT by the yeast *Saccharomyces cerevisiae* [165]. This secreted protein had high mannose-type glycosylation [166], which was thought to give rise to an immune response in humans because of non-human glycan residues, an adverse effect shared by active recombinant AAT protein expressed in the insect cell baculovirus expression vector system [167]. In an attempt to overcome the issue of glycosylation, a method of hyper glycosylation of the protein was introduced. This was achieved by adding terminal sialic acids to the existing glycans on the human AAT molecule. Such modification conferred increased protein half-life while maintaining the anti-NE capacity of the protein when injected into a mouse model [168]. In a further attempt to prepare fully glycosylated human AAT, Blanchard *et al* employed a human neuronal cell line (AGE1.HN®) to produce a recombinant AAT protein which retained biological activity and displayed a similar glycosylation patterns to native AAT [169]. Moreover, the recombinant AAT protein was biologically active and maintained anti-elastase activity and anti-inflamma-tory capacity, including modulation of TNFα production in neutrophils and monocytes [169]. *In vitro* testing of this protein revealed that the inhibitory effect of the recombinant AAT was comparable to that of Prolastin, however this has yet to be confirmed *in vivo*. More recently, AAT has been successfully produced and purified from the human PER.C6 cell line. The resultant protein shares the same primary, secondary and tertiary structures and *N*-linked glycosylation sites as AAT derived from human plasma and exhibits equivalent anti-NE capacity [170, 171]. While these studies strengthen the argument for the therapeutic use of recombinantly produced AAT, issues still remain with regards to the safety and efficacy of protein produced in this manner.

Subsequently, it was envisaged that sources of recombinant AAT from transgenic animals might overcome this posttranslational glycosylation challenge and fulfil the demand for mass production of AAT. To this end rabbits [172], mice [173] and sheep transgenic for a fusion of the ovine beta-lactoglobulin gene promoter to the human AAT genomic sequences were generated [174]. Human AAT purified from the milk of these animals appeared to be fully *N*-glycosylated and biologically active. While the use of transgenic sheep certainly tackled the issue of cost effectiveness, 5,000kg of AAT could be produced in one year, unfortunately however, a trial of inhaled AAT derived from sheep milk proved disappointing and observa-tions of a systemic antibody response in recipients to residual native sheep AAT and alpha-1 antichymotrypsin were observed [175]. Thus it is clear that transgenic preparations of AAT will only be of therapeutic value if they are of high purity in order to avoid immunogenicity.

While enhancing production of AAT seems promising from a cost and mass production point of view, significant challenges remain for the development of recombinant and transgenic AAT and they cannot compete with the current source of AAT from pooled human plasma for safety and efficacy in the treatment of AAT deficiency.

4.3. Aerosolized AAT augmentation therapy

Interest in the administration of AAT in aerosolized form has increased in recent years due to the advantageous properties provided such as a direct route to the lungs, avoidance of systemic deliver and a reduction in costs. Aerosolization of AAT has been shown to increase AAT levels and to restore anti-NE capacity in lung epithelium lining fluid of both COPD and cystic fibrosis individuals [176]. AAT administered in aerosolized form was found to positively impact upon neutrophil mediated killing of *Pseudomonas* [177], possibly by preventing cleavage of neutro-phil complement receptors by serine proteases, a previously reported adverse effect of NE [178] or by preventing cleavage of CXC chemokine receptor 1 (CXCR1) [179]. In addition, the presence of increased AAT in serum post aerosolization supports the hypothesis that aug-mented AAT is capable of diffusing across the pulmonary interstitium after administration [180] and affords anti-NE protection to the interstitial compartment [176]. Measurements of the rate of transfer of AAT from the lung and of the rate of appearance of AAT in plasma resulted in a calculated permeability of the alveolar-capillary membrane to AAT of 3.49-6.39 X 10^{-10} cm/s. In a canine model, levels of AAT rose to a maximum value at 48 hours after administration, remained elevated from 48-72 hours, and then declined slowly by 144 hours after administration [180]. Comparable results were reported by Hubbard *et al.* who evaluated aerosol administration of recombinant AAT to COPD individuals with AAT deficiency. Post aerosolization of single doses of 10-200mg of AAT, AAT anti- NE defences in ELF were augmented and aerosolized AAT was detectable in serum indicating that recombinant AAT was capable of gaining access to lung interstitium [176].

Further support for the use of aerosolized AAT in treatment of COPD was provided by Griese and colleagues who examined the effect of four weeks of plasma purified AAT inhalation on lung function, protease–antiprotease balance and airway inflammation in patients with cystic fibrosis [181]. The authors reported an increased concentration of aerosolized AAT accumulation in the airways. Post treatment, levels of NE activity, numbers of infiltrating neutrophils, pro-inflammatory cytokines levels and the numbers of bacteria (*P. aeruginosa*) were reduced culminating in a marked reduction in airway inflammation. In a second study by this research group, the authors documented that the inability of neutrophils to eradicate *Pseudomonas* infection despite the abundance of neutrophils in the cystic fibrosis lung was due to cleavage of CXCR1 from the neutrophil. *In vivo* administration of aerosolized AAT was shown to restore CXCR1 expression and improve the killing capacity of neutrophils as assessed by sputum levels of *P. aeruginosa*, thus supporting the beneficial effects of aerosolized AAT therapy [179]. In a further study employing a mouse model of smoke induced emphysema, inhaled AAT resulted in reductions in airspace enlargement of up to 73%. The results of this investigation indicated that delivery of AAT directly to the lung can prevent NE mediated tissue damage. Moreover, further evidence of the ability of aerosolised AAT to directly protect the lung tissue from proteolytic breakdown was demonstrated as aerosolised AAT abrogated NE-induced expression of cathepsin B and MMP-2 in BAL fluid, thus indirectly protecting key anti-inflammatory and antimicrobial peptides including SLPI and lactoferrin from cathepsin mediated proteolysis within the milieu of the COPD lung [36]. In terms of clinical efficacy of aerosolised AAT, a phase III trial of inhaled Kamada AAT is currently on-going with results on outcome measures including safety and efficacy, exacerbation frequency and progression of emphysema to be released presently. The outcome of this study will be pivotal to shaping the future development of aerosolised AAT augmentation therapy (NCT01217671).

4.4. Naturally occurring antiproteases elafin and SLPI as therapies for COPD

A number of studies have generated data to support the use of naturally occurring antiproteases, other than AAT, as potential anti-inflammatory therapies to modulate the high level of inflammatory within the lungs of COPD patients. Within the literature reports suggest that serine protease inhibitors may potentially be used as a treatment option for COPD. One such antiprotease is elafin, a small cationic protein (6kDa) which is a member of the chelonianin family. Throughout the literature it is often referred to as skin derived anti-leukoprotease (SKALP) due to its first identification in psoriatic epidermis [182]. More recently however, it has been shown to be produced and released by epidermal keratinocytes [183], lung derived epithelia [184], T-cells [185], macrophages [186] and also neutrophils [187].

Elafin is a subunit derived from the precursor molecule trappin-2 which has a molecular weight of 12.3 kDa [188]. The conversion of trappin-2 into elafin can occur by cleavage by several proteases including cathepsin L, cathepsin K, plasmin, trypsin but the most efficient protease at releasing elafin is tryptase [189]. The mature form of trappin-2 consists of two domains; the first domain is unique to only trappin-2, the *N*-terminal cementoin domain. This domain aids as a transglutaminase substrate which allows trappin-2 to interact and bind to extracellular matrix proteins such as fibronectin, collagen IV, fibrinogen, laminin V, vitronectin, thus prolonging its presence within in the lung [188]. The second domain, which is present in both trappin-2 and elafin, is the whey acidic protein (WAP) domain. The WAP domain provides antiprotease activity with specificity against NE [18] and PR3 [17], two key proteases that play a role in the lung pathophysiology associated with COPD [56, 190].

Several studies have demonstrated that elafin is produced under inflammatory conditions suggesting it to be an acute phase reactant [191]. Interestingly, NE can impact on elafin expression and it has been demonstrated that exposing human alveolar epithelial cells to NE can result in increased protein expression and secretion of elafin [192]. Additional studies have demonstrated that pro-inflammatory mediators such as TNFα and IL-1β increase elafin expression in lung derived cell lines, indicating that in response to cytokine induced inflammation, epithelial cells can increase their antiprotease shield [191]. This induced increase in elafin expression is not limited to only host derived inflammatory mediators as it has been shown that bacterial LPS can increase elafin expression in murine airways [193] and in macrophages from transgenic mice expressing human elafin [194].

The immuno-modulatory impact of elafin on inflammation has been established in a number of studies and animal models. For example, Vachon and colleagues utilised a murine model and following intranasal administration of LPS, pre-treatment with recombinant human elafin was shown to diminish neutrophil infiltration into the airways [195]. In the same study elafin was shown to reduce gelatinase activity, macrophage inflammatory protein-2 (MIP-2), keratinocyte chemoattractant and significantly reduced mRNA levels of three members of the IL-1 ligand family [195]. Conversely, in an earlier study involving a transgenic murine model expressing human trappin-2, an increase in neutrophil recruitment to the lungs of LPS challenged mice was observed [193]. The discrepancy between these two latter studies could in part be due to differences in the mode of elafin administration and the murine models employed. Of interest, the positive impact of elafin on COPD related complications such as pulmonary hypertension has been reported [196]. Moreover, in a hypoxia associated pulmonary hypertension murine model the protease activity, muscularization of pulmonary arteries and right ventricular pressure were reduced in transgenic mice that over expressed elafin [197]. Indeed, both elafin and its precursor molecule trappin-2 have anti-inflammatory properties, as evident by the inactivation of key inflammatory signalling pathways and immune cell activity associated with COPD pathogenesis. In a study using a human myelomonocytic cell line, elafin was shown to exert its anti-inflammatory effect intracellularly [198]. The mode of action involved direct impact on the ubiquitin-proteasome pathway, delaying turnover of polyubiquitinated proteins thus affecting NFκB activation and the AP-1 pathway leading to reduced MCP-1 expression in response to LPS [198]. Moreover, in transfection studies it was demonstrated that the impact of elafin on chemokine production was cell specific [199]. Results demonstrated that elafin reduced TNFα secretion by human macrophages and IL-8 release by human umbilical cord endothelial cells (HUVECs) in response to TNFα, LPS and oxidized LDL, through modulation of NFκB signalling. In contrast, in the same study transfecting an alveolar epithelial cell line with elafin had no significant effect on LPS induced IL-8 production [199].

In addition to possessing antiprotease and anti-inflammatory properties, elafin also demonstrates anti-microbial properties which may prove beneficial in the treatment of infective exacerbations in COPD patients. In a study carried out by Simpson *et al.*, the anti-bacterial capability of elafin was evaluated and the results demonstrated that elafin maintained bactericidal effect against both *P. aeruginosa* and *S. aureus* [200]. This effect could in part be due to the cationic charge of elafin which may destabilize bacterial membranes similar to classical antimicrobial proteins [201]. Moreover, a study by Baranger *et al.*, demonstrated that trappin-2 had antibacterial properties against other clinically important bacteria including *Klebsiella pneumoniae, Haemophilus influenzae, Streptococcus pneumoniae* and *Branhamella catarrhalis* [202]. Furthermore, this study highlighted the novel anti-fungal effect of trappin-2 against *Aspergillus fumigatus*, with the outcome of this study demonstrating the anti-microbial properties of trappin-2 to be independent of its antiprotease property. Aside from direct activity against microbes, trappin-2 in turn has been shown to enhance the clearance of *P. aeruginosa* from the lungs of infected mice [203], an effect mediated via opsonisation of bacteria with trappin-2 for more efficient CD14-dependent clearance by macrophages [197]. In additional studies it has been shown that elafin can modulate inflammation associated with LPS, through inhibition of AP-1 and NFκB activation [198], possibly by direct interaction with this microbial inflammatory mediatory [204].

These innate attributes of elafin make it an ideal candidate for a replacement therapy in treatment of inflammatory lung diseases such as COPD which is associated with excess protease burden and/or infection. However caution must be exercised, as like many other endogenous protease inhibitors, elafin is susceptible to inactivation by neutrophil-derived oxidants resulting in loss of its antiprotease activity [205]. Moreover, elafin can be cleaved by NE [206], which is present in high concentrations in the COPD lung [207] and cleavage can result in diminished ability of elafin to bind LPS and its capacity to be immobilized by transglutamination [206]. A similar observation was made in regard to the *P. aeruginosa* derived proteases pseudolysin and aeruginolysin which can cleave elafin thereby negatively impacting on its biological functions [208]. Collectively, these findings suggest that within an environment of high protease burden, as found in the COPD lung, this could have a negative impact upon the clinical efficacy of elafin.

An additional native antiprotease that has been well documented for its potential as a therapy for COPD is human SLPI, which was originally identified in parotid secretions [20]. Being a member of the antileukoprotease family, SLPI shares 40% homology with elafin. A number of cell types have been documented to produce SLPI including macrophages [186], monocytes, neutrophils [187] and lung epithelial cells [209]. It is well accepted that SLPI is a potent inhibitor of an array of serine proteases including NE, cathepsin G, trypsin and chymotrypsin. Similar to elafin, SLPI expression levels are increased post inflammatory mediator exposure; for example TNFα and IL-1β treatment of lung epithelial cells [191]. Other host derived inflammatory proteins including proteases from neutrophils (e.g. NE and defensins [184]) can increase and induce SLPI expression in bronchial epithelial cells. In more recent studies, aside from host derived inflammatory mediators, bacteria have also been shown to induced SLPI expression in macrophages by a TLR2-dependent but MyD88-independent signalling pathway [210]. Additionally, bacterial products such as LPS can increase SLPI expression in macrophages and neutrophils [211], suggesting that SLPI functions as an acute phase reactant.

SLPI exhibits an array of anti-inflammatory properties including inhibition of monocyte production of MMPs [212, 213] which play an important pathophysiological role in tissue remodelling and are observed to be in high abundance in COPD [95, 107, 214]. The range of anti-inflammatory properties of SLPI includes inhibition of nitric oxide and TNFα production in macrophages in response to LPS [215] and inhibition of IFN-γ induced cathepsin S expression in macrophages [216]. In monocytes it has been demonstrated that SLPI can cross the plasma membrane and enter the cell cytoplasm and nucleus [217]. Localization to these cell compartments facilitates the ability of SLPI to inhibit degradation of key proteins that activate NFκB and to competitively compete with p65 binding to NFκB consensus sequences thereby preventing NFκB binding to promoter regions of inflammatory genes [217]. In a more recent study involving neutrophils from COPD patients, the intracellular inhibitory activity of SLPI was further expanded as it was shown that SLPI modulated calcium flux and inositol 1,4,5-triphosphate generation thereby reducing cell migration [218] Additionally, SLPI possesses anti-microbial capabilities against *P. aeruginosa, S. aureus, S. epidermidis, E. coli and S. aureus* [219, 220]. SLPI's antifungal properties have been observed against *A. fumigatus* and *Candida albicans* [221] and in this latter study SLPIs fungicidal and fungistatic activity were shown comparable to that of human defensins and lysozyme.

Despite the potential advantages, delivery of SLPI to the lungs has proven unimpressive [222]. Aerosolisation of recombinant SLPI (100mg) twice daily to individuals with cystic fibrosis was associated with reduced NE activity on the respiratory epithelial surface, as well a reduction in the level of IL-8 and neutrophil numbers [223]. However, a greater concentration of recombinant SLPI compared to AAT is required to suppress NE activity in individuals with lung disease. Furthermore accumulation of recombinant SLPI on respiratory epithelial surfaces does not occur and SLPI does not penetrate significantly into the interstitium following aerosolization. Further drawbacks include the fact that most of the anti-NE effects are gone within 12 hours of administration. Reasons for this latter phenomenon have been proposed and may be due to uptake of SLPI by epithelial cells and macrophages, and/or binding of recombinant SLPI to molecules in the interstitium after passing through the epithelium [222, 224].

More recently, it has also been shown that SLPI is vulnerable to degradation and inactivation by cysteinyl cathepins [225] and NE [21], and thus the utilization of SLPI as effective therapy for COPD presents some challenges. One approach to this challenge is delivery of recombinant SLPI via a liposomal carrier which protects the activity of SLPI against cathepsin L mediated degradation, whilst having no adverse effect on SLPI access to intracellular sites of action *in vitro* [226]. Alternatively, co-treatment of SLPI with surfactant protein A has been proposed, which aids in the preservation of SLPI and protects it from cleavage by matrix metalloproteases [227].

4.5. Synthetic and semi-synthetic engineered protease inhibitors as alternative therapies for COPD

In a COPD animal model, ADAM-17 (a membrane bound MMP) has been shown to contribute to progression of COPD lung disease through activation of TNFα [228]. Recent studies have demonstrated that AAT, a natural serine protease inhibitor, also acts as an ADAM-17 inhibitor thereby regulating soluble immune complex induced neutrophil chemotaxis [148] and TNFα production in lung endothelial cells [229]. However, other therapeutic options for the modulation of inflammation associated with excessive protease activity is the use of synthetic or semi synthetic protease inhibitors. These molecules, for example the non-peptide inhibitor ONO-5046 or sivelestat, offer better accessibility into the lung milieu due to their reduced size. Sivelestat is a specific inhibitor of NE and in LPS animal studies was shown to significantly reduce the number of infiltrating neutrophils and elastase activity levels, thereby decreasing lung tissue damage [230-232]. Moreover, sivelestat has been reported to reduce neutrophil-mediated endothelial cell injury by inactivating extracellular elastase and by suppressing release of this serine protease by neutrophils [231]. A recent study demonstrated the ability of sivelestat to inhibit bleomycin induced pulmonary fibrosis and apoptosis in human epithelial cells [233]. The authors of this study also verified that sivelestat reduced pulmonary neutrophil counts by decreasing BAL fluid levels of cytokine-induced neutrophil chemoattractant (CINC)-1. So far there have been no *in vitro* or *in vivo* investigations on the potential use of sivelestat in COPD, but studies involving other pulmonary conditions including post-cardiopulmonary bypass lung injury [234], acute lung injury with sepsis [235] and adult respiratory distress syndrome [236] have shown some therapeutic success with this synthetic inhibitor. To date, Japan has been the only country to approve sivelestat for the above conditions [237].

An alternative synthetic inhibitor that has been utilized in several studies is the cyclic thiol compound MR889. This synthetic inhibitor demonstrated inhibition against several serine proteases *in vitro* and in sputum from patients with chronic bronchitis [238]. When used in clinical studies however, although MR889 was considered safe for COPD patients, the results demonstrated that there was no significant reduction in the level of biomarkers of lung disease except for a small subset of individuals who had a short disease duration [239]. Other synthetic elastase inhibitors such as ZD0892 and FR134043 have been shown to reduce lung inflammation associated with cigarette smoke [240, 241] or NE [242] in animal models and in cultured cells [243]. ZD0892 was shown not to exert an adverse effect on neutrophil function including uptake and killing of *S. aureus*, but use of this compound in clinical studies in humans has not been documented.

More recently, the synthetic selective inhibitor of elastase, AZD9668, has attracted a lot of attention and was shown to have significant impact on NE activity *in vitro* [244]. In rodent models, AZD9668 was shown to prevent NE-induced lung injury, cigarette smoke induced inflammatory responses, airspace enlargement and small airways remodelling [244]. Despite these positive findings however, results of a recent clinical trial involving AZD9668, queried the efficiency of this inhibitor in COPD patients as no significant change in lung function and clinical measurements was observed [245]. Although these later results suggest that targeting NE activity alone may not be an effective treatment option in COPD, a subsequent smaller study indicated the potential clinical efficacy of AZD9668 in the treatment of bronchiectasis [246].

Aside from serine proteases, and as already mentioned, MMPs also play a key role in the development of COPD. TIMPs are endogenous MMP inhibitors and in COPD, MMP activity levels associated with lung disease are not counteracted by TIMPs [247]. To date no native TIMPs have been used as potential therapeutics, but synthetic and selective MMP inhibits have been well documented. The orally administered MMP-9 and MMP-12 inhibitor AZD1236 was well tolerated by patients in two separate clinical trials but overall it was deemed to have no effect on clinical parameters [248] or disease related biomarkers in COPD patients [249]. In a recent study by Wu *et al.*, several potential MMP-12 inhibitors were analysed *in vivo*, with one specific inhibitor, Compound 26, modulating cell infiltration into the lungs of mice with MMP-12 induced inflammation [250]. Similar findings were observed for a second MMP-12 inhibitor, Compound 14 [251]. An additional *in vivo* study involved the use of the broad spectrum MMP inhibitor RS113456, which possessed comparable anti-inflammatory properties to AAT [252]. In the latter study the authors noted multi-facetted attributes of RS113456, whereby this MMP inhibitor reduced neutrophil influx, modulated NFκB activity and reduced MCP-1 and MIP-2 expression in the short term [252].

Other synthetic MMP inhibitors evaluated in cigarette smoke induced models of COPD have shown significant reductions in lung macrophage numbers [126], neutrophilia [253, 254], elastase/ MMP levels [254], air space enlargement [126, 254] and inflammatory markers [90, 126]. To date the benefits of MMP inhibitors has only been assessed in animal models and their successful use as therapeutics for treatment of COPD in humans has not been reported. Thus caution needs to be exercised due to the potential for tumour growth promotion as a result of inhibition of angiogenesis factors [255].

An alternative to synthetic inhibitors is the production of semi-synthetic protease inhibitors. These agents are created through the chemical modification of naturally occurring protease inhibitors. One such semi-synthetic inhibitor is the engineered protein inhibitor of human NE (EPI-HNE-4) which is derived from the Kunitz type domain from the naturally occurring inter α inhibitor. EPI-HNE-4 has been shown resistant to degradation by both human and bacterial MMPs and its antiprotease activity was reported impervious to oxidative inhibition [256]. Further studies involving the use of a rat model and sputum from cystic fibrosis patients demonstrated the anti-NE capacity of EPI-HNE-4 along with its ability to decrease neutrophil migration towards the bacterial peptide *N*-formyl-L-methionyl-L-leucyl-phenylalanine [257]. Subsequently however, contrary data on the immuno-regulatory effects of this inhibitor have been documented as Honoré *et al.*, demonstrated that EPI-HNE-4 had little effect on neutrophil migration or impact on bacterial clearance in a *P. aeruginosa* model of pneumonia [258].

http://dx.doi.org/10.5772/57455

Within this expanding field of potential antiprotease therapies lies the development of novel chimeras that are active against NE, PR3 and CathG. A study by Zani *et al.*, reported on the development of a chimera consisting of domains from both elafin and SLPI and a trappin-2 variant (A62L) [259]. The authors demonstrated that both A62L and the elafin-SLPI chimera retained their polypotent inhibition of protease activity while covalently cross-linked to fibronectin or elastin by a tissue transglutaminase, in a similar fashion to wild-type elafin and trappin-2 [188]. A recent extensive study on A62L in an epithelial cell line demonstrated that this engineered trappin-2 molecule prevented neutrophil and protease induced epithelial cell injury by inhibiting cell detachment, tight junction disruption and ultimately reducing apoptosis [260]. Although the preliminary data has been generated for these engineered antiproteases, overall their effect on the inflammatory status and clinical parameters in COPD patients remains to be investigated.

5. Conclusion

Extensive studies have been performed to extend our knowledge of the involvement of proteases in respiratory manifestations of COPD, the outcome of which has served to illustrate the multifactorial complexity of the disease (Figure 2). Nevertheless, this clinical and scientific knowledge has advanced the design of both fundamental and novel therapeutic strategies, directed at relieving the protease burden associated with this disorder (Table 2). There have been major advances in the evaluation of AAT augmentation therapy in the treatment of the lung disease associated with AAT deficiency with newer focus on aerosolization approaches. These studies will inevitably show within the next number of years whether this approach works clinically. No single treatment that effectively prevents activity of the broad spectrum of proteases present in the airways is available as yet. Such pharmacological approaches including the development of antiprotease chimeras would essentially correct lung disease processes and conceivably exert anti-inflammatory effects. However, this would require a more complete understanding of the mechanism of disease and of the action of presently accessible and newly discovered drugs.

Protease	Role in COPD pathogenesis	Inhibitors and inactivators	Clinical trials and evidence for antiproteases as therapeutics
Neutrophil Elastase	Elastolysis/destruction of extracellular matrix proteins including elastin, collagens, fibronectin, proteoglycans & laminin Cleaves epithelial cell surface receptors Cleaves signalling cytokines	Alpha-1 antitrypsin (AAT) Monocyte neutrophil elastase inhibitor (MNEI/ Serpin B1) Elafin Secretory leucocyte protease inhibitor (SLPI)	Intravenous augmentation therapy of AAT.(Multiple Clinical Trials in Humans, see Table 1) Clinical effects of IV AAT in AATD: Slows rate of FEV1 decline Reduces elastin degradation Reduces exacerbation frequency

Protease	Role in COPD pathogenesis	Inhibitors and inactivators	Clinical trials and evidence for antiproteases as therapeutics
	Induces IL-8 expression in bronchial epithelial cells Upregulates TGF-β in airway smooth muscle Impairs T-cell function Induces macrophage production of cathepsin B and MMP-2 Induces expression of MUC5AC leading to hypersecretion of mucus. Decreases ciliary beat frequency of bronchial epithelial cells	Sivelestat (synthetic non-peptide inhibitor) MR889 (synthetic cyclic thiol compound) ZD0892 (synthetic elastase inhibitor) FR134043 (synthetic elastase inhibitor) AZD9668 (synthetic selective elastase inhibitor)	Attenuates loss of lung density Clinical effects of aerosolized AAT: Restores anti-NE capacity (176, 177) Improved neutrophil killing of *P. aeruginosa* (179) Outcome of phase III clinical trial pending (NCT 0217671) SLPI – Reduced NE activity and reduced IL-8 levels in CF patients (223) Sivelestat – Reduced number of neutrophils in BAL. Has shown therapeutic benefit in acute lung injury and ARDS, but no trials in COPD to date (230-232, 235, 236) MR889 – Safe but no significant reduction in the level of biomarkers of lung disease in COPD patients (239) ZD0892 & FR134043 – Reduce cigarette induced lung inflammation, but no human trials to date (240,2410) AZD9668 – Decreased NE activity *in vitro* (244) No change in clinical parameters in COPD (245)
Proteinase-3 (PR3)	Elastolysis/destruction of extracellular matrix proteins including elastin, collagens, fibronectin, proteoglycans & laminin. Less destructive than NE Pro-inflammatory, activates TNFα and IL-1β Hypersecretion of mucus Cellular apoptosis	Alpha-1 antitrypsin (AAT)	See above for clinical effects of AAT therapy in AATD and COPD

Protease	Role in COPD pathogenesis	Inhibitors and inactivators	Clinical trials and evidence for antiproteases as therapeutics
Cathepsin G	Proteolysis and destruction of extracellular matrix of the lung Induces mucus secretion Impairs T-cell function	Alpha-1 antitrypsin (AAT) Secretory leucocyte protease inhibitor (SLPI)	See above for clinical effects of AAT therapy in AATD and COPD
Other Cathepsins (Cathepsin B, D, H, K, L and S)	Parenchymal destruction and emphysema development Proteolytic degradation of beta-defensins thus impairing bacterial killing Induce airway inflammation	Cystatins are a group of endogenous reversible, tight-binding competitive cysteine protease inhibitors for cathepsins B, H, and L. SLPI inhibits cathepsin S expression in macrophages	
Matrix Metalloprotease-12 (MMP-12)	Degradation of collagen and elastin Monocyte recruitment Activates TNFα Induces IL-8 production Can degrade AAT	Tissue inhibitors of metalloproteases (TIMP) Secretory leucocyte protease inhibitor (SLPI) AZD1236 (synthetic inhibitor of MMP-12 and MMP-9) Compound 26 (synthetic compound) Compound 14 (synthetic compound) RS113456 (synthetic MMP-12 inhibitor)	SLPI – Anti-inflammatory properties and specifically inhibits monocyte production of MMPs (212, 213) AZD1236 – Well tolerated in COPD but not effect on clinical parameters (248,249) Compound 26, Compound 14, RS113456 – Reduced neutrophilic inflammation but no human trial data (250-252)
Matrix Metalloprotease-1 (MMP-1)	Degradation of collagens, elastin, gelatin, pro-MMP9, pro-MMP13 TACE (TNFα converting enzyme) like activity Induces TGFβ-1 – leading to fibrotic changes Induces mucus hypersecretion	Tissue inhibitors of metalloproteases (TIMP) Secretory leucocyte protease inhibitor (SLPI) AZD1236 (synthetic inhibitor of MMP-12 and MMP-9)	SLPI – Anti-inflammatory properties and specifically inhibits monocyte production of MMPs (212, 213) AZD1236 – Well tolerated in COPD but no effect on clinical parameters (248,249)
Other Matrix Metalloproteases (MMP-2, MMP-8, MMP 10, MMP-13)	Degradation of collagens, gelatin, pro-MMP9, pro-MMP13 TACE (TNFα converting enzyme) like activity	Tissue inhibitors of metalloproteases (TIMP)	

Protease	Role in COPD pathogenesis	Inhibitors and inactivators	Clinical trials and evidence for antiproteases as therapeutics
	Degradation of collagens, elastin, gelatin and fibronectin	Tissue inhibitors of metalloproteases (TIMP)	

Table 2. Summary table listing the various proteases, their targets, their inhibitor/inactivators, and clinical trials.

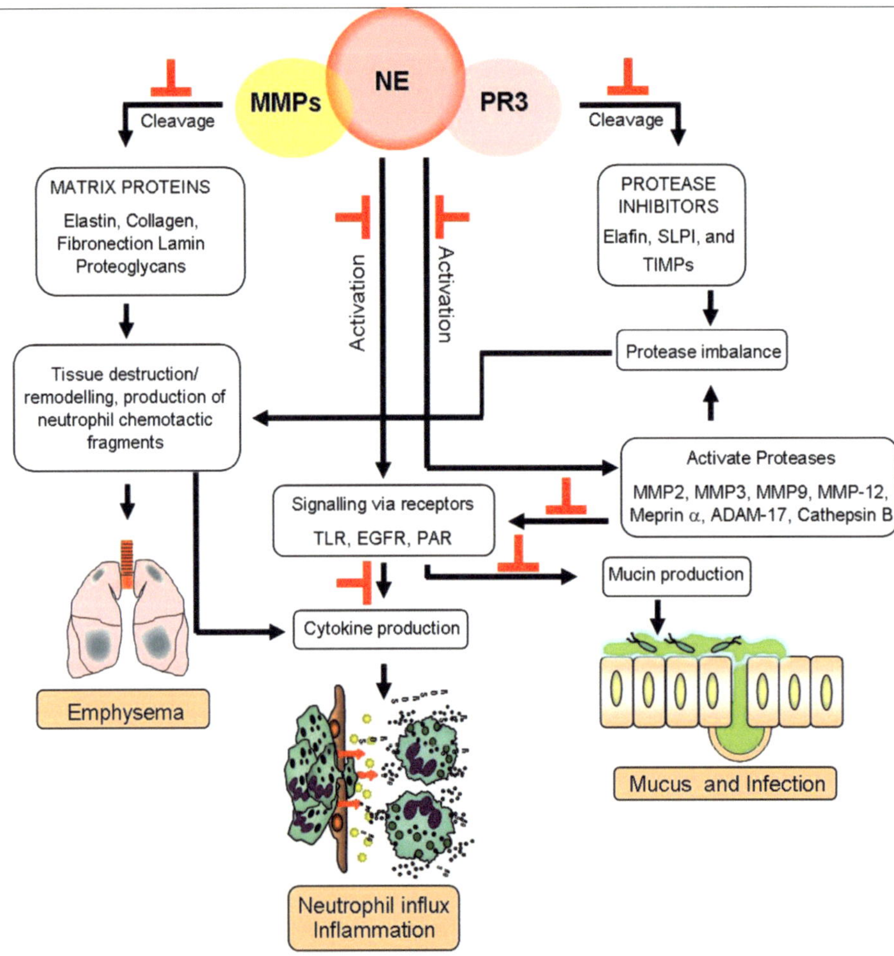

Figure 2. The effect of protease activity on the pathophysiology of COPD. A diagramatic illustration of the primary effects of excessive protease activity on inflammation in COPD. The effects include activation of signalling pathways and proteases, to cleavage and degradation of matrix proteins and antiproteases. The secondary effect of the excessive protease burden in the COPD lung can result in tissue destruction/ remodelling and excessive cytokine and mucin production. Consequenrly proteases play a key role in emphysema, neutrophil influx, inflammation, mucus production and infection. As shown by the red lines, antiprotease therapy (AAT, SLPI and elafin) can impact on several aspects of this complex and intertwined pathway and potentially modulate disease progression.

http://dx.doi.org/10.5772/57455

Acknowledgements

This work was supported by the Medical Research Charities Group/Health Research Board, Science Foundation Ireland (grant number 11/RFP/BMT/3094), the US Alpha One Foundation and the Program for Research in Third Level Institutes (PRTLI) administered by the Higher Education Authority and Science Foundation Ireland.

Author details

Cormac McCarthy, Ciara A. O'Dwyer, David A. Bergin, Noel G. McElvaney and Emer P. Reeves*

*Address all correspondence to: emerreeves@rcsi.ie

Respiratory Research Division, Department of Medicine, Royal College of Surgeons in Ireland, Education and Research Centre, Beaumont Hospital, Dublin, Ireland

References

[1] Hedstrom L. Serine protease mechanism and specificity. Chemical reviews. 2002;102(12):4501-24. Epub 2002/12/12.

[2] Rooney CP, Taggart C, Coakley R, McElvaney NG, O'Neill SJ. Anti-proteinase 3 antibody activation of neutrophils can be inhibited by alpha1-antitrypsin. American journal of respiratory cell and molecular biology. 2001;24(6):747-54. Epub 2001/06/21.

[3] Stoller JK, Aboussouan LS. Alpha1-antitrypsin deficiency. Lancet. 2005;365(9478): 2225-36. Epub 2005/06/28.

[4] Gooptu B, Ekeowa UI, Lomas DA. Mechanisms of emphysema in alpha1-antitrypsin deficiency: molecular and cellular insights. The European respiratory journal : official journal of the European Society for Clinical Respiratory Physiology. 2009;34(2): 475-88. Epub 2009/08/04.

[5] Hiemstra PS, van Wetering S, Stolk J. Neutrophil serine proteinases and defensins in chronic obstructive pulmonary disease: effects on pulmonary epithelium. The European respiratory journal : official journal of the European Society for Clinical Respiratory Physiology. 1998;12(5):1200-8. Epub 1998/12/24.

[6] Kelly E, Greene CM, McElvaney NG. Targeting neutrophil elastase in cystic fibrosis. Expert opinion on therapeutic targets. 2008;12(2):145-57. Epub 2008/01/23.

[7] Stockley RA. The role of proteinases in the pathogenesis of chronic bronchitis. American journal of respiratory and critical care medicine. 1994;150(6 Pt 2):S109-13. Epub 1994/12/01.

[8] Donnelly SC, MacGregor I, Zamani A, Gordon MW, Robertson CE, Steedman DJ, et al. Plasma elastase levels and the development of the adult respiratory distress syndrome. American journal of respiratory and critical care medicine. 1995;151(5): 1428-33. Epub 1995/05/01.

[9] Bieth JG. Elastases: catalytic and biological properties. In: RP M, editor. Regulation of Matrix Accumulation. Orlando, FL: Academic Press; 1986. p. 218–320.

[10] McElvaney NG CR. Proteases and lung injury. In: Crystal RG WJ, Barnes PJ, Weibel ER, editor. The Lung: Scientific Foundations. 2nd ed. Philadelphia, PA: Lippencott-Raven; 1997. p. 2205–18.

[11] Janoff A, Sloan B, Weinbaum G, Damiano V, Sandhaus RA, Elias J, et al. Experimental emphysema induced with purified human neutrophil elastase: tissue localization of the instilled protease. The American review of respiratory disease. 1977;115(3): 461-78. Epub 1977/03/01.

[12] Kao RC, Wehner NG, Skubitz KM, Gray BH, Hoidal JR. Proteinase 3. A distinct human polymorphonuclear leukocyte proteinase that produces emphysema in hamsters. The Journal of clinical investigation. 1988;82(6):1963-73. Epub 1988/12/01.

[13] Bode W, Meyer E, Jr., Powers JC. Human leukocyte and porcine pancreatic elastase: X-ray crystal structures, mechanism, substrate specificity, and mechanism-based inhibitors. Biochemistry. 1989;28(5):1951-63. Epub 1989/03/07.

[14] Owen CA, Campbell MA, Boukedes SS, Campbell EJ. Cytokines regulate membrane-bound leukocyte elastase on neutrophils: a novel mechanism for effector activity. The American journal of physiology. 1997;272(3 Pt 1):L385-93. Epub 1997/03/01.

[15] Carrell RW, Jeppsson JO, Laurell CB, Brennan SO, Owen MC, Vaughan L, et al. Structure and variation of human alpha 1-antitrypsin. Nature. 1982;298(5872):329-34. Epub 1982/07/22.

[16] Cooley J, Takayama TK, Shapiro SD, Schechter NM, Remold-O'Donnell E. The serpin MNEI inhibits elastase-like and chymotrypsin-like serine proteases through efficient reactions at two active sites. Biochemistry. 2001;40(51):15762-70. Epub 2001/12/19.

[17] Wiedow O, Luademann J, Utecht B. Elafin is a potent inhibitor of proteinase 3. Biochemical and biophysical research communications. 1991;174(1):6-10. Epub 1991/01/15.

[18] Wiedow O, Schroder JM, Gregory H, Young JA, Christophers E. Elafin: an elastase-specific inhibitor of human skin. Purification, characterization, and complete amino acid sequence. The Journal of biological chemistry. 1990;265(25):14791-5. Epub 1990/09/05.

[19] Boudier C, Bieth JG. The proteinase: mucus proteinase inhibitor binding stoichiometry. The Journal of biological chemistry. 1992;267(7):4370-5. Epub 1992/03/05.

[20] Thompson RC, Ohlsson K. Isolation, properties, and complete amino acid sequence of human secretory leukocyte protease inhibitor, a potent inhibitor of leukocyte elastase. Proceedings of the National Academy of Sciences of the United States of America. 1986;83(18):6692-6. Epub 1986/09/01.

[21] Weldon S, McNally P, McElvaney NG, Elborn JS, McAuley DF, Wartelle J, et al. Decreased levels of secretory leucoprotease inhibitor in the Pseudomonas-infected cystic fibrosis lung are due to neutrophil elastase degradation. J Immunol. 2009;183(12): 8148-56. Epub 2009/12/17.

[22] Gadek JE, Fells GA, Crystal RG. Cigarette smoking induces functional antiprotease deficiency in the lower respiratory tract of humans. Science. 1979;206(4424):1315-6. Epub 1979/12/14.

[23] Carp H, Miller F, Hoidal JR, Janoff A. Potential mechanism of emphysema: alpha 1-proteinase inhibitor recovered from lungs of cigarette smokers contains oxidized methionine and has decreased elastase inhibitory capacity. Proceedings of the National Academy of Sciences of the United States of America. 1982;79(6):2041-5. Epub 1982/03/01.

[24] Stone PJ, Calore JD, McGowan SE, Bernardo J, Snider GL, Franzblau C. Functional alpha 1-protease inhibitor in the lower respiratory tract of cigarette smokers is not decreased. Science. 1983;221(4616):1187-9. Epub 1983/09/16.

[25] Boudier C, Pelletier A, Pauli G, Bieth JG. The functional activity of alpha 1-proteinase inhibitor in bronchoalveolar lavage fluids from healthy human smokers and non-smokers. Clinica chimica acta; international journal of clinical chemistry. 1983;132(3): 309-15. Epub 1983/08/31.

[26] Fera T, Abboud RT, Richter A, Johal SS. Acute effect of smoking on elastaselike esterase activity and immunologic neutrophil elastase levels in bronchoalveolar lavage fluid. The American review of respiratory disease. 1986;133(4):568-73. Epub 1986/04/01.

[27] Abboud RT, Fera T, Johal S, Richter A, Gibson N. Effect of smoking on plasma neutrophil elastase levels. The Journal of laboratory and clinical medicine. 1986;108(4): 294-300. Epub 1986/10/01.

[28] Fujita J, Nelson NL, Daughton DM, Dobry CA, Spurzem JR, Irino S, et al. Evaluation of elastase and antielastase balance in patients with chronic bronchitis and pulmonary emphysema. The American review of respiratory disease. 1990;142(1):57-62. Epub 1990/07/01.

[29] Vega-Carrascal I, Reeves EP, Niki T, Arikawa T, McNally P, O'Neill SJ, et al. Dysregulation of TIM-3-galectin-9 pathway in the cystic fibrosis airways. J Immunol. 2011;186(5):2897-909. Epub 2011/01/26.

[30] Reeves EP, Williamson M, Byrne B, Bergin DA, Smith SG, Greally P, et al. IL-8 dictates glycosaminoglycan binding and stability of IL-18 in cystic fibrosis. J Immunol. 2010;184(3):1642-52. Epub 2009/12/23.

[31] Campbell EJ, White RR, Senior RM, Rodriguez RJ, Kuhn C. Receptor-mediated binding and internalization of leukocyte elastase by alveolar macrophages in vitro. The Journal of clinical investigation. 1979;64(3):824-33. Epub 1979/09/01.

[32] Betsuyaku T, Nishimura M, Takeyabu K, Tanino M, Venge P, Xu S, et al. Neutrophil granule proteins in bronchoalveolar lavage fluid from subjects with subclinical emphysema. American journal of respiratory and critical care medicine. 1999;159(6): 1985-91. Epub 1999/06/03.

[33] Damiano VV, Tsang A, Kucich U, Abrams WR, Rosenbloom J, Kimbel P, et al. Immunolocalization of elastase in human emphysematous lungs. The Journal of clinical investigation. 1986;78(2):482-93. Epub 1986/08/01.

[34] Senior RM, Tegner H, Kuhn C, Ohlsson K, Starcher BC, Pierce JA. The induction of pulmonary emphysema with human leukocyte elastase. The American review of respiratory disease. 1977;116(3):469-75. Epub 1977/09/01.

[35] Geraghty P, Rogan MP, Greene CM, Boxio RM, Poiriert T, O'Mahony M, et al. Neutrophil elastase up-regulates cathepsin B and matrix metalloprotease-2 expression. J Immunol. 2007;178(9):5871-8. Epub 2007/04/20.

[36] Geraghty P, Rogan MP, Greene CM, Brantly ML, O'Neill SJ, Taggart CC, et al. Alpha-1-antitrypsin aerosolised augmentation abrogates neutrophil elastase-induced expression of cathepsin B and matrix metalloprotease 2 in vivo and in vitro. Thorax. 2008;63(7):621-6. Epub 2008/02/06.

[37] Sommerhoff CP, Caughey GH, Finkbeiner WE, Lazarus SC, Basbaum CB, Nadel JA. Mast cell chymase. A potent secretagogue for airway gland serous cells. J Immunol. 1989;142(7):2450-6. Epub 1989/04/01.

[38] Sommerhoff CP, Nadel JA, Basbaum CB, Caughey GH. Neutrophil elastase and cathepsin G stimulate secretion from cultured bovine airway gland serous cells. The Journal of clinical investigation. 1990;85(3):682-9. Epub 1990/03/01.

[39] Takeyama K, Agusti C, Ueki I, Lausier J, Cardell LO, Nadel JA. Neutrophil-dependent goblet cell degranulation: role of membrane-bound elastase and adhesion molecules. The American journal of physiology. 1998;275(2 Pt 1):L294-302. Epub 1998/08/12.

[40] Fischer BM, Voynow JA. Neutrophil elastase induces MUC5AC gene expression in airway epithelium via a pathway involving reactive oxygen species. American journal of respiratory cell and molecular biology. 2002;26(4):447-52. Epub 2002/03/29.

[41] Voynow JA, Young LR, Wang Y, Horger T, Rose MC, Fischer BM. Neutrophil elastase increases MUC5AC mRNA and protein expression in respiratory epithelial cells. The American journal of physiology. 1999;276(5 Pt 1):L835-43. Epub 1999/05/18.

[42] Amitani R, Wilson R, Rutman A, Read R, Ward C, Burnett D, et al. Effects of human neutrophil elastase and Pseudomonas aeruginosa proteinases on human respiratory epithelium. American journal of respiratory cell and molecular biology. 1991;4(1): 26-32. Epub 1991/01/01.

[43] Nakamura H, Yoshimura K, McElvaney NG, Crystal RG. Neutrophil elastase in respiratory epithelial lining fluid of individuals with cystic fibrosis induces interleukin-8 gene expression in a human bronchial epithelial cell line. The Journal of clinical investigation. 1992;89(5):1478-84. Epub 1992/05/01.

[44] Devaney JM, Greene CM, Taggart CC, Carroll TP, O'Neill SJ, McElvaney NG. Neutrophil elastase up-regulates interleukin-8 via toll-like receptor 4. FEBS letters. 2003;544(1-3):129-32. Epub 2003/06/05.

[45] Leavell KJ, Peterson MW, Gross TJ. The role of fibrin degradation products in neutrophil recruitment to the lung. American journal of respiratory cell and molecular biology. 1996;14(1):53-60. Epub 1996/01/01.

[46] Banda MJ, Rice AG, Griffin GL, Senior RM. The inhibitory complex of human alpha 1-proteinase inhibitor and human leukocyte elastase is a neutrophil chemoattractant. The Journal of experimental medicine. 1988;167(5):1608-15. Epub 1988/05/01.

[47] Doring G, Frank F, Boudier C, Herbert S, Fleischer B, Bellon G. Cleavage of lymphocyte surface antigens CD2, CD4, and CD8 by polymorphonuclear leukocyte elastase and cathepsin G in patients with cystic fibrosis. J Immunol. 1995;154(9):4842-50. Epub 1995/05/01.

[48] Lee KY, Ho SC, Lin HC, Lin SM, Liu CY, Huang CD, et al. Neutrophil-derived elastase induces TGF-beta1 secretion in human airway smooth muscle via NF-kappaB pathway. American journal of respiratory cell and molecular biology. 2006;35(4): 407-14. Epub 2006/05/13.

[49] Yang JJ, Kettritz R, Falk RJ, Jennette JC, Gaido ML. Apoptosis of endothelial cells induced by the neutrophil serine proteases proteinase 3 and elastase. The American journal of pathology. 1996;149(5):1617-26. Epub 1996/11/01.

[50] Nahori MA, Renesto P, Vargaftig BB, Chignard M. Activation and damage of cultured airway epithelial cells by human elastase and cathepsin G. European journal of pharmacology. 1992;228(4):213-8. Epub 1992/12/01.

[51] Vandivier RW, Fadok VA, Hoffmann PR, Bratton DL, Penvari C, Brown KK, et al. Elastase-mediated phosphatidylserine receptor cleavage impairs apoptotic cell clear-

ance in cystic fibrosis and bronchiectasis. The Journal of clinical investigation. 2002;109(5):661-70. Epub 2002/03/06.

[52] Campbell EJ, Campbell MA, Owen CA. Bioactive proteinase 3 on the cell surface of human neutrophils: quantification, catalytic activity, and susceptibility to inhibition. J Immunol. 2000;165(6):3366-74. Epub 2000/09/07.

[53] Bergenfeldt M, Axelsson L, Ohlsson K. Release of neutrophil proteinase 4(3) and leukocyte elastase during phagocytosis and their interaction with proteinase inhibitors. Scandinavian journal of clinical and laboratory investigation. 1992;52(8):823-9. Epub 1992/12/01.

[54] Duranton J, Bieth JG. Inhibition of proteinase 3 by [alpha] 1-antitrypsin in vitro predicts very fast inhibition in vivo. American journal of respiratory cell and molecular biology. 2003;29(1):57-61. Epub 2003/02/26.

[55] Rao NV, Marshall BC, Gray BH, Hoidal JR. Interaction of secretory leukocyte protease inhibitor with proteinase-3. American journal of respiratory cell and molecular biology. 1993;8(6):612-6. Epub 1993/06/01.

[56] Sinden NJ, Stockley RA. Proteinase 3 activity in sputum from subjects with alpha-1-antitrypsin deficiency and COPD. The European respiratory journal : official journal of the European Society for Clinical Respiratory Physiology. 2013;41(5):1042-50. Epub 2012/09/01.

[57] Ying QL, Simon SR. Elastolysis by proteinase 3 and its inhibition by alpha(1)-proteinase inhibitor: a mechanism for the incomplete inhibition of ongoing elastolysis. American journal of respiratory cell and molecular biology. 2002;26(3):356-61. Epub 2002/02/28.

[58] Coeshott C, Ohnemus C, Pilyavskaya A, Ross S, Wieczorek M, Kroona H, et al. Converting enzyme-independent release of tumor necrosis factor alpha and IL-1beta from a stimulated human monocytic cell line in the presence of activated neutrophils or purified proteinase 3. Proceedings of the National Academy of Sciences of the United States of America. 1999;96(11):6261-6. Epub 1999/05/26.

[59] Witko-Sarsat V, Halbwachs-Mecarelli L, Schuster A, Nusbaum P, Ueki I, Canteloup S, et al. Proteinase 3, a potent secretagogue in airways, is present in cystic fibrosis sputum. American journal of respiratory cell and molecular biology. 1999;20(4): 729-36. Epub 1999/04/01.

[60] Pendergraft WF, 3rd, Rudolph EH, Falk RJ, Jahn JE, Grimmler M, Hengst L, et al. Proteinase 3 sidesteps caspases and cleaves p21(Waf1/Cip1/Sdi1) to induce endothelial cell apoptosis. Kidney international. 2004;65(1):75-84. Epub 2003/12/17.

[61] Takeyabu K, Betsuyaku T, Nishimura M, Yoshioka A, Tanino M, Miyamoto K, et al. Cysteine proteinases and cystatin C in bronchoalveolar lavage fluid from subjects with subclinical emphysema. The European respiratory journal : official journal of

the European Society for Clinical Respiratory Physiology. 1998;12(5):1033-9. Epub 1998/12/24.

[62] Lucey EC, Stone PJ, Breuer R, Christensen TG, Calore JD, Catanese A, et al. Effect of combined human neutrophil cathepsin G and elastase on induction of secretory cell metaplasia and emphysema in hamsters, with in vitro observations on elastolysis by these enzymes. The American review of respiratory disease. 1985;132(2):362-6. Epub 1985/08/01.

[63] Takahashi H, Ishidoh K, Muno D, Ohwada A, Nukiwa T, Kominami E, et al. Cathepsin L activity is increased in alveolar macrophages and bronchoalveolar lavage fluid of smokers. The American review of respiratory disease. 1993;147(6 Pt 1):1562-8. Epub 1993/06/01.

[64] Reilly JJ, Jr., Chen P, Sailor LZ, Wilcox D, Mason RW, Chapman HA, Jr. Cigarette smoking induces an elastolytic cysteine proteinase in macrophages distinct from cathepsin L. The American journal of physiology. 1991;261(2 Pt 1):L41-8. Epub 1991/08/11.

[65] Wang Z, Zheng T, Zhu Z, Homer RJ, Riese RJ, Chapman HA, Jr., et al. Interferon gamma induction of pulmonary emphysema in the adult murine lung. The Journal of experimental medicine. 2000;192(11):1587-600. Epub 2000/12/06.

[66] Zheng T, Zhu Z, Wang Z, Homer RJ, Ma B, Riese RJ, Jr., et al. Inducible targeting of IL-13 to the adult lung causes matrix metalloproteinase- and cathepsin-dependent emphysema. The Journal of clinical investigation. 2000;106(9):1081-93. Epub 2000/11/09.

[67] Bergsson G, Reeves EP, McNally P, Chotirmall SH, Greene CM, Greally P, et al. LL-37 complexation with glycosaminoglycans in cystic fibrosis lungs inhibits antimicrobial activity, which can be restored by hypertonic saline. J Immunol. 2009;183(1): 543-51. Epub 2009/06/23.

[68] Taggart CC, Greene CM, Smith SG, Levine RL, McCray PB, Jr., O'Neill S, et al. Inactivation of human beta-defensins 2 and 3 by elastolytic cathepsins. J Immunol. 2003;171(2):931-7. Epub 2003/07/09.

[69] Loffek S, Schilling O, Franzke CW. Series "matrix metalloproteinases in lung health and disease": Biological role of matrix metalloproteinases: a critical balance. The European respiratory journal : official journal of the European Society for Clinical Respiratory Physiology. 2011;38(1):191-208. Epub 2010/12/24.

[70] Gueders MM, Foidart JM, Noel A, Cataldo DD. Matrix metalloproteinases (MMPs) and tissue inhibitors of MMPs in the respiratory tract: potential implications in asthma and other lung diseases. European journal of pharmacology. 2006;533(1-3):133-44. Epub 2006/02/21.

[71] Janoff A, Raju L, Dearing R. Levels of elastase activity in bronchoalveolar lavage fluids of healthy smokers and nonsmokers. The American review of respiratory disease. 1983;127(5):540-4. Epub 1983/05/01.

[72] Russell RE, Thorley A, Culpitt SV, Dodd S, Donnelly LE, Demattos C, et al. Alveolar macrophage-mediated elastolysis: roles of matrix metalloproteinases, cysteine, and serine proteases. American journal of physiology Lung cellular and molecular physiology. 2002;283(4):L867-73. Epub 2002/09/13.

[73] Senior RM, Griffin GL, Mecham RP. Chemotactic activity of elastin-derived peptides. The Journal of clinical investigation. 1980;66(4):859-62. Epub 1980/10/01.

[74] Hunninghake GW, Davidson JM, Rennard S, Szapiel S, Gadek JE, Crystal RG. Elastin fragments attract macrophage precursors to diseased sites in pulmonary emphysema. Science. 1981;212(4497):925-7. Epub 1981/05/22.

[75] Nenan S, Planquois JM, Berna P, De Mendez I, Hitier S, Shapiro SD, et al. Analysis of the inflammatory response induced by rhMMP-12 catalytic domain instilled in mouse airways. International immunopharmacology. 2005;5(3):511-24. Epub 2005/02/03.

[76] Babusyte A, Stravinskaite K, Jeroch J, Lotvall J, Sakalauskas R, Sitkauskiene B. Patterns of airway inflammation and MMP-12 expression in smokers and ex-smokers with COPD. Respiratory research. 2007;8:81. Epub 2007/11/16.

[77] Lavigne MC, Thakker P, Gunn J, Wong A, Miyashiro JS, Wasserman AM, et al. Human bronchial epithelial cells express and secrete MMP-12. Biochemical and biophysical research communications. 2004;324(2):534-46. Epub 2004/10/12.

[78] Xie S, Issa R, Sukkar MB, Oltmanns U, Bhavsar PK, Papi A, et al. Induction and regulation of matrix metalloproteinase-12 in human airway smooth muscle cells. Respiratory research. 2005;6:148. Epub 2005/12/20.

[79] Churg A, Zhou S, Wright JL. Series "matrix metalloproteinases in lung health and disease": Matrix metalloproteinases in COPD. The European respiratory journal : official journal of the European Society for Clinical Respiratory Physiology. 2012;39(1): 197-209. Epub 2011/09/17.

[80] Churg A, Wang X, Wang RD, Meixner SC, Pryzdial EL, Wright JL. Alpha1-antitrypsin suppresses TNF-alpha and MMP-12 production by cigarette smoke-stimulated macrophages. American journal of respiratory cell and molecular biology. 2007;37(2): 144-51. Epub 2007/03/31.

[81] Raza SL, Nehring LC, Shapiro SD, Cornelius LA. Proteinase-activated receptor-1 regulation of macrophage elastase (MMP-12) secretion by serine proteinases. The Journal of biological chemistry. 2000;275(52):41243-50. Epub 2000/09/20.

[82] Botelho FM, Nikota JK, Bauer C, Davis NH, Cohen ES, Anderson IK, et al. A mouse GM-CSF receptor antibody attenuates neutrophilia in mice exposed to cigarette

smoke. The European respiratory journal : official journal of the European Society for Clinical Respiratory Physiology. 2011;38(2):285-94. Epub 2011/03/26.

[83] Lavigne MC, Eppihimer MJ. Cigarette smoke condensate induces MMP-12 gene expression in airway-like epithelia. Biochemical and biophysical research communications. 2005;330(1):194-203. Epub 2005/03/23.

[84] Leclerc O, Lagente V, Planquois JM, Berthelier C, Artola M, Eichholtz T, et al. Involvement of MMP-12 and phosphodiesterase type 4 in cigarette smoke-induced inflammation in mice. The European respiratory journal : official journal of the European Society for Clinical Respiratory Physiology. 2006;27(6):1102-9. Epub 2006/03/03.

[85] Hautamaki RD, Kobayashi DK, Senior RM, Shapiro SD. Requirement for macrophage elastase for cigarette smoke-induced emphysema in mice. Science. 1997;277(5334):2002-4. Epub 1997/09/26.

[86] Selman M, Cisneros-Lira J, Gaxiola M, Ramirez R, Kudlacz EM, Mitchell PG, et al. Matrix metalloproteinases inhibition attenuates tobacco smoke-induced emphysema in Guinea pigs. Chest. 2003;123(5):1633-41. Epub 2003/05/13.

[87] Churg A, Wang RD, Tai H, Wang X, Xie C, Dai J, et al. Macrophage metalloelastase mediates acute cigarette smoke-induced inflammation via tumor necrosis factor-alpha release. American journal of respiratory and critical care medicine. 2003;167(8):1083-9. Epub 2003/01/11.

[88] Le Quement C, Guenon I, Gillon JY, Lagente V, Boichot E. MMP-12 induces IL-8/CXCL8 secretion through EGFR and ERK1/2 activation in epithelial cells. American journal of physiology Lung cellular and molecular physiology. 2008;294(6):L1076-84. Epub 2008/04/09.

[89] Vandenbroucke RE, Dejonckheere E, Libert C. A therapeutic role for matrix metalloproteinase inhibitors in lung diseases? The European respiratory journal : official journal of the European Society for Clinical Respiratory Physiology. 2011;38(5):1200-14. Epub 2011/06/11.

[90] Le Quement C, Guenon I, Gillon JY, Valenca S, Cayron-Elizondo V, Lagente V, et al. The selective MMP-12 inhibitor, AS111793 reduces airway inflammation in mice exposed to cigarette smoke. British journal of pharmacology. 2008;154(6):1206-15. Epub 2008/05/22.

[91] Shapiro SD, Goldstein NM, Houghton AM, Kobayashi DK, Kelley D, Belaaouaj A. Neutrophil elastase contributes to cigarette smoke-induced emphysema in mice. The American journal of pathology. 2003;163(6):2329-35. Epub 2003/11/25.

[92] Woodruff PG, Koth LL, Yang YH, Rodriguez MW, Favoreto S, Dolganov GM, et al. A distinctive alveolar macrophage activation state induced by cigarette smoking.

American journal of respiratory and critical care medicine. 2005;172(11):1383-92. Epub 2005/09/17.

[93] Wallace AM, Sandford AJ, English JC, Burkett KM, Li H, Finley RJ, et al. Matrix metalloproteinase expression by human alveolar macrophages in relation to emphysema. Copd. 2008;5(1):13-23. Epub 2008/02/09.

[94] Imai K, Dalal SS, Chen ES, Downey R, Schulman LL, Ginsburg M, et al. Human collagenase (matrix metalloproteinase-1) expression in the lungs of patients with emphysema. American journal of respiratory and critical care medicine. 2001;163(3 Pt 1): 786-91. Epub 2001/03/20.

[95] Finlay GA, O'Driscoll LR, Russell KJ, D'Arcy EM, Masterson JB, FitzGerald MX, et al. Matrix metalloproteinase expression and production by alveolar macrophages in emphysema. American journal of respiratory and critical care medicine. 1997;156(1): 240-7. Epub 1997/07/01.

[96] LaPan P, Brady J, Grierson C, Fleming M, Miller D, Sypek J, et al. Optimization of total protein and activity assays for the detection of MMP-12 in induced human sputum. BMC pulmonary medicine. 2010;10:40. Epub 2010/08/04.

[97] Vernooy JH, Lindeman JH, Jacobs JA, Hanemaaijer R, Wouters EF. Increased activity of matrix metalloproteinase-8 and matrix metalloproteinase-9 in induced sputum from patients with COPD. Chest. 2004;126(6):1802-10. Epub 2004/12/15.

[98] Culpitt SV, Rogers DF, Traves SL, Barnes PJ, Donnelly LE. Sputum matrix metalloproteases: comparison between chronic obstructive pulmonary disease and asthma. Respiratory medicine. 2005;99(6):703-10. Epub 2005/05/10.

[99] Vignola AM, Riccobono L, Mirabella A, Profita M, Chanez P, Bellia V, et al. Sputum metalloproteinase-9/tissue inhibitor of metalloproteinase-1 ratio correlates with airflow obstruction in asthma and chronic bronchitis. American journal of respiratory and critical care medicine. 1998;158(6):1945-50. Epub 1998/12/16.

[100] Omachi TA, Eisner MD, Rames A, Markovtsova L, Blanc PD. Matrix metalloproteinase-9 predicts pulmonary status declines in alpha1-antitrypsin deficiency. Respiratory research. 2011;12:35. Epub 2011/03/25.

[101] Beeh KM, Beier J, Kornmann O, Buhl R. Sputum matrix metalloproteinase-9, tissue inhibitor of metalloprotinease-1, and their molar ratio in patients with chronic obstructive pulmonary disease, idiopathic pulmonary fibrosis and healthy subjects. Respiratory medicine. 2003;97(6):634-9. Epub 2003/06/20.

[102] Minematsu N, Nakamura H, Tateno H, Nakajima T, Yamaguchi K. Genetic polymorphism in matrix metalloproteinase-9 and pulmonary emphysema. Biochemical and biophysical research communications. 2001;289(1):116-9. Epub 2001/11/16.

[103] Ito I, Nagai S, Handa T, Muro S, Hirai T, Tsukino M, et al. Matrix metalloproteinase-9 promoter polymorphism associated with upper lung dominant emphysema. Ameri-

can journal of respiratory and critical care medicine. 2005;172(11):1378-82. Epub 2005/08/30.

[104] Zhou M, Huang SG, Wan HY, Li B, Deng WW, Li M. Genetic polymorphism in matrix metalloproteinase-9 and the susceptibility to chronic obstructive pulmonary disease in Han population of south China. Chinese medical journal. 2004;117(10):1481-4. Epub 2004/10/23.

[105] Lim S, Roche N, Oliver BG, Mattos W, Barnes PJ, Chung KF. Balance of matrix metalloprotease-9 and tissue inhibitor of metalloprotease-1 from alveolar macrophages in cigarette smokers. Regulation by interleukin-10. American journal of respiratory and critical care medicine. 2000;162(4 Pt 1):1355-60. Epub 2000/10/13.

[106] Russell RE, Culpitt SV, DeMatos C, Donnelly L, Smith M, Wiggins J, et al. Release and activity of matrix metalloproteinase-9 and tissue inhibitor of metalloproteinase-1 by alveolar macrophages from patients with chronic obstructive pulmonary disease. American journal of respiratory cell and molecular biology. 2002;26(5):602-9. Epub 2002/04/24.

[107] Ohnishi K, Takagi M, Kurokawa Y, Satomi S, Konttinen YT. Matrix metalloproteinase-mediated extracellular matrix protein degradation in human pulmonary emphysema. Laboratory investigation; a journal of technical methods and pathology. 1998;78(9):1077-87. Epub 1998/10/06.

[108] Segura-Valdez L, Pardo A, Gaxiola M, Uhal BD, Becerril C, Selman M. Upregulation of gelatinases A and B, collagenases 1 and 2, and increased parenchymal cell death in COPD. Chest. 2000;117(3):684-94. Epub 2000/03/14.

[109] Yu Q, Stamenkovic I. Cell surface-localized matrix metalloproteinase-9 proteolytically activates TGF-beta and promotes tumor invasion and angiogenesis. Genes & development. 2000;14(2):163-76. Epub 2000/02/01.

[110] Dallas SL, Rosser JL, Mundy GR, Bonewald LF. Proteolysis of latent transforming growth factor-beta (TGF-beta)-binding protein-1 by osteoclasts. A cellular mechanism for release of TGF-beta from bone matrix. The Journal of biological chemistry. 2002;277(24):21352-60. Epub 2002/04/04.

[111] Ferry G, Lonchampt M, Pennel L, de Nanteuil G, Canet E, Tucker GC. Activation of MMP-9 by neutrophil elastase in an in vivo model of acute lung injury. FEBS letters. 1997;402(2-3):111-5. Epub 1997/02/03.

[112] Itoh Y, Nagase H. Preferential inactivation of tissue inhibitor of metalloproteinases-1 that is bound to the precursor of matrix metalloproteinase 9 (progelatinase B) by human neutrophil elastase. The Journal of biological chemistry. 1995;270(28):16518-21. Epub 1995/07/14.

[113] Takeyama K, Dabbagh K, Lee HM, Agusti C, Lausier JA, Ueki IF, et al. Epidermal growth factor system regulates mucin production in airways. Proceedings of the Na-

tional Academy of Sciences of the United States of America. 1999;96(6):3081-6. Epub 1999/03/17.

[114] Deshmukh HS, Case LM, Wesselkamper SC, Borchers MT, Martin LD, Shertzer HG, et al. Metalloproteinases mediate mucin 5AC expression by epidermal growth factor receptor activation. American journal of respiratory and critical care medicine. 2005;171(4):305-14. Epub 2004/11/09.

[115] D'Armiento J, Dalal SS, Okada Y, Berg RA, Chada K. Collagenase expression in the lungs of transgenic mice causes pulmonary emphysema. Cell. 1992;71(6):955-61. Epub 1992/12/11.

[116] Foronjy R, D'Armiento J. The role of collagenase in emphysema. Respiratory research. 2001;2(6):348-52. Epub 2001/12/12.

[117] Finlay GA, Russell KJ, McMahon KJ, D'Arcy E M, Masterson JB, FitzGerald MX, et al. Elevated levels of matrix metalloproteinases in bronchoalveolar lavage fluid of emphysematous patients. Thorax. 1997;52(6):502-6. Epub 1997/06/01.

[118] Elshaw SR, Henderson N, Knox AJ, Watson SA, Buttle DJ, Johnson SR. Matrix metalloproteinase expression and activity in human airway smooth muscle cells. British journal of pharmacology. 2004;142(8):1318-24. Epub 2004/07/22.

[119] Mercer BA, Kolesnikova N, Sonett J, D'Armiento J. Extracellular regulated kinase/ mitogen activated protein kinase is up-regulated in pulmonary emphysema and mediates matrix metalloproteinase-1 induction by cigarette smoke. The Journal of biological chemistry. 2004;279(17):17690-6. Epub 2004/02/07.

[120] Shiomi T, Okada Y, Foronjy R, Schiltz J, Jaenish R, Krane S, et al. Emphysematous changes are caused by degradation of type III collagen in transgenic mice expressing MMP-1. Experimental lung research. 2003;29(1):1-15. Epub 2003/03/26.

[121] Selman M, Montano M, Ramos C, Vanda B, Becerril C, Delgado J, et al. Tobacco smoke-induced lung emphysema in guinea pigs is associated with increased interstitial collagenase. The American journal of physiology. 1996;271(5 Pt 1):L734-43. Epub 1996/11/01.

[122] Foronjy R, Nkyimbeng T, Wallace A, Thankachen J, Okada Y, Lemaitre V, et al. Transgenic expression of matrix metalloproteinase-9 causes adult-onset emphysema in mice associated with the loss of alveolar elastin. American journal of physiology Lung cellular and molecular physiology. 2008;294(6):L1149-57. Epub 2008/04/15.

[123] Ramos C, Cisneros J, Gonzalez-Avila G, Becerril C, Ruiz V, Montano M. Increase of matrix metalloproteinases in woodsmoke-induced lung emphysema in guinea pigs. Inhalation toxicology. 2009;21(2):119-32. Epub 2008/10/07.

[124] Gosselink JV, Hayashi S, Elliott WM, Xing L, Chan B, Yang L, et al. Differential expression of tissue repair genes in the pathogenesis of chronic obstructive pulmonary

disease. American journal of respiratory and critical care medicine. 2010;181(12): 1329-35. Epub 2010/01/16.

[125] Ilumets H, Rytila PH, Sovijarvi AR, Tervahartiala T, Myllarniemi M, Sorsa TA, et al. Transient elevation of neutrophil proteinases in induced sputum during COPD exacerbation. Scandinavian journal of clinical and laboratory investigation. 2008;68(7): 618-23. Epub 2008/01/01.

[126] Churg A, Wang R, Wang X, Onnervik PO, Thim K, Wright JL. Effect of an MMP-9/ MMP-12 inhibitor on smoke-induced emphysema and airway remodelling in guinea pigs. Thorax. 2007;62(8):706-13. Epub 2007/02/22.

[127] Lee EJ, In KH, Kim JH, Lee SY, Shin C, Shim JJ, et al. Proteomic analysis in lung tissue of smokers and COPD patients. Chest. 2009;135(2):344-52. Epub 2008/08/30.

[128] American Thoracic Society/European Respiratory Society statement: standards for the diagnosis and management of individuals with alpha-1 antitrypsin deficiency. Am J Respir Crit Care Med. 2003;168(7):818-900. Epub 2003/10/03.

[129] Turino GM, Barker AF, Brantly ML, Cohen AB, Connelly RP, Crystal RG, et al. Clinical features of individuals with PI*SZ phenotype of alpha 1-antitrypsin deficiency. alpha 1-Antitrypsin Deficiency Registry Study Group. Am J Respir Crit Care Med. 1996;154(6 Pt 1):1718-25. Epub 1996/12/01.

[130] Jones EA, Vergalla J, Steer CJ, Bradley-Moore PR, Vierling JM. Metabolism of intact and desialylated alpha 1-antitrypsin. Clin Sci Mol Med. 1978;55(2):139-48. Epub 1978/08/01.

[131] Abboud RT, Ford GT, Chapman KR. Alpha1-antitrypsin deficiency: a position statement of the Canadian Thoracic Society. Can Respir J. 2001;8(2):81-8. Epub 2001/04/26.

[132] Mordwinkin NM, Louie SG. Aralast: an alpha 1-protease inhibitor for the treatment of alpha-antitrypsin deficiency. Expert Opin Pharmacother. 2007;8(15):2609-14. Epub 2007/10/13.

[133] Stocks JM, Brantly M, Pollock D, Barker A, Kueppers F, Strange C, et al. Multi-center study: the biochemical efficacy, safety and tolerability of a new alpha1-proteinase inhibitor, Zemaira. COPD. 2006;3(1):17-23. Epub 2006/12/21.

[134] Seersholm N, Wencker M, Banik N, Viskum K, Dirksen A, Kok-Jensen A, et al. Does alpha1-antitrypsin augmentation therapy slow the annual decline in FEV1 in patients with severe hereditary alpha1-antitrypsin deficiency? Wissenschaftliche Arbeitsgemeinschaft zur Therapie von Lungenerkrankungen (WATL) alpha1-AT study group. The European respiratory journal : official journal of the European Society for Clinical Respiratory Physiology. 1997;10(10):2260-3. Epub 1997/12/05.

[135] Wencker M, Fuhrmann B, Banik N, Konietzko N. Longitudinal follow-up of patients with alpha(1)-protease inhibitor deficiency before and during therapy with IV alpha(1)-protease inhibitor. Chest. 2001;119(3):737-44. Epub 2001/03/13.

[136] Carter RI, Mumford RA, Treonze KM, Finke PE, Davies P, Si Q, et al. The fibrinogen cleavage product Aalpha-Val360, a specific marker of neutrophil elastase activity in vivo. Thorax. 2011;66(8):686-91. Epub 2011/05/28.

[137] Gottlieb DJ, Luisetti M, Stone PJ, Allegra L, Cantey-Kiser JM, Grassi C, et al. Short-term supplementation therapy does not affect elastin degradation in severe alpha(1)-antitrypsin deficiency. The American-Italian AATD Study Group. Am J Respir Crit Care Med. 2000;162(6):2069-72. Epub 2000/12/09.

[138] Campos MA, Alazemi S, Zhang G, Wanner A, Salathe M, Baier H, et al. Exacerbations in subjects with alpha-1 antitrypsin deficiency receiving augmentation therapy. Respir Med. 2009;103(10):1532-9. Epub 2009/05/26.

[139] Lieberman J. Augmentation therapy reduces frequency of lung infections in antitrypsin deficiency: a new hypothesis with supporting data. Chest. 2000;118(5):1480-5. Epub 2000/11/18.

[140] Dirksen A, Dijkman JH, Madsen F, Stoel B, Hutchison DC, Ulrik CS, et al. A randomized clinical trial of alpha(1)-antitrypsin augmentation therapy. American journal of respiratory and critical care medicine. 1999;160(5 Pt 1):1468-72. Epub 1999/11/11.

[141] Dirksen A, Piitulainen E, Parr DG, Deng C, Wencker M, Shaker SB, et al. Exploring the role of CT densitometry: a randomised study of augmentation therapy in alpha1-antitrypsin deficiency. The European respiratory journal : official journal of the European Society for Clinical Respiratory Physiology. 2009;33(6):1345-53. Epub 2009/02/07.

[142] Wewers MD, Casolaro MA, Sellers SE, Swayze SC, McPhaul KM, Wittes JT, et al. Replacement therapy for alpha 1-antitrypsin deficiency associated with emphysema. N Engl J Med. 1987;316(17):1055-62. Epub 1987/04/23.

[143] Russi EW. Alpha-1 antitrypsin: now available, but do we need it? Swiss Med Wkly. 2008;138(13-14):191-6. Epub 2008/04/05.

[144] McCarthy C, Dimitrov BD. Augmentation therapy for alpha-1 antitrypsin deficiency--not enough evidence to support its use yet! Copd. 2010;7(3):234; author reply 5-6. Epub 2010/05/22.

[145] Woolhouse IS, Bayley DL, Stockley RA. Sputum chemotactic activity in chronic obstructive pulmonary disease: effect of alpha(1)-antitrypsin deficiency and the role of leukotriene B(4) and interleukin 8. Thorax. 2002;57(8):709-14. Epub 2002/08/01.

[146] Hubbard RC, Fells G, Gadek J, Pacholok S, Humes J, Crystal RG. Neutrophil accumulation in the lung in alpha 1-antitrypsin deficiency. Spontaneous release of leukotriene B4 by alveolar macrophages. J Clin Invest. 1991;88(3):891-7. Epub 1991/09/01.

[147] Stockley RA, Bayley DL, Unsal I, Dowson LJ. The effect of augmentation therapy on bronchial inflammation in alpha1-antitrypsin deficiency. Am J Respir Crit Care Med. 2002;165(11):1494-8. Epub 2002/06/05.

[148] Bergin DA, Reeves EP, Meleady P, Henry M, McElvaney OJ, Carroll TP, et al. Alpha-1 Antitrypsin regulates human neutrophil chemotaxis induced by soluble immune complexes and IL-8. J Clin Invest. 2010;120(12):4236-50. Epub 2010/11/10.

[149] Stoller JK, Rouhani F, Brantly M, Shahin S, Dweik RA, Stocks JM, et al. Biochemical efficacy and safety of a new pooled human plasma alpha(1)-antitrypsin, Respitin. Chest. 2002;122(1):66-74. Epub 2002/07/13.

[150] group TA--adrs. Survival and FEV1 decline in individuals with severe deficiency of alpha1-antitrypsin. The Alpha-1-Antitrypsin Deficiency Registry Study Group. Am J Respir Crit Care Med. 1998;158(1):49-59. Epub 1998/07/09.

[151] Tonelli AR, Rouhani F, Li N, Schreck P, Brantly ML. Alpha-1-antitrypsin augmentation therapy in deficient individuals enrolled in the Alpha-1 Foundation DNA and Tissue Bank. Int J Chron Obstruct Pulmon Dis. 2009;4:443-52. Epub 2010/01/08.

[152] Stone PJ, Morris TA, 3rd, Franzblau C, Snider GL. Preliminary evidence that augmentation therapy diminishes degradation of cross-linked elastin in alpha-1-antitrypsin-deficient humans. Respiration. 1995;62(2):76-9. Epub 1995/01/01.

[153] Ma S, Lin YY, He J, Rouhani FN, Brantly M, Turino GM. Alpha-1 antitrypsin augmentation therapy and biomarkers of elastin degradation. Copd. 2013;10(4):473-81. Epub 2013/04/09.

[154] Gotzsche PC, Johansen HK. Intravenous alpha-1 antitrypsin augmentation therapy: systematic review. Danish medical bulletin. 2010;57(9):A4175. Epub 2010/09/08.

[155] McElvaney NG, Stoller JK, Buist AS, Prakash UB, Brantly ML, Schluchter MD, et al. Baseline characteristics of enrollees in the National Heart, Lung and Blood Institute Registry of alpha 1-antitrypsin deficiency. Alpha 1-Antitrypsin Deficiency Registry Study Group. Chest. 1997;111(2):394-403. Epub 1997/02/01.

[156] Campos MA, Kueppers F, Stocks JM, Strange C, Chen J, Griffin R, et al. Safety and Pharmacokinetics of 120 mg/kg versus 60 mg/kg Weekly Intravenous Infusions of Alpha-1 Proteinase Inhibitor in Alpha-1 Antitrypsin Deficiency: A Multicenter, Randomized, Double-Blind, Crossover Study (SPARK). COPD. 2013. Epub 2013/07/19.

[157] Schriver EE, Davidson JM, Sutcliffe MC, Swindell BB, Bernard GR. Comparison of elastin peptide concentrations in body fluids from healthy volunteers, smokers, and patients with chronic obstructive pulmonary disease. The American review of respiratory disease. 1992;145(4 Pt 1):762-6. Epub 1992/04/01.

[158] Viglio S, Iadarola P, Lupi A, Trisolini R, Tinelli C, Balbi B, et al. MEKC of desmosine and isodesmosine in urine of chronic destructive lung disease patients. The European respiratory journal : official journal of the European Society for Clinical Respiratory Physiology. 2000;15(6):1039-45. Epub 2000/07/08.

[159] Boschetto P, Quintavalle S, Zeni E, Leprotti S, Potena A, Ballerin L, et al. Association between markers of emphysema and more severe chronic obstructive pulmonary disease. Thorax. 2006;61(12):1037-42. Epub 2006/06/14.

[160] Jones PW, Agusti AG. Outcomes and markers in the assessment of chronic obstructive pulmonary disease. Eur Respir J. 2006;27(4):822-32. Epub 2006/04/06.

[161] Stockley RA. Biomarkers in COPD: time for a deep breath. Thorax. 2007;62(8):657-60. Epub 2007/08/10.

[162] Stockley RA, Parr DG, Piitulainen E, Stolk J, Stoel BC, Dirksen A. Therapeutic efficacy of alpha-1 antitrypsin augmentation therapy on the loss of lung tissue: an integrated analysis of 2 randomised clinical trials using computed tomography densitometry. Respir Res. 2010;11:136. Epub 2010/10/06.

[163] Wanner A, Arce AD, Pardee E. Novel therapeutic uses of alpha-1 antitrypsin: a window to the future. COPD. 2012;9(6):583-8. Epub 2012/12/05.

[164] Cantin AM, Woods DE, Cloutier D, Dufour EK, Leduc R. Polyethylene glycol conjugation at Cys232 prolongs the half-life of alpha1 proteinase inhibitor. American journal of respiratory cell and molecular biology. 2002;27(6):659-65. Epub 2002/11/22.

[165] Kwon KS, Song M, Yu MH. Purification and characterization of alpha 1-antitrypsin secreted by recombinant yeast Saccharomyces diastaticus. J Biotechnol. 1995;42(3): 191-5. Epub 1995/10/16.

[166] Kang HA, Nam SW, Kwon KS, Chung BH, Yu MH. High-level secretion of human alpha 1-antitrypsin from Saccharomyces cerevisiae using inulinase signal sequence. J Biotechnol. 1996;48(1-2):15-24. Epub 1996/07/18.

[167] Sandoval C, Curtis H, Congote LF. Enhanced proliferative effects of a baculovirus-produced fusion protein of insulin-like growth factor and alpha(1)-proteinase inhibitor and improved anti-elastase activity of the inhibitor with glutamate at position 351. Protein engineering. 2002;15(5):413-8. Epub 2002/05/30.

[168] Lindhout T, Iqbal U, Willis LM, Reid AN, Li J, Liu X, et al. Site-specific enzymatic polysialylation of therapeutic proteins using bacterial enzymes. Proc Natl Acad Sci U S A. 2011;108(18):7397-402. Epub 2011/04/20.

[169] Blanchard V, Liu X, Eigel S, Kaup M, Rieck S, Janciauskiene S, et al. N-glycosylation and biological activity of recombinant human alpha1-antitrypsin expressed in a novel human neuronal cell line. Biotechnol Bioeng. 2011;108(9):2118-28. Epub 2011/04/16.

[170] Ross D, Brown T, Harper R, Pamarthi M, Nixon J, Bromirski J, et al. Production and characterization of a novel human recombinant alpha-1-antitrypsin in PER.C6 cells. J Biotechnol. 2012;162(2-3):262-73. Epub 2012/10/06.

[171] Wang Z, Hilder TL, van der Drift K, Sloan J, Wee K. Structural characterization of recombinant alpha-1-antitrypsin expressed in a human cell line. Anal Biochem. 2013;437(1):20-8. Epub 2013/03/07.

[172] Massoud M, Bischoff R, Dalemans W, Pointu H, Attal J, Schultz H, et al. Expression of active recombinant human alpha 1-antitrypsin in transgenic rabbits. J Biotechnol. 1991;18(3):193-203. Epub 1991/05/01.

[173] Archibald AL, McClenaghan M, Hornsey V, Simons JP, Clark AJ. High-level expression of biologically active human alpha 1-antitrypsin in the milk of transgenic mice. Proc Natl Acad Sci U S A. 1990;87(13):5178-82. Epub 1990/07/01.

[174] Wright G, Carver A, Cottom D, Reeves D, Scott A, Simons P, et al. High level expression of active human alpha-1-antitrypsin in the milk of transgenic sheep. Biotechnology (N Y). 1991;9(9):830-4. Epub 1991/09/01.

[175] Spencer LT, Humphries JE, Brantly ML. Antibody response to aerosolized transgenic human alpha1-antitrypsin. The New England journal of medicine. 2005;352(19): 2030-1. Epub 2005/05/13.

[176] Hubbard RC, McElvaney NG, Sellers SE, Healy JT, Czerski DB, Crystal RG. Recombinant DNA-produced alpha 1-antitrypsin administered by aerosol augments lower respiratory tract antineutrophil elastase defenses in individuals with alpha 1-antitrypsin deficiency. The Journal of clinical investigation. 1989;84(4):1349-54. Epub 1989/10/01.

[177] McElvaney NG, Hubbard RC, Birrer P, Chernick MS, Caplan DB, Frank MM, et al. Aerosol alpha 1-antitrypsin treatment for cystic fibrosis. Lancet. 1991;337(8738):392-4. Epub 1991/02/16.

[178] Berger M, Sorensen RU, Tosi MF, Dearborn DG, Doring G. Complement receptor expression on neutrophils at an inflammatory site, the Pseudomonas-infected lung in cystic fibrosis. J Clin Invest. 1989;84(4):1302-13. Epub 1989/10/01.

[179] Hartl D, Latzin P, Hordijk P, Marcos V, Rudolph C, Woischnik M, et al. Cleavage of CXCR1 on neutrophils disables bacterial killing in cystic fibrosis lung disease. Nature medicine. 2007;13(12):1423-30. Epub 2007/12/07.

[180] Smith RM, Traber LD, Traber DL, Spragg RG. Pulmonary deposition and clearance of aerosolized alpha-1-proteinase inhibitor administered to dogs and to sheep. The Journal of clinical investigation. 1989;84(4):1145-54. Epub 1989/10/01.

[181] Griese M, Latzin P, Kappler M, Weckerle K, Heinzlmaier T, Bernhardt T, et al. alpha1-Antitrypsin inhalation reduces airway inflammation in cystic fibrosis patients. The European respiratory journal : official journal of the European Society for Clinical Respiratory Physiology. 2007;29(2):240-50. Epub 2006/10/20.

[182] Schalkwijk J, Chang A, Janssen P, De Jongh GJ, Mier PD. Skin-derived antileucoproteases (SKALPs): characterization of two new elastase inhibitors from psoriatic epidermis. Br J Dermatol. 1990;122(5):631-41. Epub 1990/05/01.

[183] Alkemade JA, Molhuizen HO, Ponec M, Kempenaar JA, Zeeuwen PL, de Jongh GJ, et al. SKALP/elafin is an inducible proteinase inhibitor in human epidermal keratinocytes. J Cell Sci. 1994;107 (Pt 8):2335-42. Epub 1994/08/01.

[184] van Wetering S, van der Linden AC, van Sterkenburg MA, de Boer WI, Kuijpers AL, Schalkwijk J, et al. Regulation of SLPI and elafin release from bronchial epithelial cells by neutrophil defensins. Am J Physiol Lung Cell Mol Physiol. 2000;278(1):L51-8. Epub 2000/01/25.

[185] Marischen L, Wesch D, Schroder JM, Wiedow O, Kabelitz D. Human gammadelta T cells produce the protease inhibitor and antimicrobial peptide elafin. Scand J Immunol. 2009;70(6):547-52. Epub 2009/11/13.

[186] Mihaila A, Tremblay GM. Human alveolar macrophages express elafin and secretory leukocyte protease inhibitor. Z Naturforsch C. 2001;56(3-4):291-7. Epub 2001/05/24.

[187] Sallenave JM, Si Tahar M, Cox G, Chignard M, Gauldie J. Secretory leukocyte proteinase inhibitor is a major leukocyte elastase inhibitor in human neutrophils. J Leukoc Biol. 1997;61(6):695-702. Epub 1997/06/01.

[188] Guyot N, Zani ML, Maurel MC, Dallet-Choisy S, Moreau T. Elafin and its precursor trappin-2 still inhibit neutrophil serine proteinases when they are covalently bound to extracellular matrix proteins by tissue transglutaminase. Biochemistry. 2005;44(47):15610-8. Epub 2005/11/23.

[189] Guyot N, Zani ML, Berger P, Dallet-Choisy S, Moreau T. Proteolytic susceptibility of the serine protease inhibitor trappin-2 (pre-elafin): evidence for tryptase-mediated generation of elafin. Biol Chem. 2005;386(4):391-9. Epub 2005/05/19.

[190] Carter RI, Ungurs MJ, Mumford RA, Stockley RA. Aalpha-Val360: a marker of neutrophil elastase and COPD disease activity. Eur Respir J. 2013;41(1):31-8. Epub 2012/04/24.

[191] Sallenave JM, Shulmann J, Crossley J, Jordana M, Gauldie J. Regulation of secretory leukocyte proteinase inhibitor (SLPI) and elastase-specific inhibitor (ESI/elafin) in human airway epithelial cells by cytokines and neutrophilic enzymes. Am J Respir Cell Mol Biol. 1994;11(6):733-41. Epub 1994/12/01.

[192] Reid PT, Marsden ME, Cunningham GA, Haslett C, Sallenave JM. Human neutrophil elastase regulates the expression and secretion of elafin (elastase-specific inhibitor) in type II alveolar epithelial cells. FEBS Lett. 1999;457(1):33-7. Epub 1999/09/16.

[193] Simpson AJ, Cunningham GA, Porteous DJ, Haslett C, Sallenave JM. Regulation of adenovirus-mediated elafin transgene expression by bacterial lipopolysaccharide. Hum Gene Ther. 2001;12(11):1395-406. Epub 2001/08/04.

[194] Sallenave JM, Cunningham GA, James RM, McLachlan G, Haslett C. Regulation of pulmonary and systemic bacterial lipopolysaccharide responses in transgenic mice expressing human elafin. Infect Immun. 2003;71(7):3766-74. Epub 2003/06/24.

[195] Vachon E, Bourbonnais Y, Bingle CD, Rowe SJ, Janelle MF, Tremblay GM. Anti-inflammatory effect of pre-elafin in lipopolysaccharide-induced acute lung inflammation. Biol Chem. 2002;383(7-8):1249-56. Epub 2002/11/20.

[196] Chaouat A, Naeije R, Weitzenblum E. Pulmonary hypertension in COPD. Eur Respir J. 2008;32(5):1371-85. Epub 2008/11/04.

[197] Wilkinson TS, Dhaliwal K, Hamilton TW, Lipka AF, Farrell L, Davidson DJ, et al. Trappin-2 promotes early clearance of Pseudomonas aeruginosa through CD14-dependent macrophage activation and neutrophil recruitment. Am J Pathol. 2009;174(4):1338-46. Epub 2009/03/07.

[198] Butler MW, Robertson I, Greene CM, O'Neill SJ, Taggart CC, McElvaney NG. Elafin prevents lipopolysaccharide-induced AP-1 and NF-kappaB activation via an effect on the ubiquitin-proteasome pathway. J Biol Chem. 2006;281(46):34730-5. Epub 2006/09/19.

[199] Henriksen PA, Hitt M, Xing Z, Wang J, Haslett C, Riemersma RA, et al. Adenoviral gene delivery of elafin and secretory leukocyte protease inhibitor attenuates NF-kappa B-dependent inflammatory responses of human endothelial cells and macrophages to atherogenic stimuli. J Immunol. 2004;172(7):4535-44. Epub 2004/03/23.

[200] Simpson AJ, Maxwell AI, Govan JR, Haslett C, Sallenave JM. Elafin (elastase-specific inhibitor) has anti-microbial activity against gram-positive and gram-negative respiratory pathogens. FEBS Lett. 1999;452(3):309-13. Epub 1999/07/01.

[201] Williams SE, Brown TI, Roghanian A, Sallenave JM. SLPI and elafin: one glove, many fingers. Clin Sci (Lond). 2006;110(1):21-35. Epub 2005/12/13.

[202] Baranger K, Zani ML, Chandenier J, Dallet-Choisy S, Moreau T. The antibacterial and antifungal properties of trappin-2 (pre-elafin) do not depend on its protease inhibitory function. FEBS J. 2008;275(9):2008-20. Epub 2008/03/18.

[203] Simpson AJ, Wallace WA, Marsden ME, Govan JR, Porteous DJ, Haslett C, et al. Adenoviral augmentation of elafin protects the lung against acute injury mediated by activated neutrophils and bacterial infection. J Immunol. 2001;167(3):1778-86. Epub 2001/07/24.

[204] McMichael JW, Roghanian A, Jiang L, Ramage R, Sallenave JM. The antimicrobial antiproteinase elafin binds to lipopolysaccharide and modulates macrophage responses. Am J Respir Cell Mol Biol. 2005;32(5):443-52. Epub 2005/01/26.

[205] Nobar SM, Zani ML, Boudier C, Moreau T, Bieth JG. Oxidized elafin and trappin poorly inhibit the elastolytic activity of neutrophil elastase and proteinase 3. FEBS J. 2005;272(22):5883-93. Epub 2005/11/11.

[206] Guyot N, Butler MW, McNally P, Weldon S, Greene CM, Levine RL, et al. Elafin, an elastase-specific inhibitor, is cleaved by its cognate enzyme neutrophil elastase in sputum from individuals with cystic fibrosis. J Biol Chem. 2008;283(47):32377-85. Epub 2008/09/19.

[207] D'Armiento JM, Goldklang MP, Hardigan AA, Geraghty P, Roth MD, Connett JE, et al. Increased matrix metalloproteinase (MMPs) levels do not predict disease severity or progression in emphysema. PLoS One. 2013;8(2):e56352. Epub 2013/02/27.

[208] Guyot N, Bergsson G, Butler MW, Greene CM, Weldon S, Kessler E, et al. Functional study of elafin cleaved by Pseudomonas aeruginosa metalloproteinases. Biol Chem. 2010;391(6):705-16. Epub 2010/04/08.

[209] Doumas S, Kolokotronis A, Stefanopoulos P. Anti-inflammatory and antimicrobial roles of secretory leukocyte protease inhibitor. Infect Immun. 2005;73(3):1271-4. Epub 2005/02/26.

[210] Ding A, Yu H, Yang J, Shi S, Ehrt S. Induction of macrophage-derived SLPI by Mycobacterium tuberculosis depends on TLR2 but not MyD88. Immunology. 2005;116(3): 381-9. Epub 2005/10/21.

[211] Jin FY, Nathan C, Radzioch D, Ding A. Secretory leukocyte protease inhibitor: a macrophage product induced by and antagonistic to bacterial lipopolysaccharide. Cell. 1997;88(3):417-26. Epub 1997/02/07.

[212] Wen J, Nikitakis NG, Chaisuparat R, Greenwell-Wild T, Gliozzi M, Jin W, et al. Secretory leukocyte protease inhibitor (SLPI) expression and tumor invasion in oral squamous cell carcinoma. Am J Pathol. 2011;178(6):2866-78. Epub 2011/06/07.

[213] Zhang Y, DeWitt DL, McNeely TB, Wahl SM, Wahl LM. Secretory leukocyte protease inhibitor suppresses the production of monocyte prostaglandin H synthase-2, prostaglandin E2, and matrix metalloproteinases. J Clin Invest. 1997;99(5):894-900. Epub 1997/03/01.

[214] Navratilova Z, Zatloukal J, Kriegova E, Kolek V, Petrek M. Simultaneous up-regulation of matrix metalloproteinases 1, 2, 3, 7, 8, 9 and tissue inhibitors of metalloproteinases 1, 4 in serum of patients with chronic obstructive pulmonary disease. Respirology. 2012;17(6):1006-12. Epub 2012/05/18.

[215] Yang J, Zhu J, Sun D, Ding A. Suppression of macrophage responses to bacterial lipopolysaccharide (LPS) by secretory leukocyte protease inhibitor (SLPI) is independent of its anti-protease function. Biochim Biophys Acta. 2005;1745(3):310-7. Epub 2005/08/23.

[216] Geraghty P, Greene CM, O'Mahony M, O'Neill SJ, Taggart CC, McElvaney NG. Secretory leucocyte protease inhibitor inhibits interferon-gamma-induced cathepsin S expression. J Biol Chem. 2007;282(46):33389-95. Epub 2007/09/20.

[217] Taggart CC, Cryan SA, Weldon S, Gibbons A, Greene CM, Kelly E, et al. Secretory leucoprotease inhibitor binds to NF-kappaB binding sites in monocytes and inhibits p65 binding. J Exp Med. 2005;202(12):1659-68. Epub 2005/12/15.

[218] Reeves EP BN, Ryan D, McElvaney OJ, Bergin DA, Pohl K, Molloy K, Alsaleh K, Al-jorfi A, Kandalaft O, O'Flynn E, Geraghty P, O'Neill SJ, McElvaney NG. Intracellular secretory leukoprotease inhibitor modulates inositol 1,4,5 triphosphate generation and exerts an anti-inflammatory effect on neutrophils of individuals with cystic fibrosis and chronic obstructive pulmonary disease. BioMed Research International. 2013.

[219] Hiemstra PS, Maassen RJ, Stolk J, Heinzel-Wieland R, Steffens GJ, Dijkman JH. Antibacterial activity of antileukoprotease. Infect Immun. 1996;64(11):4520-4. Epub 1996/11/01.

[220] Wiedow O, Harder J, Bartels J, Streit V, Christophers E. Antileukoprotease in human skin: an antibiotic peptide constitutively produced by keratinocytes. Biochem Biophys Res Commun. 1998;248(3):904-9. Epub 1998/08/15.

[221] Tomee JF, Hiemstra PS, Heinzel-Wieland R, Kauffman HF. Antileukoprotease: an endogenous protein in the innate mucosal defense against fungi. J Infect Dis. 1997;176(3):740-7. Epub 1997/09/18.

[222] Vogelmeier C, Buhl R, Hoyt RF, Wilson E, Fells GA, Hubbard RC, et al. Aerosolization of recombinant SLPI to augment antineutrophil elastase protection of pulmonary epithelium. J Appl Physiol. 1990;69(5):1843-8. Epub 1990/11/01.

[223] McElvaney NG, Nakamura H, Birrer P, Hebert CA, Wong WL, Alphonso M, et al. Modulation of airway inflammation in cystic fibrosis. In vivo suppression of interleukin-8 levels on the respiratory epithelial surface by aerosolization of recombinant secretory leukoprotease inhibitor. J Clin Invest. 1992;90(4):1296-301. Epub 1992/10/01.

[224] Birrer P, McElvaney NG, Rudeberg A, Sommer CW, Liechti-Gallati S, Kraemer R, et al. Protease-antiprotease imbalance in the lungs of children with cystic fibrosis. Am J Respir Crit Care Med. 1994;150(1):207-13. Epub 1994/07/01.

[225] Taggart CC, Lowe GJ, Greene CM, Mulgrew AT, O'Neill SJ, Levine RL, et al. Cathepsin B, L, and S cleave and inactivate secretory leucoprotease inhibitor. J Biol Chem. 2001;276(36):33345-52. Epub 2001/07/04.

[226] Gibbons AM, McElvaney NG, Taggart CC, Cryan SA. Delivery of rSLPI in a liposomal carrier for inhalation provides protection against cathepsin L degradation. J Microencapsul. 2009;26(6):513-22. Epub 2008/10/18.

[227] Ramadas RA, Wu L, LeVine AM. Surfactant protein A enhances production of secretory leukoprotease inhibitor and protects it from cleavage by matrix metalloproteinases. J Immunol. 2009;182(3):1560-7. Epub 2009/01/22.

[228] Ju CR, Xia XZ, Chen RC. Expressions of tumor necrosis factor-converting enzyme and ErbB3 in rats with chronic obstructive pulmonary disease. Chin Med J (Engl). 2007;120(17):1505-10. Epub 2007/10/03.

[229] Lockett AD, Kimani S, Ddungu G, Wrenger S, Tuder RM, Janciauskiene SM, et al. alpha(1)-Antitrypsin modulates lung endothelial cell inflammatory responses to TNF-alpha. Am J Respir Cell Mol Biol. 2013;49(1):143-50. Epub 2013/03/26.

[230] Iba T, Kidokoro A, Fukunaga M, Takuhiro K, Yoshikawa S, Sugimotoa K. Pretreatment of sivelestat sodium hydrate improves the lung microcirculation and alveolar damage in lipopolysaccharide-induced acute lung inflammation in hamsters. Shock. 2006;26(1):95-8. Epub 2006/06/20.

[231] Nakatani K, Takeshita S, Tsujimoto H, Kawamura Y, Sekine I. Inhibitory effect of serine protease inhibitors on neutrophil-mediated endothelial cell injury. J Leukoc Biol. 2001;69(2):241-7. Epub 2001/03/29.

[232] Yasui S, Nagai A, Aoshiba K, Ozawa Y, Kakuta Y, Konno K. A specific neutrophil elastase inhibitor (ONO-5046.Na) attenuates LPS-induced acute lung inflammation in the hamster. Eur Respir J. 1995;8(8):1293-9. Epub 1995/08/01.

[233] Song JS, Kang CM, Rhee CK, Yoon HK, Kim YK, Moon HS, et al. Effects of elastase inhibitor on the epithelial cell apoptosis in bleomycin-induced pulmonary fibrosis. Exp Lung Res. 2009;35(10):817-29. Epub 2009/12/10.

[234] Abe T, Usui A, Oshima H, Akita T, Ueda Y. A pilot randomized study of the neutrophil elastase inhibitor, Sivelestat, in patients undergoing cardiac surgery. Interact Cardiovasc Thorac Surg. 2009;9(2):236-40. Epub 2009/05/19.

[235] Miyoshi S, Hamada H, Ito R, Katayama H, Irifune K, Suwaki T, et al. Usefulness of a selective neutrophil elastase inhibitor, sivelestat, in acute lung injury patients with sepsis. Drug Des Devel Ther. 2013;7:305-16. Epub 2013/04/19.

[236] Tsuboko Y, Takeda S, Mii S, Nakazato K, Tanaka K, Uchida E, et al. Clinical evaluation of sivelestat for acute lung injury/acute respiratory distress syndrome following surgery for abdominal sepsis. Drug Des Devel Ther. 2012;6:273-8. Epub 2012/10/24.

[237] Lucas SD, Costa E, Guedes RC, Moreira R. Targeting COPD: advances on low-molecular-weight inhibitors of human neutrophil elastase. Med Res Rev. 2013;33 Suppl 1:E73-101. Epub 2011/06/18.

[238] Luisetti M, Piccioni PD, Donnini M, Peona V, Pozzi E, Grassi C. Studies of MR 889, a new synthetic proteinase inhibitor. Biochem Biophys Res Commun. 1989;165(2): 568-73. Epub 1989/12/15.

[239] Luisetti M, Sturani C, Sella D, Madonini E, Galavotti V, Bruno G, et al. MR889, a neutrophil elastase inhibitor, in patients with chronic obstructive pulmonary disease: a double-blind, randomized, placebo-controlled clinical trial. Eur Respir J. 1996;9(7): 1482-6. Epub 1996/07/01.

[240] Churg A, Wang RD, Xie C, Wright JL. alpha-1-Antitrypsin ameliorates cigarette smoke-induced emphysema in the mouse. Am J Respir Crit Care Med. 2003;168(2): 199-207. Epub 2003/04/12.

[241] Wright JL, Farmer SG, Churg A. A neutrophil elastase inhibitor reduces cigarette smoke-induced remodelling of lung vessels. Eur Respir J. 2003;22(1):77-81. Epub 2003/07/29.

[242] Shinguh Y, Yamazaki A, Inamura N, Fujie K, Okamoto M, Nakahara K, et al. Biochemical and pharmacological characterization of FR134043, a novel elastase inhibitor. Eur J Pharmacol. 1998;345(3):299-308. Epub 1998/05/20.

[243] Numanami H, Koyama S, Nelson DK, Hoyt JC, Freels JL, Habib MP, et al. Serine protease inhibitors modulate smoke-induced chemokine release from human lung fibroblasts. Am J Respir Cell Mol Biol. 2003;29(5):613-9. Epub 2003/05/10.

[244] Stevens T, Ekholm K, Granse M, Lindahl M, Kozma V, Jungar C, et al. AZD9668: pharmacological characterization of a novel oral inhibitor of neutrophil elastase. J Pharmacol Exp Ther. 2011;339(1):313-20. Epub 2011/07/28.

[245] Vogelmeier C, Aquino TO, O'Brien CD, Perrett J, Gunawardena KA. A randomised, placebo-controlled, dose-finding study of AZD9668, an oral inhibitor of neutrophil elastase, in patients with chronic obstructive pulmonary disease treated with tiotropium. COPD. 2012;9(2):111-20. Epub 2012/03/31.

[246] Stockley R, De Soyza A, Gunawardena K, Perrett J, Forsman-Semb K, Entwistle N, et al. Phase II study of a neutrophil elastase inhibitor (AZD9668) in patients with bronchiectasis. Respir Med. 2013;107(4):524-33. Epub 2013/02/26.

[247] Mocchegiani E, Giacconi R, Costarelli L. Metalloproteases/anti-metalloproteases imbalance in chronic obstructive pulmonary disease: genetic factors and treatment implications. Curr Opin Pulm Med. 2011;17 Suppl 1:S11-9. Epub 2012/01/11.

[248] Magnussen H, Watz H, Kirsten A, Wang M, Wray H, Samuelsson V, et al. Safety and tolerability of an oral MMP-9 and -12 inhibitor, AZD1236, in patients with moderate-to-severe COPD: a randomised controlled 6-week trial. Pulm Pharmacol Ther. 2011;24(5):563-70. Epub 2011/06/01.

[249] Dahl R, Titlestad I, Lindqvist A, Wielders P, Wray H, Wang M, et al. Effects of an oral MMP-9 and -12 inhibitor, AZD1236, on biomarkers in moderate/severe COPD: a randomised controlled trial. Pulm Pharmacol Ther. 2012;25(2):169-77. Epub 2012/02/07.

[250] Wu Y, Li J, Wu J, Morgan P, Xu X, Rancati F, et al. Discovery of potent and selective matrix metalloprotease 12 inhibitors for the potential treatment of chronic obstructive pulmonary disease (COPD). Bioorg Med Chem Lett. 2012;22(1):138-43. Epub 2011/12/14.

[251] Li W, Li J, Wu Y, Wu J, Hotchandani R, Cunningham K, et al. A selective matrix metalloprotease 12 inhibitor for potential treatment of chronic obstructive pulmonary

disease (COPD): discovery of (S)-2-(8-(methoxycarbonylamino)dibenzo[b,d] furan-3-sulfonamido)-3-methylbutanoic acid (MMP408). J Med Chem. 2009;52(7):1799-802. Epub 2009/03/13.

[252] Churg A, Dai J, Zay K, Karsan A, Hendricks R, Yee C, et al. Alpha-1-antitrypsin and a broad spectrum metalloprotease inhibitor, RS113456, have similar acute anti-inflammatory effects. Lab Invest. 2001;81(8):1119-31. Epub 2001/08/15.

[253] Morris A, Kinnear G, Wan WY, Wyss D, Bahra P, Stevenson CS. Comparison of cigarette smoke-induced acute inflammation in multiple strains of mice and the effect of a matrix metalloproteinase inhibitor on these responses. J Pharmacol Exp Ther. 2008;327(3):851-62. Epub 2008/09/23.

[254] Pemberton PA, Cantwell JS, Kim KM, Sundin DJ, Kobayashi D, Fink JB, et al. An inhaled matrix metalloprotease inhibitor prevents cigarette smoke-induced emphysema in the mouse. COPD. 2005;2(3):303-10. Epub 2006/12/07.

[255] Gross NJ. Novel antiinflammatory therapies for COPD. Chest. 2012;142(5):1300-7. Epub 2012/11/08.

[256] Attucci S, Gauthier A, Korkmaz B, Delepine P, Martino MF, Saudubray F, et al. EPI-hNE4, a proteolysis-resistant inhibitor of human neutrophil elastase and potential anti-inflammatory drug for treating cystic fibrosis. J Pharmacol Exp Ther. 2006;318(2):803-9. Epub 2006/04/22.

[257] Delacourt C, Herigault S, Delclaux C, Poncin A, Levame M, Harf A, et al. Protection against acute lung injury by intravenous or intratracheal pretreatment with EPI-HNE-4, a new potent neutrophil elastase inhibitor. Am J Respir Cell Mol Biol. 2002;26(3):290-7. Epub 2002/02/28.

[258] Honore S, Attalah HL, Azoulay E, Soussy CJ, Saudubray F, Harf A, et al. Beneficial effect of an inhibitor of leukocyte elastase (EPI-hNE-4) in presence of repeated lung injuries. Shock. 2004;22(2):131-6. Epub 2004/07/17.

[259] Zani ML, Baranger K, Guyot N, Dallet-Choisy S, Moreau T. Protease inhibitors derived from elafin and SLPI and engineered to have enhanced specificity towards neutrophil serine proteases. Protein Sci. 2009;18(3):579-94. Epub 2009/02/26.

[260] Tanga A, Saidi A, Jourdan ML, Dallet-Choisy S, Zani ML, Moreau T. Protection of lung epithelial cells from protease-mediated injury by trappin-2 A62L, an engineered inhibitor of neutrophil serine proteases. Biochem Pharmacol. 2012;83(12):1663-73. Epub 2012/04/03.

Chapter 5

Sleep and Chronic Obstructive Pulmonary Disease – the Role of Oxidative Stress in Overlap Syndrome

Radostina Vlaeva Cherneva,
Ognian Borisov Georgiev,
Daniela Stoichkova Petrova, Emil Ivanov Manov and
Julia Ivanova Petrova

Additional information is available at the end of the chapter

http://dx.doi.org/10.5772/57220

1. Introduction

Chronic obstructive pulmonary diseasese (COPD) is the fourth leading cause of mortality and its prevalence continues to increase. While the debilitating effects of COPD on daytime functioning are well known, COPD's effects on sleep have been less fully investigated. Sleep problems affect as many as 50% of patients with COPD. The mild hypoventilation that is physiologically observed during sleep is heightened in this patient group and is often accompanied by ventilation/perfusion mismatch. Significant hypoxemia ensues that is often accompanied by hypercapnia. These gas exchange abnormalities (particularly nocturnal oxygen desaturation, NOD) place COPD patients at increased risk of pulmonary hypertension, arrhythmias, and possibly cardiovascular death. Approximately 50% of COPD patients with mild daytime hypoxaemia experience NOD which suggests that NOD may be a frequent occurrence with devastating consequences in individuals with COPD.

The increased prevalence of obesity worldwide is associated with a subsequent increase in the occurrence of sleep disordered breathing, particularly obstructive sleep apnea (OSA). The co-existence of OSA and COPD, known as the overlap syndrome, has been estimated to occur in 1% of the general population. The presence of one of the disorders, however, potentiates the occurrence of the other by more than 10%. Overlap patients are a unique group of COPD patients who experience complex sleep disordered breathing, with nocturnal hypoxaemia and hypercapnia that is often disproportionately worse than their ventilatory impairments, pulmonary hypertension, and significant cardiovascular comorbidity. Evidence of systemic inflammation and oxidative stress in both COPD and OSA provides a common pathophysiologic link between these disorders which may predispose these individuals to increased cardiovascular morbidity and mortality. Further studies of the overlap syndrome are required to provide information on the additive and/or synergistic effects of these disorders at the molecular, physiological, and clinical level. Current, ongoing, long-term studies will provide information on the clinical consequences of the overlap syndrome, especially regarding cardiovascular mortality.

Despite the lack of understanding of the pathophysiologic processes mediating the development and effects of the overlap syndrome, treatment with continuous positive airway pressure (CPAP) reduces hypoxaemia, pulmonary and systemic hypertension, and improves survival. Furthermore, CPAP reduces exacerbations and lung decline in patients with the overlap syndrome.

Thus, a more aggressive approach in diagnosing OSA in COPD patients is strongly recommended. This chapter will acquaint you with the physiology of breathing in normal subjects and those with COPD, OSA, and overlap syndrome. We will review the effects of these disorders on sleep quality, gas exchange, and cardiovascular comorbidity. The current diagnostic and treatment options will be introduced. The role of oxidative stress in cardiovascular and metabolic comorbidity in OSA and overlap will also be discussed from our research perspective. The effect of bilevel positive pressure ventilation for one month on sleep quality, gas exchange, and ventilatory parameters, insulin resistance, and oxidative stress in overlap syndrome will also be reviewed.

2. Sleep and ventilation

2.1. Sleep and ventilation in normal physiology

Based upon the electroencephalographic characteristics, sleep can be divided into non-rapid eye movement sleep (NREM) and rapid eye movement sleep (REM) which have unique physiological characteristics. The four stages of NREM sleep are categorized by the presence of sleep spindles, K-complexes, and distinctive electro-occulogram and electromyogram findings. REM sleep is characterized by bursts of rapid eye movement, muscle atonia, and shallow and irregular breathing. It is subdivided into two periods: tonic and phasic. Four to five cycles of recurring NREM and REM episodes occur throughout the night. The duration of REM sleep increases during the night, being longest in the last part of nocturnal sleep. Sleep profoundly affects breathing by altering respiratory drive, minute ventilation, and ventilation/perfusion matching.

2.1.1. Respiratory drive

The physiological mechanisms of breathing during sleep are similar to those in wakefulness except for the fact that feedback mechanisms are blunted. This dampening effect is mostly attributed to the slight decrease in the metabolic rate during sleep which attenuates the response to mechanical, cortical, and metabolic stimuli [1,2]. The ventilatory and arousal responses to hypercapnia are much more robust than for hypoxia, with only slight changes in PaCO2 causing recognizable alterations of minute ventilation [3]. However, under normal conditions in sleep and especially during periods of REM, the responses to hypoxaemia and hypercapnia are blunted in comparison to wakefulness. The diminished ventilatory responses to hypercapnia and hypoxia are more profound during REM compared with NREM sleep [1, 4]. These attenuated feedback mechanisms stress the respiratory system which in individuals with COPD is already deranged and dysfunctional. The combinations of sleep disordered breathing, impaired respiratory function, and dampened feedback interactions may cause significant reductions in minute ventilation and precipitate respiratory failure

2.1.2. Minute ventilation

Compared to wakefulness, minute ventilation decreases during NREM sleep and declines even further during REM sleep when minute ventilation may be 15% less than occurs during wakefulness. The minute ventilation decrease is caused by a reduction in tidal volume due to muscle atonia and cephaloid displacement of the diaphragm that is not fully compensated by an increase in respiratory frequency [5]. The consequence is sleep related hypoventilation which causes a significant reduction (2-8 mmHg) in the partial pressure of oxygen in arterial blood (PaO_2) and an increase in the partial pressure of carbon dioxide (3-10mmHg) in arterial blood ($PaCO_2$) [6]. The decreased muscle tone during sleep increases respiratory resistance and the inability to compensate for these changes probably contributes to attenuated physiologic responses [7]. During NREM sleep, the phasic electromyographic activity of the genioglossus and geniohyoid muscles is well-maintained [8], but tonic activity of upper airway dilator muscles decreases [9]. During REM sleep, breathing is shallow and irregular and upper airway resistance increases due to full skeletal-muscle atonia [10].

2.1.3. Ventilation-perfusion mismatch

During NREM sleep, lung volume decreases leading to a reduction in the functional residual capacity (FRC) [11]. Reduction in lung compliance and reduced respiratory muscle tone, have been suggested as potential causal factors in the reduction in FRC [12]. It has been hypothesized that reduced FRC during sleep may contribute to the airway closure, causing ventilation–perfusion mismatch and, thus, contributing to the small changes in arterial oxygen saturation especially during REM sleep [13].

2.2. Sleep and ventilation in COPD patients

The control of breathing in patients with COPD follows the same basic principles as in normal subjects. The lower baseline oxygenation and abnormal respiratory mechanics in patients with COPD become clinically important when combined with the normal physiologic alterations in ventilatory control and respiratory muscle tone that occur during sleep. In COPD patients, the more profound decrease in oxygen saturation during sleep is mainly attributed to the lower PaO_2 during wakefulness. This PaO_2 level is on a steeper section of the O_2 dissociation curve; thus, a slight decline in oxygenation leads to a more profound reduction in oxygen saturation.

Thus, nocturnal oxygen desaturation (NOD) is the most significant sleep abnormality associated with COPD [14,15]. Even without any upper-airway contribution, various studies have reported that 27–70% of patients with COPD with awake oxygen saturation levels of 90 –95% can experience substantial desaturation at night, particularly during REM sleep [16-18].

2.2.1. Definition of NOD

The definition of NOD varies depending on various studies. At least three different definitions have been used: 1) Mean nocturnal oxygen saturation (SaO_2) < 90%; 2.) SaO_2 < 90% for more than 30% of recording time (total time in bed); 3) SaO_2 < 90% for more than 5 minutes of recording time with a nadir <=85%. Most studies use either definition 2 or 3 [19]. Similarly, the definition for the amount of desaturation dip is not universal. Wynee and colleagues [20] defined a desaturation dip by a fall in SaO_2 by more than 4% from baseline during quiet breathing just before the episode of hypoxemia. Flenley's group [6,21] defined a dip as a 10% or greater drop in SaO_2.

The nocturnal oxygen desaturation in COPD patients presents specific characteristics. It takes place at the end of the night during REM sleep [22] and may be variable from one night to the other, especially in patients with moderate-to-severe COPD [23]. The desaturations are significantly related to daytime hypoxaemia and hypercapnia [24]-the more pronounced daytime hypoxaemia and hypercapnia, the more severe nocturnal desaturation [25].

2.2.2. Mechanisms of NOD

Flenley [25] identified three mechanisms that might contribute to nocturnal oxygen desaturation: 1) alveolar hypoventilation; 2) decreased ventilation/perfusion matching; 3) decreased end-expiratory lung volume. Subsequent research confirmed much of his hypothesis. The description of sleep disordered breathing, particularly, obstructive sleep apnea, led to the introduction of the overlap syndrome in 1985 as an independent phenomenon in COPD patients [25].

2.2.2.1. Alveolar Hypoventilation

Alveolar hypoventilation plays a significant role in NOD, especially during REM sleep. The exact mechanism causing alveolar hypoventilation in COPD patients is arguable. This may be due to the type of measurements performed, the stage of sleep (REM vs. NREM), and the status of subjects-normocapnic or hypercapnic COPD patients. Becker et al [5] observed a drop in minute ventilation of 16% and 32% during non-REM and REM sleep, respectively. This reduction was predominantly due to a decrease in tidal volume measured by a pneumotachograph. The greater drop in minute ventilation in subjects with COPD may reflect increased dependence on accessory muscles that become hypotonic during sleep, particularly during REM sleep, as well as the presence of blunted chemical respiratory drive. Ballard and coworkers [10] showed a decrease in minute ventilation in COPD patients which was associated with an increase in upper airway resistance as well as a decrease in neuromuscular output to the respiratory muscles rather than a decrease in lung volumes. O'Donoghue et al [26] noted a decline in minute ventilation in NREM sleep in hypercapnic COPD patients due to a decrease in tidal volume and an increase in upper airway resistance. Although the exact mechanism is unknown, current evidence suggests that alveolar hypoventilation during sleep contributes to NOD in COPD patients.

2.2.2.2. Ventilation-perfusion (V/Q) mismatch

V/Q mismatch has not been directly measured during sleep. However, for a mild and similar increase in $PaCO_2$ (and thereby alveolar hypoventilation), some COPD patients had more significant decreases in nocturnal PaO_2 than others, suggesting a role for V/Q mismatch as a mechanism for NOD [24]. This may be due to reduced lung volumes (particularly functional residual capacity-FRC) caused by declines in respiratory muscle tone leading to atelectasis at the lung bases. It is likely that in COPD patients, especially during REM, the ventilation/perfusion mismatch may be due to the dissociation between intercostal and diaphragmatic activity on one hand [22] and the cephaloid displacement of the diaphragm and decreased FRC on the other [27].

2.2.2.3. Impact of oxyhemoglobin dissociation curve

Hypoxaemic patients at baseline are more likely to drop their SaO_2 with hypoventilation during sleep, compared to normoxic patients due to the effect of the oxyhemoglobin dissociation curve [22]. Mild decreases in oxygenation change the location on the oxygen-hemoglobin dissociation curve from the plateau to the edge of the slope where a slight decrease in oxygenation will cause a profound decline in oxygen saturation. This effect is not an independent mechanism but contributes to the NOD in collaboration with other factors.

2.2.2.4. Obstructive sleep apnea (Overlap syndrome)

Patients with coexisting obstructive sleep apnea (overlap syndrome) may be hypoxaemic at the commencement of an apnea and thus are more likely to desaturate compared to patients with only OSA who may be able to recover to a normal SaO_2 after the apneic episode. Overlap syndrome and its mechanisms and consequences will be discussed in detail.

2.2.3. Consequences of NOD

Potential consequences of NOD are mainly related to cardiovascular mortality and morbidity and affect pulmonary haemodynamics mainly.

2.2.3.1. Pulmonary hypertension

Alveolar hypoxemia is the major mechanism that triggers pulmonary arterial vasoconstriction and leads to pulmonary hypertension [28]. In a study of 12 patients with COPD, an acute increase in pulmonary artery pressure was noted in all sleep stages, most significantly in REM. The increase corresponded much more to the decrease in PaO_2 compared to the rise in $PaCO_2$ [29]. Although highly persuasive, there is still not enough evidence for a causational link between sleep oxygen desaturation episodes and the development of pulmonary hypertension in COPD patients.

Pulmonary haemodynamic studies during sleep in COPD patients have been scarce as the invasive nature of their investigation is not compatible with normal sleep [30]. Moreover almost all of them are in severe COPD patients with daytime hypoxaemia, marked nocturnal hypoxaemia, and daytime pulmonary hypertension (pulmonary artery pressure (PAP) > 20 mm Hg) [31-33]. Nocturnal elevation of PAP appears to correlate with NOD in this patient population [33]. Whether this correlation stays true in patients with mild and moderate COPD with less diurnal hypoxaemia is elusive.

In patients with mild and moderate COPD, studies on the relationship between pulmonary hypertension and NOD are not conclusive and their interpretation depends on the type of definition used for NOD, as well as the amount of decrease in PaO_2 [34,35,36]. Fletcher et al [34] studied 36 COPD patients who had daytime PaO_2 > 60 mm Hg and NOD during REM sleep (a drop in SaO_2 < 90% for 5 minutes or more and a nadir of at least 85%). They measured an increase in systolic and mean pulmonary artery pressures, as well as pulmonary vascular resistance. In forty COPD patients with a daytime PaO_2 of 60-70 mm Hg, Levi-Valensi et al [35] detected higher mean pulmonary artery pressures in those individuals with NOD compared with those who did not have NOD (defined as SaO_2 < 90% for > 30% of total time in bed (TIB)). In a larger group of 66 COPD patients with a daytime PaO_2 >60 mm Hg, Chaouat et al [16] found no difference in the mean pulmonary artery pressure measured by right heart catheterization. NOD was defined by the same criteria used by Levi-Valensi.

In conclusion, acute nocturnal oxygen desaturation is associated with increases in both systemic and pulmonary blood pressures [34]. It is very likely that the repetitive, transient nocturnal oxygen desaturations that appear in some COPD patients can cause pulmonary hypertension [37]. Which patients are more likely to be affected by NOD and what clinical factors predict the hemodynamic effects of NOD are unknown. It is, however, generally assumed that patients with COPD and daytime normoxia who have **only nocturnal oxygen desaturation** generally do not develop substantial pulmonary hypertension. This assumption is supported by the lack of efficacy of nocturnal supplemental oxygen in treatment trials in this patient population [38]

2.2.3.2. Cardiac arrhythmias

Various arrhythmias are reported during episodes of nocturnal desaturation [4]. These consequences might explain why nocturnal oxygen desaturation is a marker of increased mortality and why COPD patients are reported to die more frequently at night than expected [39]. Though some studies have shown increased frequency of premature supraventricular and ventricular contractions (PVC) during sleep in COPD patients, overall there appears to be no correlation between PVC's and nocturnal SaO_2 [40,41].

2.2.3.4. Polycythemia

Daytime hypoxaemia in COPD patients is a well known cause of polycythemia. However, NOD without daytime hypoxaemia has not been associated with polycythemia [35,42]. In addition, there is no clear evidence that erythropoetin is increased in COPD patients with primary NOD [43].

2.2.3.5. Sleep quality

NOD can also affect sleep quality. Arousals may be related to episodes of desaturation [44] and, consistent with this observation, some (but not all) studies have shown that supplemental oxygen improves sleep quality [6].

2.2.3.6. Mortality

While some COPD patients die due to respiratory failure, they more frequently die from cardiovascular disease or malignancy [45]. There is some evidence that these deaths occur predominantly at night. McNicholas reported that patients admitted to the hospital with chronic bronchitis or emphysema were more likely to die at night than other hospital patients. Deaths occurred more frequently among so called "blue-bloaters" [39]. Although these data relate to patients with daytime hypoxaemia, the effect of NOD on survival of COPD patients without significant daytime hypoxemia is not well established. Fletcher et al [34] performed a retrospective study in 169 COPD patients without daytime hypoxemia. NOD was define-deither as a drop in SaO_2 below 90% for 5 or more minutes reaching a nadir of 85% or as SaO_2 <90% for > 30% of TIB. Although patients with NOD had improved survival compared to the non-NOD group, correcting NOD has not shown to improve survival. In 97 COPD patients, Connaughton et al [46] found no survival advantage when they followed them for a median of 70 months, performing nocturnal SaO2 measurement.

Comorbid OSA was recently reported to increase mortality in patients with COPD. Marin et al, published outcome data on patients with COPD and patients with the overlap syndrome, both with and without CPAP treatment [47]. Subjects were initially screened because of a clinical suspicion of sleep-disordered breathing. Then, a diagnostic polysomnogram and spirometry were performed. After a median follow-up of over 9 years, all-cause mortality was higher in the untreated (without CPAP) overlap group (42.2%) than in the COPD-only group (24.2%). Even after adjustment for COPD severity, comorbid OSA remained a risk factor for death. In this study, death in the untreated overlap group was most commonly attributed to cardiovascular disease. In the overlap group, OSA contributed to an increased incidence of COPD exacerbations, which may accelerate lung-function decline and, hence, augment mortality [48,49]

The exact mechanism(s) for the increased mortality risk in overlap syndrome is not established. Increased risk of death may be due to more prolonged hypoxia. Nighttime hypercapnia may also be important. The systemic consequences of both COPD and OSA should also be considered. They both cause inflammation and oxidative stress. Whether these mechanisms are additive or synergistic is, however, unknown.

3. Sleep quality in copd

3.1. Characteristics of sleep disturbances

Insomnia and other sleep problems are increased in patients with COPD [44]. Elderly COPD patients experience more morning tiredness and early awakenings [50]. The most commonly reported sleep disturbances are insomnia, poor sleep maintenance, early morning awakenings and headaches, and daytime sleepiness. These symptoms occur in approximately 30-70% of patients with COPD [44, 50, 52]. When surveyed for a broad range of symptoms, "sleep difficulties" were mentioned as occurring "almost always" or "always" in 43% of subjects with either chronic bronchitis or emphysema and were the third (after dyspnea and fatigue) most common complaint [53]. The sleep architecture of individuals with COPD is notable for many arousals. These arousals were attributed not just to the diagnosis of COPD, but largely due to the presence of related symptoms-cough, sputum production, or wheezing. These symptoms correlated most with difficulty falling or staying asleep [53]. Many COPD patients report use of hypnotics (28% compared to controls-10%) to combat sleep disturbances [44].

Subjective complaints of sleep disturbances appear to be associated with the presence of objective evidence for disturbed sleep quality in patients with COPD (predominantly in small cohorts of patients with **severe** COPD) as documented by overnight polysomnograms (PSGs). These findings include increased sleep latency, decreased total sleep time, decreased sleep efficiency, increased nocturnal arousals, decreased slow-wave sleep, and decreased REM sleep [6,20,44,54]. Cormick et al found significant agreement between subjective complaints of initiating and maintaining sleep and objective findings of poor sleep quality as shown by a decreased total sleep time of 208 minutes and increased arousal index [44].

Sleep disturbances may not be as pervasive in patients with mild/moderate COPD. The Sleep Heart Health Study (SHHS) did not show altered sleep quality in mild COPD patients (FEV_1/FVC 63.81±6.56%) [55]. Sanders et al observed that COPD only patients had minimally perturbed sleep and found no correlation between the decline in FEV_1 and sleep architecture. In a community-based study, Redline et al [56] showed that sleep structure variables did not change in subjects with a history of lung disease. In addition, they found that sleep stage distributions varied in accordance with AHI level.

3.1.1. Mechanisms of sleep disturbances in COPD patients

Various reasons for sleep disturbances in COPD patients exist. The most common are cough, dyspnea, nocturnal oxygen desaturation (NOD), hypercapnia, degree of airway obstruction (measured by FEV_1), and medication side effects [6,20,44,54,57]. Although SHHS suggests a lesser degree of effect on sleep quality in patients with milder COPD, no clear relationship between sleep quality measures and FEV_1 is established [50]. Poor-quality of sleep may be associated with hypoxaemia and increased superficial sleep [58].

http://dx.doi.org/10.5772/57220

3.1.2. Consequences of sleep disturbances

The poor sleep quality in COPD patients may lead to decreased daytime functioning due to excessive daytime sleepiness, altered neurocognition, and psychomotor vigilance. There are no studies that address whether neurocognition or psychomotor vigilance are affected in COPD patients. COPD patients often complain of daytime sleepiness. However Orr et al [59] found no objective evidence for daytime sleepiness based on multiple sleep latency testing in 14 severe COPD patients who had poor sleep quality based upon decreased total sleep time and increased arousal index.

4. Predictors of nod in copd patients

Approximately 27–70% of patients with COPD with awake SaO_2, 90–95%, can experience substantial desaturation at night, especially during REM sleep [20,24]. The high prevalence of NOD and its consequences on haemodynamics are a challenge for many researchers who have attempted to determine daytime physiological parameters that might help in predicting NOD in COPD. Although NOD is more pronounced in COPD patients with daytime hypoxaemia, it is established that an additional quarter of patients with adequate oxygenation during wakefulness can experience NOD [20,24].

4.1. Severe COPD

In severe COPD, the 'blue bloater' rather than the 'pink puffer' phenotype is more likely to have NOD [60]. Various studies showed that the blue bloaters had lower baseline oxygen saturations, more episodes of NOD, larger falls in NOD, and spent more time at low levels of oxygen saturation while asleep, than the pink puffers [6,20,21]. A significant relationship between waking values of low PaO_2 and high $PaCO_2$ with NOD was also established [42,44,61]. Moreover, although there was a good correlation between mean sleep SaO_2 and mean exercise SaO_2, the awake PaO_2 appeared to be a better predictor for NOD than exercise desaturation [24]. The desaturation nadir was lower during sleep than during exercise, with oxygen saturation falling an average of 6 ± 4% during peak exercise and 13 ± 9% during sleep [62]. Pulmonary function testing correlated poorly with nocturnal hypoxaemia[55].

In summary, most evidence suggests that awake oxygen saturation is a better predictor for NOD in severe COPD patients than PFT parameters or exercise desaturations [24,63]. Increased daytime PaCO2 also carries an increased risk for NOD [55].

4.2. Mild and moderate COPD

The clinical approach to NOD detection in COPD is more difficult in patients with mild/ moderate COPD (GOLD I-II) and mild daytime hypoxaemia. Approximately one quarter of these individuals have NOD, which is independent of the co-existence of OSA [42]. Current guidelines for evaluation of nocturnal oxyhemoglobin saturation in COPD patients without significant daytime hypoxaemia, however, are restrictive. Measuring nocturnal oxyhemoglo bin saturation in COPD patients who have daytime PaO2-55–59 mm Hg is not recommended [64]. Polysomnography should be performed in COPD patients whose symptoms are suggestive of coexistent OSA.. Other high risk groups include is COPD patients with daytime hypercapnia and only moderately reduced FEV_1; obese snorers, those who develop headache after nocturnal oxygen therapy, and patients with mild hypoxaemia and unexplained polycythemia, pulmonary hypertension, and cor pulmonale [64]. Witnessed apneas while asleep and daytime sleepiness are also highly suspective of OSA [65]. However, the presence of concomitant OSA is often difficult to predict from daytime symptoms in patients with mild/moderate COPD. They do not have daytime hypercapnia, headache, or daytime sleepiness. Classic sleep complaints and daytime sleepiness are not common. COPD alone, when moderate, does not disturb sleep quality, and OSA may not always present with sleep complaints. So if sleep complaints are the trigger for polysomnography in mild/moderate COPD, a large number of patients will not be tested.

5. Diagnostic approaches to detecting nod in copd patients

Nocturnal oximetry alone is probably not helpful diagnostically in COPD patients, as nocturnal oxygen desaturation may reflect only COPD or some combination of COPD and OSA, and treatment will differ (see below). Definitions of nocturnal oxygen desaturation differ, and physician decision and management based on nocturnal oximetry results differ greatly. Finally, there is little evidence that correction of nocturnal hypoxemia in COPD with only nocturnal desaturation improves outcomes [38].

Epidemiological data suggest that nocturnal oxyhemoglobin desaturation either related or unrelated to OSA is present in at least 50% of COPD patients without significant daytime hypoxaemia. Considering that approximately half of these patient have coexistent OSA, clinicians should establish the diagnosis of OSA in these patients. Nocturnal oxymetry should be performed in severe COPD, in mild and moderate COPD patients with the clinical characteristics listed in table 1. Patients with COPD who are diagnosed with nocturnal hypoxaemia by nocturnal oxymetry should undergo attended nocturnal polysomnography to exclude coexistent OSA.

Mild COPD	Severe COPD
Daytime hypoxemia disproportionate to FEV_1	Blue boaters
Daytime Hypercapnia disproportionate to FEV_1	Daytime hypoxemia $PaO_2 < 55$ mmHg
Pulmonary hypertension disproportionate to FEV_1	
FEV_1<65%	
Obese snorers	
Sleep complaints	
Witnessed apneas, hypopneas	

Table 1. Indications for performing a nocturnal oxymetry in mild/severe COPD

6. Osa as a mechanism for nod

Obstructive sleep apnea (OSA) is an independent phenomenon, leading to sleep-disordered breathing that is characterized by a cessation (apnea) or limitation (hypopnea) of airflow accompanied by a desaturation (Figure 1). OSA is diagnosed when more than 5 apneas and hypopneas occur per hour of sleep and are associated with excessive daytime sleepiness. OSA and COPD are two common respiratory diseases whose combination was first noted by Flenley [25] and is now recognized as the classic overlap syndrome (Figure 2). Both OSA and COPD have systemic inflammatory consequences that are responsible for increased cardiovascular morbidity and mortality. Moreover, until recently, OSA itself was categorized as an inflammatory consequence of COPD [66]. For this, as well as many other reasons, OSA and the overlap syndrome will be discussed separately in this chapter. Although they share common manifestations, COPD and OSA are united in the overlap syndrome, presenting a unique combination of upper and lower airway resistance and a blunted respiratory drive. In overlap patients, these disorders have more than an additive or synergistic effect, but rather present as an independent sleep-related breathing abnormality.

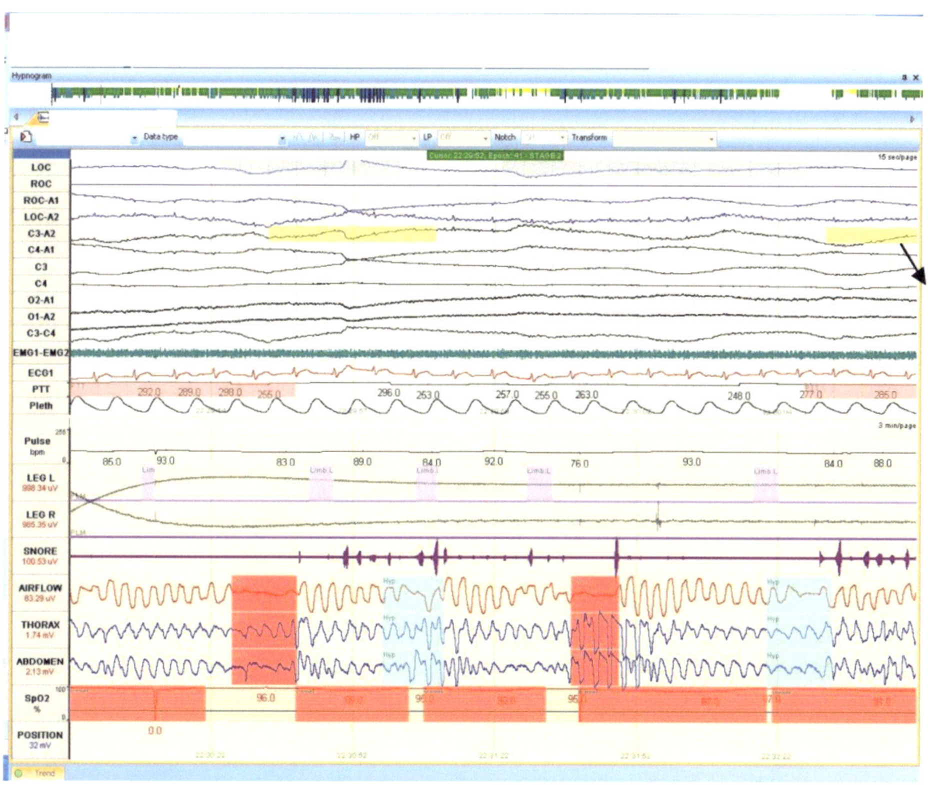

Figure 1. Polysomnogram of a patient with OSA only (note the desaturations highlighted by the circles and arrows)

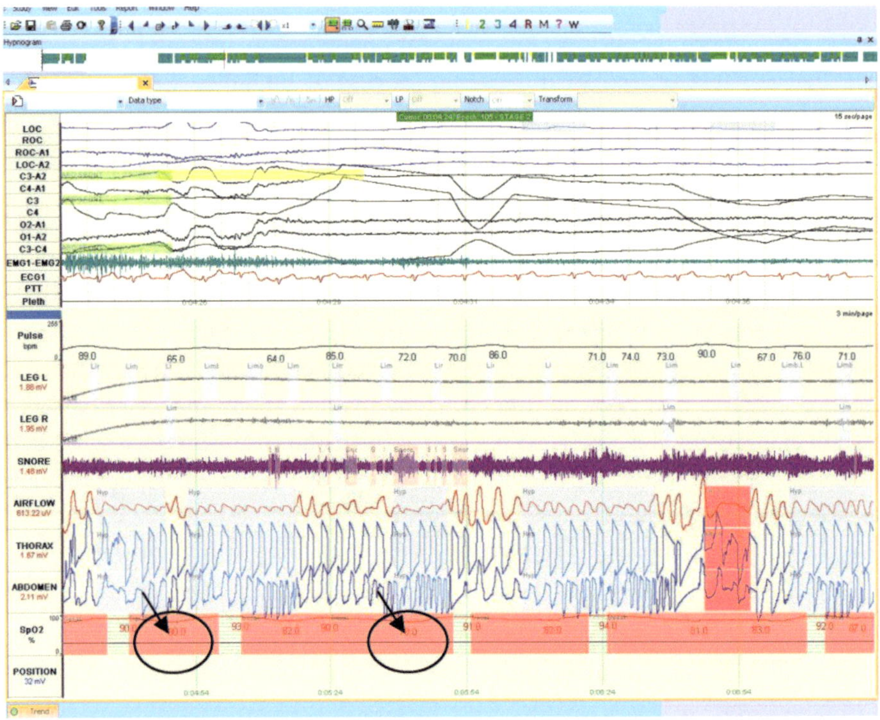

Figure 2. Polysomnogram of a patient with overlap syndrome (the desaturation is more severe; desaturations are highlighted by the circles and arrows)

6.1. Sleep and respiration in OSA

During apneas, the collapsed pharynx impedes airflow in spite of the respiratory effort. The obstruction leads to progressive asphyxia, which additionally stimulates breathing against the collapsed airway and usually continues until the person awakens [67]. Various factors-upper airway anatomy, central respiratory control mechanisms etc., contribute to the development of the clinical syndrome of OSA. The primary defect might be an anatomically small or collapsible pharyngeal airway, in combination with sleep-induced upper airway muscle atonia [68,69]. Instability of ventilatory control [70,71] or inefficiency of the central respiratory drive that modulates upper airway resistance in OSA may be other factors responsible for this disorder [72]. Abnormal hypoxic and hypercapnic respiratory response has also been reported in hypercapnic OSA patients [73,74]. The role of reduced chemical feedback is, however, still under debate. It is not clear whether the abnormal hypoxic and/or hypercapnic respiratory response is secondary to sleep apnea or is an inherited abnormality in ventilatory control [75, 76]. The improvement in the ventilatory feedback to CO_2 in hypercapnic OSA patients after CPAP therapy suggests that this dysregulation is acquired and not genetic [77,78].

6.2. OSA and COPD – predisposing factors and prevalence

Whether any pathophysiological link exists between OSA and COPD is still unknown, but they share common risk factors and pathophysiological processes that contribute to the genesis and exacerbation of each other. The relationship between COPD and OSA may be influenced by smoking and BMI. Neck obesity contributes to upper airway narrowing while truncal obesity promotes ventilatory disturbances by reduced chest wall compliance and muscle strength. Visceral obesity is responsible for reduced residual capacity and contributes to ventilation/perfusion mismatch. BMI may be lower in some patients with COPD, especially those with advanced disease and may be protective against OSA [27,65].

Smoking is another risk factor for COPD that, in addition, predisposes to sleep apnea. It increases airway resistance due to local inflammation and edema. Besides BMI and smoking, OSA and COPD may by themselves contribute to the onset of each other.

Redolfi et al [79] demonstrated that, even in healthy subjects, there is an overnight fluid shift from the legs that increases neck circumference. In COPD patients with cor pulmonale and peripheral edema, rostral fluid shifts that occur during supine positioning may contribute to pharyngeal narrowing and favour the onset of obstructive apneas/hypopneas. The corticosteroid induced myopathy or the cachexia that occurs in advanced COPD stages may be the reason for blunted inspiratory force. Local pharyngeal muscle edema associated with steroid inhalations might contribute to upper airways narrowing, thus facilitating sleep/disordered breathing [80]. Increased end-expiratory lung volume within an individual improves upper-airway mechanics, probably via tracheal traction. In emphysematous COPD patients, although end-expiratory lung volume may be elevated, the loss of lung recoil may not be protective for upper-airway mechanics. It is assumed that the decreased tethering of airways by destruction of parenchyma may actually produce a more collapsible upper airway [81]. Repetitive upper-airway collapse increases lower-airway resistance in an animal model suggesting that OSA might itself promote COPD [82]. Finally, in order to lose or maintain weight, or to fight excessive daytime sleepiness, patients with OSA might smoke more frequently than those without it [83].

6.3. Epidemiology

Initial studies may have overestimated the prevalence of overlap syndrome [84]. Patients with obstructive lung disease, referred mostly for evaluation of excessive daytime sleepiness, were determined to frequently have OSA as well [85]. In early studies, a high prevalence of OSAS was found in individuals with COPD. Guilleminault et al [86] studied 26 COPD patients while sleeping and found that 92% of all abnormal respiratory events during sleep contained an obstructive component. Conversely, patients with known OSA were evaluated with spirometry and 11% were found to have an $FEV_1/FVC < 0.60$ l [87]. Another study found the prevalence of the overlap syndrome to be 29%, although the data were gathered in a retrospective chart study of patients who had been refered for polysomnography and who also had an interpretable pulmonary function test [88]. The seemingly very high prevalence prompted speculation that OSA and COPD were linked by a common mechanism or common pathophysiology.

Recently, however, data from the Sleep Heart Health Study, a prospective multicenter cohort study showed that overlap syndrome has a prevalence of 14% among patients with mild COPD which is not different from those without COPD (18.6%) [55]. The presence of airway obstruction did not seem to affect the respiratory disturbance index. The Multinational Monitoring of Trends and Determinants in Cardiovascular Disease [MONICA-II]) also found no increased risk between the two disorders [89]. The major limitation of these studies, however, is that most subjects had very mild airway obstruction on spirometry.

Although there may be no increased association between relatively mild COPD and OSA because of the rising prevalence of these diseases, a patient with one of the disorders will often have the other disease. For example, in the Sleep Heart Health Study and the MONICA-II study, GOLD stage II COPD was found in 19% and 11% of the subjects with OSA, respectively. Sleep-disordered breathing was seen in 14% of subjects in the Sleep Heart Health Study (respiratory disturbance index > 15 events/h) and 11% of subjects (AHI > 5 events/h and excessive daytime sleepiness) in the MONICA-II cohort [55,89]. A patient with one of the disorders has a greater than 10% chance of also having the other. Thus, when seeing a patient with either OSA or COPD, it is reasonable to screen for the other disorder.

Our experience generally confirms the findings from the SHHS and MONICA II cohorts. From January–December, 2011, we performed a prospective study of patients with complaints of daytime sleepiness, witnessed apneas and/or hyponeas who were referred to the Sleep Lab, Division of Pulmonology, Clinic of Internal Medicine, University Hospital Alexandrovska, Sofia. Only patients who signed informed consent participated in the study. The aim of the study was to compare the anthropometric, metabolic, cardiovascular, and respiratory characteristics of patients with OSA and overlap syndrome. Gas exchange and ventilatory parameters were also compared. The level of oxidative stress, measured by the urinary concentration of 8-isoprostanes was of special interest. A correlation between oxidative stress and cardiovascular and metabolic comorbidity was investigated. Patients were followed for a month after the initiation of bilevel positive pressure ventilation (BiPAP). The effect of this treatment modality on the level of oxidative stress, gas exchange, and ventilatory parameters measured by pulmonary function testing was studied.

Patients who agreed to participate in the study underwent a full polysomnography (Compumedics, Australia). Continuous recordings were taken with electrode positions C3/A2-C4/A1-Cz/01 of the international 10–20 Electrode Placement System; eye movements, chin electromyogram, and ECG modified V2 lead were also recorded. Sleep was scored manually according to standard criteria. Airflow was measured using nasal pressure associated with the sum of buccal and nasal thermistor signals. Respiratory efforts were monitored with abdominal and thoracic bands. Arterial oxygen saturation (SpO_2) was measured using a pulse oximeter. An apnoea was defined as a complete cessation of airflow for >10 s, and a hypopnoea as a > 50% reduction in the nasal pressure signal or a 30–50% decrease associated with either oxygen desaturation of >3% or an arousal (defined according to the Chicago report or by autonomic activations on pulse transit time), lasting for at least 10 s. Apnoeas were classified as obstructive, central, or mixed according to the presence or absence of respiratory efforts. The diagnosis of OSA was established if the AHI was > 5 events/h [90].

For the period of the study, 265 patients with newly diagnosed OSA signed an informed consent to participate in the study. COPD was determined in accordance with the GOLD criteria, 2011 – FEV_1/FVC <70% after administration of a bronchodilator [91]. 26 (9.8%) patients (23 men; 3 women) were diagnosed with overlap syndrome. All patients had stage II COPD (80%> FEV_1<50%). These findings corroborate the results of larger epidemiological studies measuring the prevalence of overlap syndrome in patients with moderate COPD.

6.4. Overlap syndrome and physiological consequences

6.4.1. Gas exchange

The majority of patients with OSAS are eucapnic during wakefulness. Daytime hypercapnia is usually associated with mechanical impairment of the respiratory system related to obesity and/or COPD [92,93]. It is also associated with the severity of OSA, higher BMI levels, or degree of restrictive chest wall mechanics. Hypoxaemia is also described in OSA. It is closely related to apneas and hypopneas and is a result of alveolar hypoventilation.

In overlap syndrome, however, there is a predisposition to daytime hypercapnia and hypoxaemia that is independent of lung function [16]. Nocturnal desaturation severity varies within the wide spectrum of sleep-disordered breathing and the severity of COPD. In overlap patients, the nocturnal desaturation is greater and lasts longer than in patients with either OSAS or COPD. OSA seems to be an important cause of hypercapnia and hypoxemia in some COPD patients that is disproportionate to their lung function impairment. Chan et al [94] showed that hypercapnic COPD patients have higher BMI and smaller airway cross sectional areas when compared with lung function matched eucapnic controls. Furthermore, it is known that overlap patients have more nocturnal desaturation events than patients with either COPD or OSA alone [55]. Sanders and colleagues examined the degree to which COPD and OSAS independently and jointly contribute to desaturations during sleep [55]. After adjusting for confounding factors, the odds ratio for nocturnal oxyhemoglobin desaturation (SpO_2 < 85% for more than 20% of total sleep time) was 20 times greater in OSA and 30 times greater in overlap syndrome. Bednarek et al [89] demonstrated that patients with overlap syndrome had lower mean arterial blood oxygen saturations and spent more time in desaturation than the OSAS group when polysomnography variables were compared.

These observations are confirmed by our own investigations. We compared overlap syndrome patients to patients with OSA alone. Patients with OSA had a moderate degree of sleep disordered breathing with an average AHI – 24.11± 5.34 events/h. They were compared to AHI and age matched patients with overlap syndrome. The overlap patients had an average AHI – 28.14±5.47 events/h. 21(80%) patients had moderate OSA (AHI 15-30 events/h); 5 (20%) had mild OSA (AHI 5-15 events/h). The average desaturation in overlap and OSA was 12.3% vs 6.9% (p=0.037), respectively. The proportion of sleep time with SaO_2<90% in the overlap group was greater, 57.21%, in comparison with the OSA only group, 34.8 %, p=0.042.

The nighttime respiratory disturbances reflected the daytime gas exchange parameters. In overlap patients, the average daytime $PaO_2$2 was 61.67±5.78 mmHg vs 75.59±8.43mmHg in OSA. The prevalence of hypercapnic patients was greater in the overlap (19.2%) with an average daytime $PaCO_2$ in the group – 52.14±11.39 mmHg. In the OSA only group, hypercapnia was detected in 1 patient (4%) and the average $PaCO_2$ was 36.25±6.11 mmHg. Thus, our investigation shows that patients with overlap syndrome experience longer and more severe nighttime desaturations that disturb gas exchange parameters in comparison to OSA patients with similar AHI

The mechanisms responsible for the gas exchange abnormalities in overlap syndrome are complex. Radwan et al [95] compared the breathing pattern and CO_2 response in 11 obese male overlap syndrome patients, 20 obese male OSAS patients with normal lung function, and 13 healthy nonobese controls. Overlap patients with hypercapnia had both blunted ventilatory and mouth occlusion pressure responses to CO_2 and their ventilatory response may also be disturbed. The repetitive inspiratory effort against an occluded airway and intermittent hypoxia may be deleterious for the inspiratory muscles in severe OSA. In overlap syndrome patients, this increased fatiguability is even more accentuated, which is related to the mechanical disadvantage of chest wall hyperinflation and reduced functional residual capacity [96].

Moreover, it is established that overlap syndrome patients hypoventilate not only during the night but also during the day. The reason is still unknown. When measured, their chemosensitivity is reduced compared to those with OSA alone. It is elusive whether this is a cause or an effect of the overlap syndrome [95]. It is interesting to speculate that overlap syndrome patients have a genetic predisposition to hypercapnia, or that the higher $PaCO_2$ reflects the increased muscle load in those with both increased upper and lower airway resistance. Inflammation, nocturnal $PaCO_2$ elevations, and/or obesity (for example, leptin has been implicated as a modulator of respiratory drive) may be the triggers changing the $PaCO_2$ set-point [97].

In summary, the pathophysiology of sleep disordered breathing is complex in overlap syndrome and mainly associated with upper and lower airway obstruction and a reduction in respiratory drive. Hyperinflation may cause fatigue of respiratory muscles. Moreover, the functional residual capacity is reduced because of the supine posture and sleep state which predisposes the patient to ventilation/perfusion mismatch.

6.4.2. Pulmonary haemodynamics and right heart failure

OSAS patients may have sustained pulmonary hypertension (PH) [98,99,100] and the risk for its development increases further in the presence of COPD, obesity or both [101,102]. Chaouat et al [87] observed that the prevalence of PH was 42% in overlap syndrome compared with OSA alone (13%). They found that the main determinants of pulmonary hypertension in overlap syndrome were daytime arterial blood gases and FEV_1. Moreover, overlap patients often have relatively mild abnormalities (spirometry or oxygenation), especially when compared to COPD-only patients with pulmonary hypertension. Overlap patients with pulmonary hypertension have an average FEV_1 of 1.8 L, FEV_1/FVC of 0.64, and awake PaO_2 of 64 mm Hg. COPD-only patients with pulmonary hypertension have more severe obstructive disease, with $FEV_1 < 1$ L, $FEV_1/FVC < 0.50$, and awake $PaO_2 < 55$ mmHg. Fletcher [17] demonstrated that in overlap syndrome, FEV_1/FVC was 60%. Patients with COPD and daytime normoxia who have only nocturnal oxygen desaturation generally do not develop substantial pulmonary hypertension [38]. PH is usually observed in COPD patients with daytime PaO_2<55±5 mmHg. According to Chaouat et al [87], PH develops in patients with overlap syndrome at even higher daytime PaO_2 levels (PaO_2>66±10mmHg) than in patients with COPD.The mean PaO_2 in sleep is certainly lower due to the synergistic effect that both disorders have on pulmonary haemodynamics and gas exchange. Hawrylkiewicz and colleagues observed that 16% of OSA patients had pulmonary hypertension compared with 86% of those with overlap syndrome [103]. In regression analysis, traditional markers of OSA severity, such as the AHI or oxygen saturation nadir, have generally not correlated with the presence of pulmonary hypertension. Even patients with severe OSA alone do not tend to develop marked pulmonary hypertension if they are free from other cardiopulmonary diseases [102]. The degree of pulmonary hypertension if any, is mild and of uncertain clinical importance [37,103,104].

In our overlap group, pulmonary hypertension was detected in 84.6% of patients who had an average systolic pulmonary pressure of 38.87 mmHg. In the group of patients with OSA, pulmonary hypertension was found in only 47.8% with an average systolic pulmonary pressure of 34.16 mmHg. Both the time spent at SaO_2<90% (57.2% vs. 34.8%) and the average desaturation index (12.3% vs 6.9%) were greater in the overlap vs OSA group. In overlap patients, the average daytime PaO_2 was 61.67±5.78 mmHg vs 75.59±8.43 mmHg in those with OSA; the average daytime $PaCO_2$ was 52.14±11.39 mmHg vs 36.25±6.11 mmHg in the OSA only group.

The ventilatory parameters in overlap patients were disproportionate to the level of gas exchange parameters and poorer than in the OSA only group. Comparing those with overlap syndrome to those with OSA, forced vital capacity (FVC) was 55.5±24.5% vs 77.25± 19.6%; forced expiratory volume in 1 s (FEV_1) was 53.5±10.87% vs 62.25±20.22; FEV_1/FVC was 64.46±9.19% vs 86.9±8.85%, respectively.

According to our results, the degree of PH was of similar range in both patient groups. The prevalence of pulmonary hypertension in the overlap syndrome was almost two fold greater than in the OSA only group. It is, however, disproportionate to what should be expected from the gas exchange and ventilatory parameters. Before making final conclusions, we should point out that our study was performed in patients with extreme obesity and that pulmonary hypertension was determined by echocardiography which may not be the most accurate measure of pulmonary pressures. The cardiovascular comorbidity, smoking status as well as the higher BMI in overlap syndrome prevented the precise analysis of the clinical factors associated with PAP in overlap and OSA patients.

In summary, in overlap patients, nocturnal desaturation is greater, lasts longer, and is associated with more pronounced daytime hypoxemia and hypercapnia. The combination of OSA and COPD may be associated with increased pulmonary and systemic blood pressures as well as greater cardiovascular morbidity.

6.4.3. Mortality

Mortality in patients with the overlap syndrome has not been well studied until recently. COPD patients frequently die from cardiovascular disease predominantly at night. It can be speculated that some of these patients may have had the overlap syndrome. Similarly, OSA patients have also been shown to die disproportionately at night, compared to control groups, who are at greatest risk during the morning hours [105]. Tachyarhythmias are very likely to be responsible for nighttime deaths in both patient groups. In COPD patients, ventricular premature contractions occur commonlyin sleep when the SaO2 is < 80%. In OSA patients, the entire spectrum of cardiac arrhythmias may be observed. Olmetti et al [106] showed that in COPD patients with concomitant OSA, tachyarrhythmias are more common.

The diagnosis of concomitant COPD and reduced FEV_1 or smoking history are markers for increased mortality in OSA patients [107-109]. In a univariate analysis, COPD conferred a 7-fold risk of death in OSA patients [108]. Vice versa, comorbid OSA was recently reported to increase mortality in patients with COPD. Marin et al [47] presented outcome data on patients with COPD and patients with the overlap syndrome. After a median follow-up of over 9 years, all-cause mortality was higher in the untreated (no CPAP) overlap group (42.2%) than in the COPD-only group (24.2%). After adjustment for COPD severity, comorbid OSA remained a risk factor for death. An intriguing issue in that study is that OSA may also contribute to an increased incidence of COPD exacerbations, which may accelerate lung-function decline and lead to increased mortality [48,49].

Mermigkis et al demonstrated that, in addition to the increased morbidity and mortality, patients with the overlap syndrome also have significantly worse quality of life (measured with the St George's Respiratory Questionnaire), when compared to COPD-only controls [110]. The overlap syndrome patients in their study were COPD patients with habitual snoring but without excessive daytime sleepiness or elevated Epworth sleepiness score which underscores how difficult clinical diagnosis and screening of snoring in non-sleepy COPD patients may be.

6.5. Inflammation, oxidative stress and cardiovascular and metabolic comorbidity in overlap

The exact mechanisms that account for the increased morbidity and mortality risk in overlap syndrome are not known exactly. Increased risk of death may be due to prolonged hypoxia. Nighttime hypercapnia may also be important. There is enough evidence that both COPD and OSA have systemic consequences since both cause inflammation and oxidative stress.

6.5.1. Inflammation and oxidative stress

Systemic inflammation is being recognized as a risk factor for a number of complications including atherosclerosis [111]. It is a well-established factor in the pathogenesis of cardiovascular disease (CVD) [112]. There is growing recognition that COPD is a systemic disease [113,114] with multiple effects on end-organs including those in the cardiovascular system [115,116].

Patients with OSA experience persistent low grade inflammation, mainly attributed to repetitive episodes of hypoxia/ reoxygenation during apneas and hypopneas while asleep.

This inflammation is associated with increased arterial stiffness, blood pressure [117,118] and increased risk for hypertension, heart failure, stroke, and cardiovascular mortality. The molecular pathways of systemic inflammation in OSA and COPD may be similar, suggesting a multiplicative effect in overlap syndrome.

CRP is an acute phase protein that contributes to atherosclerosis. Its plasma levels are elevated in OSA, but obesity is the major confounder because there is no evidence for an independent relationship between OSA and CRP [119,120]. IL-6, another inflammatory marker, is increased in OSA even after adjustment for BMI [121]. Further, IL-6 and CRP are elevated in stable COPD patients and increase during exacerbations [122,123].

NF-kB is a regulator of inflammatory gene expression and controls the synthesis of cytokines (TNF-α, IL-8) [112] that increase expression of adhesion molecules and contribute to atherosclerosis [124]. Hypoxia is the major trigger for the activation of both adaptive and maladaptive transcription factors. Ryan et al [125] showed that sustained hypoxia is responsible for the expression of adaptive hypoxia inducible factor (HIF)-a molecule promoting the expression of genes which stimulate tissue perfusion and oxygenation. Intermittent hypoxia (apnea/hypopnea events in OSA, NOD in REM induced hypoventilation of COPD patients and overlap patients) is a trigger for NF-kB activation [112]. Thus, we hypothesize that, in OSAS as well as in COPD with overlap, there may be synergistic activation of "overlapping" pathways leading to inflammation. This hypothesis explains the evidence of increased inflammation observed in both COPD and OSA. TNF-α and IL-8 are elevated in COPD and OSA when compared to control subjects [126]. Both molecules are well established risk factors for coronary artery disease and heart failure [127].

Furthermore, oxidative stress occurs in COPD and OSAS and is associated with increased ROS [128,129] which are produced by intrapulmonary leukocytes in COPD and circulating leukocytes in OSA [128,130]. Although ROS are important physiologic regulators in many signaling pathways, their increased production may cause abnormal oxidation of DNA, proteins and lipids and may contribute to vascular endothelial dysfunction [131].

In our investigation, we tried to compare the degree of oxidative stress, measured by the urinary concentration of 8-isoprostanes. The study was performed in 26 overlap patients and 23 age and AHI matched OSA patients. None of them had been treated with CPAP or oxygen. An overnight urine sample was collected and the levels of urinary 8-isoprostane were determined by HRAM (high resolution accurate mass) mass spectrometry on a LTQ Orbitrap® Discovery (ThetmoScientific Co, USA) mass spectrometer equipped with a Surveyor® Plus HPLC system and IonMax® electrospray ionization module. The analyses were performed using the stable isotope dilution method in negative ionization mode with a HESI II (heated electrospray ionization) source type. The concentration and purification of 8-isoprostane from urine samples was processed by affinity sorbent (Cayman Chemical, USA), according to the manufacturer's protocol. The urinary isoprostane levels were standardized to the levels of urinary creatinine which were measured using the enzyme method (Creatinine plus version 2 (CREP2), Cobas Integra (Roche)). In overlap patients, the average values were higher than in OSA patients, 0.251±0.10 pg/mkmol/cre vs. 0.185±0.06 pg/mkmol/cre, $p<0.05$. The urinary isoprostane levels did not correlate with the respiratory disturbance parameters (AHI, average desaturation, time of sleep at SaO2<90%), gas exchange parameters (PaO2/PaCO2) or with the ventilatory parameters (FVC, FEV_1, FEV_1/FVC).

We confirmed that in overlap patients the degree of oxidative stress is higher irrespective of the parameters mentioned above. The exact mechanisms of oxidative stress as well as its consequences were not determined in our study.

Abnormally activated leucocytes in COPD and OSA may also be a mechanism for atherosclerosis [112]. A systemic metaanalysis has shown that circulating neutrophils are elevated in COPD patients [132]. In vivo studies demonstrate decreased neutrophil apoptosis in OSA patients and increased expression of adhesion molecules [133]. The adhesion of these cells to endothelium is a key step in atherosclerosis and endothelial dysfunction.

In summary, the ''overlapping pathways'' activating inflammation and oxidative stress in overlap patients are poorly understood and further investigations at the molecular level are required for a better understanding of these processes and their abrogation in clinical practice.

6.5.2. Cardiovacular comorbidity and oxidative stress in overlap vs OSA

6.5.2.1. Hypertension, target organ damage, and oxidative stress

Large scale epidemiological studies have demonstrated an independent relationship between OSAS and cardiovascular disorders, particularly systemic hypertension [134,135], but also coronary heart disease, congestive heart failure, and stroke [136,137]. The presence of moderate to severe OSA as indicated by an AHI>15 events/h leads to a relative risk of 2,89 of developing hypertension over 8 years, after adjustment for potential confounders. The prevalence of hypertension is over 50% in OSAS patients. Hypertension in OSAS patients is particularly nocturnal and potentially driven by sleep disordered breathing.

We performed BP monitoring in 20 (77%) of the overlap and 12 (52%) of the OSA patients in our study. We compared the haemodynamic characteristics and clinical factors associated with them. BP was measured according to European Society of Hypertension (ESH)/European Society of Cardiology (ESC) guidelines. The following parameters were measured: systolic BP (SBP) and diastolic BP (DBP). Hypertension was defined as a SBP >140 mmHg and/or a DBP > 90 mmHg. Ambulatory BP monitoring (ABPM) was performed with a BOSO device (Bosch &Sons, Gruningen, Germany). The measurements were made every 20 min over 24 h. Daytime (07:00–22:00 h) hypertension was defined as daytime SBP > 135 mmHg and/or daytime DBP >85 mmHg, and nocturnal (22.00–07:00 h) hypertension as SBP >120 mmHg and/or nocturnal DBP > 70 mmHg. Dipper pattern was defined by a nocturnal fall of BP >10%. Twenty of the overlap patients and 12 of those with OSA agreed to undergo the procedure.

In the overlap group, 75% (15) were non-dippers and 25% dippers. Nocturnal hypertension was found in 12 (60%) patients. The daytime systolic and diastolic BP's were 121.93±17.09 mmHg and 70.93±8.12 mmHg. The nocturnal SBP and DBP were 112.76±5.38 mmHg and 68.16±3.34 mmHg. In OSA patients, 58% (7) were non-dippers and 42% dippers. Nocturnal hypertension was found in 7 (58%) patients. The daytime systolic and diastolic BP were 138.3±13.64 mmHg and 84.38±8.20 mmHg. The nocturmal SBP and DBP were 133.90±18.89

mmHg and 76.80±11.65 mmHg. We could not find an association between any of the studied parameters; anthropometric (age, BMI, waist and neck circumference), sleep (AHI, average desaturation, time of sleep at SaO_2<90%), gas exchange (PaO_2 and $PaCO_2$) and ventilatory (FEV_1, FVC) and daytime/nighttime systolic/diastolic BP in any of the groups. Though the level of urinary isoprostanes was higher in the overlap group, they did not correlate with the haemodynamic characteristics either.

An echocardiogram and carotid ultrasonography were also performed to compare the degree of target organ damage in overlap and OSA patients and to explore the role of urinary 8-isoprostanes. The echocardiogram was performed using a PhilipsiE33 machine. The examination was performed in M-mode with two-dimensional (2D) guidance in the long axis of the left parasternal view. LV internal end-diastolic and end-systolic diameters, as well as interventricular septum and posterior wall thicknesses were measured over five consecutive cycles. Systolic function was assessed by the LVEF according to the Teicholz formula. LV mass (LVM) was measured according to the Penn convention using the Devereux formula and was normalised for body surface area (BSA) to derive the LVM index (LVMI). LVH was defined as an LVMI of >111 g/m^2 in males and of >106 g/m^2 in females. The relative wall thickness (RWT) was calculated as the ratio (2xPWT)/LVIDd. All echocardiograms were performed by the same experienced echocardiographer.

In OSA and overlap patients, LVMI and RWT were, respectively: LVMI 123.97 vs 142.1 g/m2, p=0.013; RWT – 0.44 vs 0.46, p=0.045. The LVMI and RWT were significantly higher in the overlap patients, even after adjustment for AHI, BMI, SBP and DBP. Microalbumiuria was measured and standardized to creatinine excretion and given as ratio – mg/mkmol/l Creat. The micralbuminuria level in OSA was 5.69mg/mkmol/creat. In the overlap patients, it was significantly higher, 26.17mg/mkmol/creat, irrespective of confounding variables (p=0.041). 8-Urinary isoprostane levels correlated with neither LVMI nor the degree of microalbuminuria.

6.5.2.3. Atherosclerosis and oxidative stress

Patients with severe OSA are more likely to die of cardiovascular causes than those without OSAS [45]. While the absolute risk attributable to SDB is relatively small at an individual level, the high OSA prevalence makes it an important contributor to cardiovascular morbidity and mortality at populational levels. Several reports have stated that OSA may also contribute to coronary heart disease [138]. Studies utilizing carotid ultrasonography have shown severe OSA to be associated with increased intima-media thickness (IMT) which is a marker of atherosclerosis [139]

In our investigation, we assessed carotid artery IMT by B-mode ultrasound scanning with an 11-MHz linear phase array transducer. Bilateral IMT measurements were obtained in the distal 10 mm of the common carotid artery. The IMT was defined as the distance between the leading edge of the luminal echo to that of the media/adventitia echo and analyzed with a computerized edge-detection system. Three end-diastolic frames were selected, digitized, and analyzed for the mean IMT, and the average reading from these 3 frames was calculated for both right and left carotid arteries. The sole carotid scan operator was blinded to the clinical status of the studied subjects and was not involved in the clinical assessment. IMT was almost similar in both groups. In the overlap patients the average IMT was 0.90 while in the overlap group it was 0.89.

In our study, nocturnal blood pressure abnormalities were similar in overlap and OSA only patients. Those with overlap syndrome had greater target organ damage (cardiac-left ventricular hypertrophy and renal – microalbuminuria) in comparison with age and AHI matched OSA patients, even after adjustment for confounders (BMI, average desaturation, time of sleep at SaO_2<90%, duration of hypertension, current therapy). Giving this statement we should point out that it refers to OSA of moderate severity and overlap patients with moderate SDB and airflow obstruction. Both patient groups had extreme obesity. A disadvantage of the study is that the historical information for the management of hypertension was self reported and thus subjective.

6.5.2.4. Metabolic disorders in overlap and OSA patients

Many studies confirm the greater prevalence of metabolic syndrome in OSA patients. Both glucose and lipid metabolism abnormalities have been reported [140]. The role of intermittent hypoxia, sympathetic activation and sleep fragmentation has been reviewed [141]. Comparative data regarding the metabolic disturbances in overlap syndrome, COPD, and OSA are still lacking. The effect of both disorders in overlap syndrome, their additive and/or synergistic interaction, and physiological pathways on metabolism is not well understood.

In our investigation, we measured parameters of glucose metabolism in the overlap and OSA patients. A correlation analysis with oxidative stress markers (8-isoprostanes) was performed. Using enzymatic colorimetry plasma levels of total cholesterol, triglycerides, high-density lipoprotein cholesterol, low-density lipoprotein cholesterol (using the Friedwald formula), glucose, immuno-reactive insulin, and HOMA-index were measured. An oral glucose tolerance test (OGTT) was performed to detect glucose metabolism abnormalities.

Diabetes was found in 30% of the overlap patients, 50% were healthy, and 20% had an impaired glucose tolerance. In OSA patients, 33% were diabetic, 44% were healthy, and an impaired glucose tolerance was found in 23%. Although the average parameters tended to be higher in overlap vs OSA patients resp-IRI-21.04±15.46 mU/l vs 18.37±9.95 mU/l; average fasting blood glucose-6.19±2.86 mmol/l vs 5.73±2.03 mmol/l, HOMA-I 5.52±4.03 vs 4.84±2.64; there were no statistically significant differences. Only the glycosylated hemoglobin was significantly higher-6.51±1.24 vs 5.91±1.07, $p<0.05$ and remained significantly different after adjusting for confounders (age, BMI, AHI). FEV_1, PaO_2, and $PaCO_2$ did not correlate any of the glucometabolic parameters. A positive correlation between HbA1c and urinary 8-isoprostanes was established, p=0.023. The lipid profiles in both groups were similar. Dyslipidemia was present in 50% of overlap and 47% of OSA patients. In OSA and overlap patients, they were respectively-HDL 1.24±0.4 mmol/l vs 1.20±0.23 mmol/l; LDL 3.13±0.81 mmol/l vs 3.14±1.00 mmol/l; Tot chol – 5.30±0.95 vs 5.27± 1.6 mmol/l; Triglycerides – 2.82±1.24 vs 2.06±1.03 mmol/l. FEV_1, PaO_2, $PaCO_2$ and urinary isoprostanes did not correlate with any of the lipid profile parameters.

In conclusion, our study showed that the prevalence of glucometabolic abnormalities in the overlap and OSA patients was similar. The glucometabolic parameters for patients with overlap syndrome, however, were worse in comparison with OSA only. HbA1C levels were associated with the level of oxidative stress-urinary 8-isoprostanes. The prevalence of dyslipidemia and lipid profile parameters in both groups were almost identical and were not associated with the marker of oxidative stress. Our OSA subjects had moderately severe OSA and overlap syndrome patients had moderate SDB and airflow obstruction. Both patient groups had extreme obesity.

6.6. Sleep quality in overlap

In OSAS patients, one of the most common symptoms is excessive daytime somnolence, which results from disrupted sleep or/and nighttime oxygen desaturation [142,143]. Mild to moderate COPD patients usually do not have significant daytime sleepiness. Fatigue and tiredness are more common [59,144].

Sanders et al [55] studied 1132 patients with mild COPD and observed that COPD only patients had minimally perturbed sleep in the absence of OSA. Sleep architecture did not correlate with the level of airflow obstruction. There were small but not statistically significant differences between patients with or without COPD with regards to Epworth Sleepiness Scale (ESS), total sleep time, arousal index, lower total sleep time, and sleep efficiency. Only small differences were found between patients with OSA alone or those with both disorders, suggesting that sleep quality in overlap patients is mainly influenced by the presence of OSA. This is confirmed by Redline et al [56]. They demonstrated that sleep structure characteristics did not change in subjects with a history of lung disease but sleep stage distributions varied according to AHI level.

Analysing the data from our investigation, we found that the ESS was the same in patients with overlap syndrome and OSA only. The average ESS score in the overlap group was 15±4.3 while in the OSA only patients, it was 14±5.8. The sleep study characteristics in OSA and overlap were respectively – stage 1-30.1±9.59/27.04±7.7 min; stage 2-27.5±11.3/33.7±716.5 min; stage 3+4-28.35±17.12/31.87±16.43 min; AI – 31.6 vs 36.4 apneas/h; sleep efficiency was 69% in OSA and 64% in overlap patients. Though the duration of sleep with SaO_2<90% was much longer for the overlap patients, it correlated neither to the level of 8-isoprostanes (oxidative stress) nor to the ESS. The degree of airway obstruction (measured by FEV_1) did not correlate with sleep stage distribution, AHI, AI, or ESS.

6.7. Clinical presentation

The most common symptoms of OSA patients are snoring, excessive daytime sleepiness, and deterioration of quality of life [145,146]. COPD patients, on the other hand, may present with cough, sputum production, and/or dyspnea [64]. Nevertheless, overlap patients possess a unique characteristic, which sets them apart from either COPD or OSA patients. A number of studies compare the clinical presentation of overlap patients to those of OSAS-only patients.

Chaouat et al [87] stated that compared to the OSA only group, the overlap patients tended to be older, had hypoxemia and hypercapnia more frequently and had higher mean pulmonary artery pressures but similar body mass index (BMI). O'Brien and Whitman [147] found that overlap patients were older and less obese. Resta et al [148] showed that overlap patients had higher $PaCO_2$, but similar apnea–hypopnea indices (AHI).

Kessler noted that in OSAS patients exhibiting permanent pulmonary hypertension, bronchial obstruction is generally not severe and the level of hypoxemia and hypercapnia is modest. Therefore, chronic airway obstruction in these patients may be asymptomatic. These findings suggest that the performance of pulmonary function tests in all patients diagnosed with OSAS by a polysomnogram might be beneficial to detect occult airflow obstruction [149].

In our investigation, we observed 26 patients with overlap syndrome and compared them to 23 age and AHI matched patients with OSA only. In the overlap group, the mean FEV_1 was – 53.5±10.87%; FVC-55.5±24.5% ; FEV_1/FVC-64.46±9.19% The average daytime PaO_2 was 61.67±5.78 mmHg. Five (19%) patients had daytime hypercapnia and their average daytime $PaCO_2$ was 52.14±11.39 mmHg. The patients had the following anthropometric charactersistics: mean age-46.83±8.62 y; BMI-41.89±4.57 kg/m2; waist circumference – 133.11±10.94 cm; neck circumference – 48.54±3.92 cm. One (3%) was a non-smoker. In our overlap group, pulmonary hypertension was detected in 84.6% with an average systolic pulmonary pressure-38.87 mmHg.

A group of 23 age and AHI matched OSA patients were selected from the registry of sleep lab patients. The average daytime PaO_2 was 75.59±8.43 mmHg. None of the patients had hypercapnia and the average daytime $PaCO_2$ was 36.25±6.11 mmHg. The patients had the following anthropometric charactersistics: mean age-49.95±10.54 y; BMI-37.47±7.98 kg/m2; waist circumference – 126.43±11.28 cm; neck circumference – 45.46±4.49 cm; Four (17%) were non-smokers. The ventilatory parameters in the OSA only group were: FVC-77.25± 19.6%; FEV_1-62.25±20.22%; FEV_1/FVC-86.9±8.85%. In the group of patients with OSA only, pulmonary hypertension was found in 47.8% with average systolic pulmonary pressure – 34.16 mmHg. The Epworth sleepiness score (ESS) was similar in both groups-overlap-15±4.3 vs OSA only 14±5.8.

According to our results the overlap patients were younger, had increased BMI, waist and neck circumferences in comparison to the OSA only patients. The AHI, AI, the duration of sleep with SaO_2<90% as well as the daytime gas exchange abnormalities were more severe in the overlap group. The sleep complaints however were almost identical. The degree of PH was similar in both patient groups. The prevalence of pulmonary hypertension in the overlap syndrome was almost two fold greater than in the OSA only group. It was, however, disproportionate to what should be expected from the gas exchange parameters. As our results are not in agreement to those mentioned above, we should point out that our investigation was performed in patients with extreme obesity, which more or less reflects the respiratory drive, respiratory mechanics and pulmonary haemodynamics. They should be compared to patients with a moderate degree of sleep disordered breathing and excessive sleepiness and/or disturbed sleep.

http://dx.doi.org/10.5772/57220

6.8. Current guidelines and recommendations in the diagnostic approach to overlap syndrome in OSA patients

Nocturnal polysomnography is recommended in COPD patients whose symptoms suggest coexistent OSA. This encompasses COPD patients with daytime hypercapnia and moderately reduced FEV_1; COPD snorers, or those who develop headache after nocturnal oxygen therapy [25,64]. Apneas while asleep and daytime sleepiness are highly suggestive of OSA [65]. However, the presence of concomitant OSA is often difficult to predict. A large number of patients with OSA do not have daytime hypercapnia or headache and some of them are not obese. Daytime sleepiness is often absent. The significant cardiovascular morbidity and mortality related to untreated OSA and its reversibility with CPAP treatment strongly demands a more aggressive approach in diagnosing coexistent OSA among patients with COPD [150,151].

The recognition and diagnosis of COPD may be challenging in patients with OSA. Smoking history should always be obtained. COPD among OSA patients should be suspected if daytime hypercapnia, pulmonary hypertension, and nocturnal tachyarrhythmias are present. [42,87,106,148]. Chaouat et al [87] performed a study in 265 patients. They found that the prevalence of daytime hypercapnia was 27% in the 30 patients with associated COPD and 8% in the 235 patients without COPD. Daytime hypercapnia was observed in 11% of 1141 OSA patients who were free of COPD and was related to the severity of obesity [152]. Pulmonary hypertension is observed in 75% of patients with coexistent OSA and COPD [42] and in only 12%–20% of unselected OSA patients [102]. Patients with coexistent OSA and COPD are 2.53 times more likely to experience tachyarrhythmias during sleep than patients with OSA alone [106].

In summary, patients with OSA who do not carry a diagnosis of COPD but have daytime hypercapnia, pulmonary hypertension, and/or nocturnal tachyarrhythmias should undergo pulmonary function testing (table 2). On the other hand, COPD patients with witnessed apneas, daytime sleepiness, obese snorers, those who have daytime hypercapnia and/or pulmonary hypertension, and/or daytime hypoxaemia disproportionate to their FEV_1 should undergo a polysomnography study.

OSA
Daytime hypercapnia disproportionate to obesity
Pulmonary hypertension
Tachyarrhythmias

Table 2. Indications for performing a pulmonary function testing in OSA

7. Treatment of nod in copd patients

7.1. Medications – bronchodilators, corticosteroids, hypnotics

7.1.1. Effect on sleep quality

Ipratropium improves sleep quality [153] in patients with moderate to severe COPD, while tiotropium has no effect [154], at least not in patients with severe COPD. Data regarding theophylline have been variable, with some studies showing sleep disturbances [155], and others showing no changes [156-58]. 28% of COPD patients use hypnotics because of insomnia and other sleep disorders. Benzodiazepines are not recommended as they worsen nocturnal hypoxemia [159]. Non-benzodiazepine compounds like Zolpidem are safer [160].

7.1.2. Effect on NOD

Bronchodilators have variable effects on sleep quality but they significantly improve NOD. Theophylline [155,157], ipratropium [153], and tiotropium inhalers [154] have shown improvements in NOD. Martin et al studied the effect of ipratropium, taken 4 times a day in 36 patients with moderate to severe COPD (FEV_1 <65%) [153]. After a month of treatment, nocturnal oxygen saturation decreased, subjective sleep complaints improved, and total REM time increased. Tiotropium also improved nocturnal oxygen saturation but sleep quality remained unchanged [154]. Long-acting β2 agonists have similar benefits [161]. Oral steroids in stable COPD improve nocturnal oxygen desaturation and increase total sleep time [162]. Despite the lack of data, we might suggest that inhaled corticosteroids may have a similar effect.

7.2. Oxygen

7.2.1. Effect on sleep quality

A limited number of studies have examined the effect of oxygen therapy on sleep. A decrease in sleep latency, increase in total sleep duration, and REM were noted by Calverley et al [6]. Fleetham et al [57] noted no improvements in total sleep time (TST), sleep stages or frequency of arousals with the addition of oxygen.

7.2.2. Effect on NOD

In COPD patients with severe daytime hypoxemia (49-52 mm Hg), and nocturnal desaturations, it has been clearly established in both the British Medical Research Council (MRC) Long-Term Domiciliary Oxygen Therapy Trial [164] and the Nocturnal Oxygen Therapy Trial (NOTT) [165] that continuous oxygen therapy improves survival. This improvement was seen in comparison to supplemental oxygen administered only at night. COPD patients with hypoxemia only during sleep may also have increased mortality risk [166]. The correction of nocturnal hypoxaemia alone in patients with daytime normoxia does not significantly improve pulmonary haemodynamics or mortality [38], but it may improve sleep quality and is frequently prescribed [6].

Oxygen therapy for COPD patients with moderate daytime hypoxaemia and nocturnal desaturations remains very controversial. After a 3 year follow-up, no difference in survival among COPD patients with moderate hypoxaemia (PaO_2 56 and 69 mm Hg) was noted between the supplemental oxygen therapy group (average use of 14 h/d) and the control when [167]. Fletcher et al [168] found no survival benefit in COPD patients with NOD and an awake $PaO_2 > 60$ mm Hg, when randomized to 3 L/minute of oxygen or sham control for 36 months. Pulmonary hemodynamics, however, improved in the oxygen therapy group. In a 5-year follow up study, Chaouat et al [39] found no survival advantage in COPD patients with PaO_2 56-69 mm Hg who were randomized to oxygen therapy versus a control group. They found no difference in the progression of COPD to respiratory failure or the development of pulmonary hypertension.

The effect of long-term oxygen therapy on mortality in COPD patients with isolated nocturnal oxyhemoglobin desaturation remains unclear. Pooling together COPD patients with and without nocturnal oxyhemoglobin desaturation may mask the benefit of long-term oxygen therapy on survival in COPD patients with nocturnal oxyhemoglobin desaturation only.

In summary, survival benefit of long term oxygen therapy is attained in COPD patients with severe daytime hypoxaemia. Based on current data, oxygen therapy is unproven in COPD patients with moderate daytime hypoxemia and NOD, or in COPD patients who experience only NOD. Improvement of pulmonary haemodynamics and sleep quality with oxygen is also unproven.

7.3. Non-invasive positive pressure ventilation (NIPPV)

The role of NIPPV has been clearly established in COPD patients with an acute exacerbation. Data about its role in stable COPD patients is missing. Studies present mixed results and vary depending on the design. A recent systematic review of NIPPV in severe stable COPD patients was conducted by Kolodziej et al. [169]. They reviewed 9 randomized controlled trials (RCTs) and nine non-RCTs. No improvement in gas exchange with NIPPV among the RCTs was found. In the non-RCTs a reduction in lung hyperinflation and diaphragmatic work of breathing was noted. Improvement in gas exchange was also established [169]. Although NIPPV may have favorable effects, its therapeutic role has not been firmly stated for stable COPD patients. Despite this, the application of NIPPV in medical centres has been increasing. Recommendations from the American College of Chest Physicians (ACCP) were published to help clinicians in guiding therapy with NIPPV in stable COPD patients. According to ACCP guidelines, NIPPV may be considered in stable COPD when symptoms (fatigue, morning headache, daytime hypersomnolence) and one of the following is present: 1. $PaCO_2 > 55$ mm Hg; (OR) 2. $PaCO_2$ – 50-54 mmHg and NOD (overnight oximetry with $SaO_2 < 88\%$ for 5 min while on oxygen therapy > 2 L/minute; (OR) 3. $PaCO_2$ 50-54 mm Hg and hospitalization related to recurrent episodes (>two in a 12-month period) of hypercapnic respiratory failure [170].

Two recent results deserve attention. McEvoy et al [171] performed a randomized controlled trial of NIV in patients with stable hypercapnic COPD which showed a significant improvement in adjusted mortality. Little or no change in pulmonary function or daytime blood gases was detected. The improvement in mortality was associated with a worse quality of life with NIV. A second study by Windisch et al [172] also reported mortality improvements with NIV, although compared to historical controls. They used "high-intensity NIV" with very high driving pressures (average inspiratory pressure 28cm H_2O, average expiratory pressure 5 cm H_2O) and a high respiratory rate (21 breaths/min). Under these settings, there were also improvements in spirometry and blood gases.

8. Treatment of nod in copd patients with osa – the overlap syndrome

The aim of the treatment of patients with overlap is to avoid desaturations and sleep-disordered breathing. Treatment should be individualized according to the degree of OSA and/or COPD severity and in consideration of the co-existing illnesses – obesity, heart failure, pulmonary hypertension. All patients should however be advised about the potential benefits of therapy and the risks of going without it. Although CPAP therapy is a well-established treatment for OSA, it is not suitable for all overlap patients [173,174]. Auto-titrating CPAP is not recommended in COPD and overlap patients. Treatment options may also include oral appliances, additional supplement of oxygen or non-invasive positive pressure ventilation (NPPV).

8.1. General recommendations and medications

All patients should be advised of the importance of avoiding factors that increase the severity of upper-airway obstruction such as use of alcohol, smoking, hypnotic agents, and increased weight [175]. Data suggest that treatment of COPD in overlap syndrome will ameliorate nocturnal oxygen desaturation, and may decrease the need for supplemental oxygen in addition to CPAP [83]. Whether treatment of COPD in the overlap syndrome also improves OSA is not known.

8.2. Oxygen

The benefit of supplemental oxygen therapy alone in OSA is lacking [176]. After two-weeks of oxygen administration, nocturnal oxygen desaturation is improved, but sleep architecture, arousals, and subjective sleepiness are not. Alford et al applied 4 L/min supplemental oxygen to 20 overlap patients; NOD improved, but the duration of obstructive events increased which resulted in an increase of end-apneic PCO2 from 52.8 mm Hg to 62.3 mm Hg. Thus, oxygen alone should not be used for the treatment of the overlap syndrome.

8.3. Continuous positive airway pressure

CPAP remains the standard treatment for OSA and is the accepted therapy for overlap syndrome. Its effect however depends on the severity of OSA/COPD and on the presence of comorbidities. In some patients CPAP alone may not fully correct hypoxaemia and supplemental oxygen may be required [177]. In hypercapnic COPD patients however it is not recommended.

COPD patients with mild sleep-disordered breathing and severe nocturnal hypoxaemia may not tolerate CPAP. They may be better managed with oxygen. As most of the oxygen trials were performed at the time when polysomnography was not widely used, further evaluation of its benefits in COPD patients with mild sleep apnea should be performed.

CPAP is better tolerated in COPD patients with moderate/severe OSA. Data about its effects on daytime lung function is controversial. Some authors suggest that upper-airway irritation increases lower-airway resistance and correction of repetitive airway collapse might improve pulmonary function [177]. Others postulate that CPAP off-loads the respiratory muscles, decreases hypoventilation, oxygen consumption, and carbon dioxide production. During sleep these muscles may be alleviated by CPAP, since it prevents the increase of upper-airway resistance that occurs in sleep [178]. In severe COPD, CPAP may offset intrinsic PEEP in severe COPD. In 8 COPD-only patients, Mezzanotte et al, [179] applied CPAP for 1–3 weeks. They assessed inspiratory force and endurance and found significant improvements in maximum inspiratory force and 12-min walk test. Improvements have also been observed in daytime oxygenation and hypercapnia, [180,181] and in the number of COPD-related hospital admissions following the start of CPAP treatment for OSA [182].

Conflicting spirometry results have been seen when CPAP is used in the overlap syndrome. A few non-randomized studies have shown improvements in FEV_1, PaO_2, $PaCO_2$, after CPAP initiation [84,103,180]. The largest study (55 patients), by de Miguel et al [84] observed significant improvements in FEV_1, FVC, and $PaCO_2$ after 6 months of CPAP therapy. Both spirometry and gas exchange parameters remained improved for 18 months after CPAP cessation.

The addition of long-term CPAP therapy to standard treatment of COPD patients may also improve gas exchange while reducing hospitalization rates in patients with COPD and OSA [84,180]. The improvement in gas exchange with CPAP has important implications when assessing the necessity of long term oxygen therapy in patients with coexistent COPD and OSA. Among 55 middle-aged men with daytime hypoxaemia and coexistent COPD and OSA, only 22% continued to have daytime PaO_2<60 mmHg after 6 months of CPAP therapy [84]. Furthermore, CPAP therapy reduces elevated pulmonary and systemic arterial pressures in OSA [103,183] which emphasizes the importance of timely diagnosis and treatment of coexistent COPD and OSA. A substantial weight loss in that trial (mean weight loss approximately 15 pounds) could also explain part of the improvement. A negative study by O'Brien found that the overlap patients who were most adherent to CPAP had the greatest decline in lung function [151]. This could reflect bias, since those patients with the most progressive disease and symptoms may have used CPAP the most (or were urged to do so by their physicians). The small number of patients (35), the fact that only one third of them were included in the final analysis, the lack of precise timing of baseline and follow-up pulmonary function testing, makes these data difficult to interpret.

Long-term follow-up and outcomes of CPAP therapy in the overlap syndrome have only recently been reported. In an observational study, Machado et al [184] evaluated 95 patients with moderate-to-severe OSA and hypoxaemic COPD. Patients were hypoxaemic and hypercapnic at rest. They received long term oxygen therapy (LTOT). 61 patients received CPAP, the remainder were not adherent to ventilatory treatment. The five-year survival was 71% in the CPAP treated and 26% in the non-treated group. The adjustment for confounding factors showed that patients treated with CPAP had a significantly lower risk of death.

Marin et al [150] studied 441 patients with overlap syndrome (228 patients were treated with CPAP and 213 not treated) and 210 patients with COPD only for almost ten years. The co-existence of OSA/COPD was associated with an increased mortality (particularly cardiovascular) compared to COPD alone. Secondly, effective CPAP treatment of OSA reduces mortality in overlap patients. Finally, patients with overlap not treated with CPAP were more likely to suffer severe COPD exacerbations and hospitalizations in comparison to the COPD only group. In both studies, however, CPAP was not provided in a randomized, blinded manner.

8.4. Non-invasive ventilation

While CPAP therapy is effective in most OSA patients with or without coexistent COPD, bilevel positive airway pressure (PAP) may be useful when overlap patients experience difficulty exhaling against pressure or when, despite the adequate airflow during CPAP titration, intermittent nocturnal hypoxemia persists [185]. This is usually observed in severe COPD patients who hypoventilate during the night. In such cases bilevel devices should be considered. Bilevel PAP delivers a lower expiratory PAP and higher inspiratory PAP thereby augmenting ventilation [186,187]. In overlap patients who experience persistent intermittent nocturnal hypoxemia despite the adequate airflow during CPAP or BiPAP the positive airway pressure can be increased to ameliorate possible residual upper airway resistance. If increased PAP is ineffective or poorly tolerated, supplemental oxygen can be added [188].

The current guidelines suggest initial follow-up within 1 month after the start of PAP treatment. Subsequent visits should be annually or as needed The objective monitoring of PAP compliance is strongly recommended [185]. The close follow-up of patients includes patient education, adjustment of facial interfaces, and treatment of nasal conditions [185].

The effects of bilevel PAP on overlap syndrome have not been evaluated.

In our investigation, we followed 21 overlap patients who were adherent to BiPAP therapy after a period of one month. A slight improvement in ventilatory parameters was detected: FEV_1 53.5±10.87% vs 62.1± 9.18; FVC-55.5±24.5% vs 64.8±17.19% (Figure 3). A minor correction of blood exchange abnormalities was also observed (Figure 3). The average daytime PaO_2 increased from 61.67±5.78 mmHg to 69.32±7.18 mmHg (Figure 3). Hypercapnia was compensated in 43% of the patients and decreased from 52.14±11.39 mmHg to 48.32±8.17 mmHg. Though not of statistical significance, oxidative stress, as measured by urinary 8-isoprostanes, was also lower after one month of BiPAP therapy – 0.251±0.10 vs 0.214±0.12. The subjective sleepiness (ESS) improved from 15±4.3 to 12±3.8; this is related to an improvement of sleep disordered breathing. A reduction of IRI was also detected 21.04±15.46 vs 19.13±9.21 mU/l. Our data suggests that BiPAP therapy improves gas exchange and ventilatory parameters in overlap partients. It reduces the oxidative stress level and alleviates sleep complaints. Comparative data with CPAP is however missing. Whether long-term NIV would improve outcomes in the overlap syndrome, compared to CPAP is also unknown.

	Before BiPAP treatment	After BiPAP ventilation
FVC (l)	1.52	1.61
FEV_1 (l)	1.12	1.18
pH	7.41	7.46
PaO_2 (mmHg)	66.8	69.9
$PaCO_2$ (mmHg)	39.5	35.9

Figure 3. Representative spirometric and gas exchange parameters before and after treatment with BiPAP for one month from a single patient.

9. Conclusions

Sleep disturbances and NOD are common in COPD patients. Those patients with severe disease have both subjective and objective complaints of poor sleep quality and are easily suspected to experience NOD. The challenge to clinicians is to detect NOD among COPD subjects with mild daytime hypoxaemia where the clinical parameters predisposing patients to NOD are not as well recognized.

OSA is an independent, contributing mechanism to NOD in almost half of COPD patients who experience nighttime desaturations. The overlap syndrome though highly prevalent is frequently unrecognized in clinical practice. Daytime sleepiness and naps are not universal for OSA patients and the failure of clinicians to consider SDB in COPD is the reason for its poor detection. Overlap syndrome is associated with greater hypoxaemia and hypercapnia than COPD and OSA alone, which may have cardiovascular implications. Its early recognition and treatment with positive pressure ventilation may reduce morbidity and mortality and is strongly recommended.

According to our investigation, overlap patients have a higher prevalence of metabolic and cardiovascular disorders in comparison to OSA alone. Even after adjustment for confounding variables, the level of oxidative stress (measured by urinary 8-isoprostanes) is significantly higher in the overlap syndrome compared to OSA alone. One month treatment with BiPAP improved the ventilatory and gas exchange parameters and decreased the oxidative stress level in overlap patients. Despite the lack of weight reduction, a significant improvement in glucometabolic parameters was established.

10. Future directions

The new definitions of OSA proposed by the American Association of Sleep Medicine (AASM), based on epidemiological data sets are a major change of perspective that may facilitate the diagnostic approach to overlap [92]. The data regarding the prevalence of OSA in the general population and in COPD must be re-analysed. This is especially important to reestablish clinical phenotypes of both diseases in order to acquaint clinicians with the signs and symptoms that are highly suggestive of OSA in mild/moderate COPD and those suggestive of COPD in OSA patients.

'Molecular" and "physiological" studies are needed to evaluate the role of oxidative stress and inflammation in overlap syndrome as well as its possible additive and/or synergistic effects on cardiovascular morbidity. Biomarkers, indicative of increased cardiovascular risk are also demanded.

The introduction of more standardized therapeutic approaches is mandatory. The effects of oxygen therapy in COPD patients with only nighttime hypoxaemia and/or mild daytime hypoxaemia are unknown, especially those regarding gas exchange and pulmonary haemodynamics outcomes.

Overlap patients have severe daytime hypoxaemia than is expected based on lung mechanics. The effect of CPAP on dayime hypoxaemia in overlap syndrome has not, however, been investigated. It is obvious from the study of Machado et al, that some indications for LTOT should be reconsidered in a group of overlap patients; follow-up visits and reevaluation of ventilatory therapy should also be performed in detail. CPAP is the first choice in a phenotype of overlap patients where "OSA is prevalent". The optimal therapy for patients with mild OSA and moderate/severe COPD or for those with mild OSA and COPD remains a challenge.

It is obvious that CPAP is not as safe in COPD as is generally supposed. Holanda et al stated that in COPD, CPAP increased lung volume and worsened the baseline level of alveolar hyperinflation [189]. The AASM has proposed non-invasive ventilation for treatment of patients with overlap syndrome, especially for those intolerant of CPAP, or those with severe nocturnal hypoxia and/or hypoventilation. Pressure support ventilation stabilizes the upper airways in patients with OSA or overlap, as it changes the level of effective pressure between inspiration and expiration. It is also the most common mode of ventilation for the management of COPD related nocturnal hypoventilation.

Comparative follow-up mortality studies in overlap patients treated with either CPAP or BiPAP modality are required to determine the optimal therapeutic management.

Author details

Radostina Vlaeva Cherneva[1*], Ognian Borisov Georgiev[1], Daniela Stoichkova Petrova[1], Emil Ivanov Manov[2] and Julia Ivanova Petrova[3]

http://dx.doi.org/10.5772/57220

*Address all correspondence to: cherneva_radost@yahoo.com

1 Department of Internal Medicine, Division of Pulmonary Medicine, Medical University, Sofia, Bulgaria

2 Department of Internal Medicine, Division of Cardiology, Medical University, Sofia, Bulgaria

3 Department of Neurology, Medical University, Sofia, Bulgaria

References

[1] Douglas NJ, White DP, Pickett CK, et al.Respiration during sleep in normal man. *Thorax*,1982a; 37:840–4.

[2] White DP, Weil JV, Zwillich CW. Matabolic rate and breathing during sleep. J Appl. Physio 1985;58:384-91.

[3] Morrel MJ, Harty HR, Adams L, et al. Changes in total pulmonary resistance and PCO2 between wakefulness and slepp in normal human subjects. J Appl. Physiol. 1995;78:1339-49.

[4] Douglas NJ, White DP, Weil JV, et al. Hypercapnic ventilatory response in sleeping adults. Am. Rev Respir Dis 1982:126:758-62.

[5] Becker HF, Piper AJ, Flynn WE, et al. Breathing during sleep in patients with nocturnal desaturation. Am J Resp Crit Care Med 1999;159:112-8

[6] Calverley PM, Brezinova V, Douglas NJ, et al. The effect of oxygenation on sleep quality in hronic bronchitis and amphysema. Am Rev Resp Dis. 1982;126:206-10.

[7] Wiegand DA, Latz B, Zwillich CW, et al. Geniohyoid muscle activity in normal men during wakefulness and sleep. J Appl. Physiol 1990;60:1262-9.

[8] Basner RC, Ringler J, Schawartzstein RM, et al. Phasic electromyographic activity of the genioglossus increases in normals during slow wave sleep.Respir Physiol, 1991;83:189-200.

[9] Tangel DJ, Mezzanotte WS, Sandberg EJ, et al. Influences of NREM sleep on the activity of tonic vs. inspiratory phasic muscles in normal men.J Appl Phisiol 1992; 73:1058-66.

[10] Ballard RD, Clover CW, Suh BY. Influence of sleep on respiratory function in emphysema. Am J Resp Crit Care Med 1995;151:945-51.

[11] Hudgel DW, Dewadatta P. Decrease in functional residual capacity in normal humans. J Appl Physiol 1984;57:1319-22.

[12] Bryan AC, Muller NL. Lung mechanucs and gas exchange during sleep.Sleep 1980; 3:401-6.

[13] Block AJ, Boysen PG, Wynne JW, et al. Sleep apnea, hypopnea and oxygen desaturation in normal subjects. A strong male predominance. N Engl J Med 1979;300:513-7.

[14] Trask CH, Cree EM. Oximeter studies on patients with chronic obstructive emphysema, awake and during sleep. N Engl J Med. 1962; 266:639–642.

[15] Pierce AK, Jarrett CE, Werkle G Jr, Miller WF. Respiratory function during sleep in patients with chronic obstructive lung disease. J Clin Invest. 1966; 45(5):631–636.

[16] Chaouat A, Weitzenblum E, Kessler R, Charpentier C, Ehrhart M, Levi-Valensi P, et al. Sleep related O2 desaturation and daytime pulmonary haemodynamics in COPD patients with mild hypoxaemia. Eur Respir J. 1997; 10(8):1730–1735.

[17] Fletcher EC, Schaaf JW, Miller J, Fletcher JG. Long-term cardio-pulmonary sequelae in patients with sleep apnea and chronic lung disease. Am Rev Respir Dis. 1987; 135(3):525–533.

[18] Lewis CA, Fergusson W, Eaton T, Zeng I, Kolbe J. Isolated nocturnal desaturation in COPD: prevalence and impact on quality of life and sleep. Thorax. 2009; 64(2):133–138.

[19] Ramar K. Sleep Problems in Chronic Obstructive Pulmonary Disease. Tur Toraks Der 2008;9:117-23.

[20] Wynne JW, Block AJ, Hemenway J, et al. Disordered breathing and oxygen desaturation during sleep in patients with chronic obstructive lung disease (COLD). Am J Med 1979;66:573-9.

[21] Catterall JR, Douglas NJ, Calverley PM, et al. Transienthypoxemia during sleep in chronic obstructive pulmonary disease is not a sleep apnea syndrome. Am Rev Respir Dis 1983;128:24-9.

[22] Catterall JR, Calverley PM, MacNee W, et al.Mechanism of transient nocturnal hypoxemia in hypoxic chronic bronchitis and emphysema. J Appl Physiol, 1985;59:1698–703.

[23] Lewis CA, Eaton TE, Fergusson W, et al. Home overnight pulse oximetry in patients with COPD: more than one recording may be needed. Chest,2003;123:1127–33.

[24] Mulloy E, McNicholas WT.Ventilation and gas exchange during sleep and exercise in severe COPD. Chest,1996; 109:387–94.

[25] Flenley DC.Sleep in chronic obstructive lung disease. Clin Chest Med,1985;6:651–61.

[26] O'Donoghue FJ, Catcheside PG, Eckert DJ, McEvoy RD. Changes in respiration in NREM sleep in hypercapnic chronic obstructive pulmonary disease. J Physiol 2004;559:663-73.

[27] Pronzato C. Chronic Obstructive Pulmonary disease and obstructive sleep apnea. Association, consequences and treatment.Monaldi Arch Chest Dis,2010;73:155-161.

[28] Bonsignore MR, Marrone O, Insalaco G, et al. The cardiovascular effects of obstructive sleep apnoeas: analysis of pathogenic mechanisms. *Eur Respir J*, 1994;7:786–805.

[29] Coccagna G, Lugaresi E. Arterial blood gases and pulmonary and systemic arterial pressure during sleep in chronic obstructive pulmonary disease. Sleep 1978;1:117-24.

[30] Weitzenblum E, Chaouat A. Sleep and chronic obstructive pulmonary disease. *Sleep Med Rev*, 2004;8:281–94.

[31] Boysen PG, Block AJ, Wynne JW, et al. Nocturnal pulmonary hypertension in patients with chronic obstructive pulmonary disease. Chest 1979;76:536-42.

[32] Fletcher EC, Levin DC. Cardiopulmonary hemodynamics during sleep in subjects with chronic obstructive pulmonary disease. The effect of short-and long-term oxygen. Chest 1984;85:6-14.

[33] Weitzenblum E, Muzet A, Ehrhart M, et al. Nocturnal changes in blood gases and pulmonary arterial pressure in chronic bronchitis patients with respiratory insufficiency. Nouv Presse Med 1982;11:1119-22.

[34] Fletcher EC, Luckett RA, Miller T, et al. Pulmonary vascular hemodynamics in chronic lung disease patients with and without oxyhemoglobin desaturation during sleep. Chest 1989;95:757-64.

[35] Levi-Valensi P, Weitzenblum E, Rida Z, et al. Sleep-related oxygen desaturation and daytime pulmonary haemodynamics in COPD patients. Eur Respir J 1992;5:301-7.

[36] Wright JL, Levy RD, Churg A. Pulmonary hypertension in chronic obstructive pulmonary disease: current theories of pathogenesis and their implications for treatment. *Thorax*, 2005;60:605–9.

[37] Sajkov D, McEvoy RD. Obstructive sleep apnea and pulmonary hypertension. Prog Cardiovasc Dis. 2009; 51(5):363–370.

[38] Chaouat A, Weitzenblum E, Kessler R, Charpentier C, Enhart M, Schott R, et al. A randomized trial of nocturnal oxygen therapy in chronic obstructive pulmonary disease patients. Eur Respir J. 1999; 14(5):1002–1008.

[39] McNicholas WT, Fitzgerald MX. Nocturnal deaths among patients with chronic bronchitis and emphysema. BMJ (Clin Res Ed). 1984; 289(6449):878.

[40] Flick MR, Block AJ. Nocturnal vs diurnal cardiac arrhythmias in patients with chronic obstructive pulmonary disease. Chest 1979;75:8-11.

[41] Shepard JW Jr., Schweitzer PK, Keller CA, et al. Myocardial stress. Exercise versus sleep in patients with COPD. Chest 1984;86:366-74

[42] Fletcher EC, Miller J, Divine GW, et al. Nocturnal oxyhemoglobin desaturation in COPD patients with arterial oxygen tensions above 60 mm Hg. Chest 1987;92:604-8.

[43] Fitzpatrick MF, Mackay T, Whyte KF, et al. Nocturnal desaturation and serum erythropoietin: a study in patients with chronic obstructive pulmonary disease and in normal subjects. Clin Sci (Lond) 1993;84:319-24.

[44] Cormick W, Olson LG, Hensley MJ, Saunders NA. Nocturnal hypoxaemia and quality of sleep in patients with chronic obstructive lung disease. Thorax. 1986; 41(11): 846–854

[45] Sin DD, Man SF. Chronic obstructive pulmonary disease: a novel risk factor for cardiovascular disease. Can J Physiol Pharmacol. 2005; 83(1):8–13.

[46] Connaughton JJ, Catterall JR, Elton RA, et al. Do sleep studies contribute to the management of patients with severe chronic obstructive pulmonary disease? Am Rev Respir Dis 1988;138:341-4.

[47] Marin JM, Soriano JB, Carrizo SJ, Boldova A, Celli BR. Outcomes in patients with chronic obstructive pulmonary disease and obstructive sleep apnea: the overlap syndrome. Am J Respir Crit Care Med. 2010; 182(3):325–33

[48] Donaldson GC, Seemungal TA, Bhowmik A, Wedzicha JA. Relationship between exacerbation frequency and lung function decline in chronic obstructive pulmonary disease. Thorax. 2002; 57(10):847–852.

[49] Soler-Cataluna JJ, Martinez-Garcia MA, Roman Sanchez P, Salcedo E, Navarro M, Ochando R. Severe acute exacerbations and mortality in patients with chronic obstructive pulmonary disease. Thorax. 2005; 60(11):925–931.

[50] Bellia V, Catalano F, Scichilone N, et al. Sleep disorders in theelderly with and without chronic airfl ow obstruction: the SARA study.*Sleep*, 2003;26:318–23.

[51] Klink M, Quan SF. Prevalence of reported sleep disturbancesin a general adult population and their relationship toobstructive airways diseases. Chest 1987;91:540-6

[52] Kinsman RA, Yaroush RA, Fernandez E, Dirks JF, Schocket M, Fukuhara J. Symptoms and experiences in chronic bronchitis and emphysema. Chest. 1983; 83(5):755–761.

[53] Klink ME, Dodge R, Quan SF. The relation of sleep complaints to respiratory symptoms in a general population. Chest. 1994; 105(1):151–154.

[54] Krachman SL, Chatila W, Martin UJ, et al. Effects of lungvolume reduction surgery on sleep quality and nocturnal gasexchange in patients with severe emphysema. Chest, 2005;128:3221-8.

[55] Sanders MH, Newman AB, Haggerty CL, et al. Sleep and sleep-disordered breathing in adults with predominantlymild obstructive airway disease. Am J Respir Crit Care Med 2003;167:7-14.

[56] Redline S, Kirchner HL, Quan SF, et al. The effects of age, sex, ethnicity, and sleep-disordered breathing on sleep architecture. *Arch Intern Med,*. 2004;164:406–18.

[57] Fleetham J, West P, Mezon B, et al. Sleep, arousals, and oxygen desaturation in chronic obstructive pulmonary disease. The effect of oxygen therapy. Am Rev Respir Dis 1982;126:429-33.

[58] Sandek K, Andersson T, Bratel T, et al.Sleep quality, carbon dioxide responsiveness and hypoxaemic patterns in nocturnal hypoxaemia due to chronic obstructive pulmonary disease (COPD) without daytime hypoxaemia. *Respir Med,* 1999;93:79–87.

[59] Orr WC, Shamma-Othman Z, Levin D, et al. Persistent hypoxemia and excessive daytime sleepiness in chronic obstructive pulmonary disease (COPD). Chest 1990;97:583-5.

[60] DeMarco FJ Jr., Wynne JW, Block AJ, et al. Oxygen desaturation during sleep as a determinant of the "Blue and Bloated" syndrome. Chest 1981;79:621-5.

[61] Bradley TD, Mateika J, Li D, et al. Daytime hypercapnia in the development of nocturnal hypoxemia in COPD. Chest 1990;97:308-12.

[62] Mulloy E, Fitzpatrick M, Bourke S, O'Regan A, McNicholas WT. Oxygen desaturation during sleep and exercise in patients with severe chronic obstructive pulmonary disease. Respir Med. 1995; 89(3):193–198.

[63] Krachman S, Minai OA, Scharf SM. Sleep abnormalities and treatment in emphysema. Proc Am Thorac Soc. 2008; 5(4):536–542

[64] Celli BR, MacNee W; ATS/ERS Task Force. 2004. Standards for the diagnosis and treatment of patients with COPD: a summary of the ATS/ERS position paper. *Eur Respir J,* 2004;23:932–46.

[65] Hiestand DM, Britz P, Goldman M, et al. Prevalence of symptoms and risk of sleep apnea in the US population: Results from the national sleep foundation sleep in America 2005 *Chest,* 2006; 130:780–6.

[66] Carratu P and Resta O. Is obstructive sleep apnea a comorbidity of COPD and is it involved in systemic inflammatory syndrome? ERJ, 2008:31:1381-1382.

[67] Wiegand L, Zwillich CW.. Obstructive sleep apnea. *Dis Mon,* 1994;40:197–252

[68] Fogel RB, Malhotra A, White DP. Sleep. 2: pathophysiology of obstructive sleep apnoea/hypopnoea syndrome. *Thorax,* 2004;59:159–63.

[69] Liistro G. Pathophysiology of upper airway obstruction during sleep. *Acta Otorhinolaryngol Belg,*. 2002;56:101–6.

[70] Hudgel DW, Gordon EA, Thanakitcharu S, et al. Instability of ventilatory control in patients with obstructive sleep apnea. *Am J Respir Crit Care Med,* 1998;158:1142–9.

[71] Younes M, Ostrowski M, Thompson W, et al.. Chemical control stability in patients with obstructive sleep apnea. *Am J Respir Crit Care Med*, 2001;163:1181–90.

[72] Series F, Cormier Y, Desmeules M, et al. Effects of respiratory drive on upper airways in sleep apnea patients and normal subjects. *J Appl Physiol*, 1989; 67:973–9.

[73] Garay SM, Rapoport D, Sorkin B, et al.. Regulation of ventilation in the obstructive sleep apnea syndrome. *Am Rev Respir Dis*, 1981;124:451–7.

[74] Soto Campos JG, Cano GS, Fernandez GJ, et al.. Hypercapnic stimulation and ventilation response in the syndrome of sleep obstructive apnea. Comparison of reinhalation and steady state. *Arch Bronconeumol*, 1996;32:341–7.

[75] El Bayadi S, Millman RP, Tishler PV, et al.. A family study of sleep apnea. Anatomic and physiologic interactions. *Chest*, 1990;98:554–9.

[76] Redline S, Leitner J, Arnold J, et al.. Ventilatory-control abnormalities in familial sleep apnea. *Am J Respir Crit Care Med*, 1997;156:155–60.

[77] Berthon-Jones M, Sullivan CE. Time course of change in ventilatory response to CO2 with long-term CPAP therapy for obstructive sleep apnea. *Am Rev Respir Dis*, 1987;135:144–7.

[78] Lin CC.Effect of nasal CPAP on ventilatory drive in normocapnic and hypercapnic patients with obstructive sleep apnoea syndrome. *Eur Respir J*, 1994;7:2005–10.

[79] Redolfi S, Yumino D, Ruttanaumpawn P, et al. Relationship between overnight rostral fluid shift and obstructive sleep apnea in non-obese men. Am j respire Crit Care Med 2009;179:241-246.

[80] Eckert DJ, Saboisky JP, Jordan AS, Malhotra A. Upper airway myopathy is not important in the pathophysiology of obstructive sleep apnea. J Clin Sleep Med. 2007; 3(6):570–573.

[81] Owens RL, Malhotra A, Eckert DJ, White DP, Jordan AS. The influence of end-expiratory lungvolume on measurements of pharyngeal collapsibility. J Appl Physiol. 2010; 108(2):445–451.

[82] Nadel JA, Widdicombe JG. Reflex effects of upper airway irritation on total lung resistance andblood pressure. J Appl Physiol. 1962; 17:861–865.

[83] Owens RL, Malhtora A. Sleep-Disordered Breathing and COPD: The Overlap Syndrome Respir Care. 2010;55(10): 1333–1346.

[84] De Miguel J, Cabello J, Sanchez-Alarcos JM, et al. Long-term effects of treatment with nasal continuous positive airway pressure on lung function in patients with overlap syndrome. *Sleep Breath*, 2002.;6:3–10.

[85] Young T, Palta M, Dempsey J, et al. The occurrence of sleepdisordered breathing among middle-aged adults. *N Engl J Med*, 1993;328:1230–5.

[86] Guilleminault C. Obstructive sleep apnea. The clinical syndrome and historical perspective. *Med Clin North Am*, 1985;69:1187–203.

[87] Chaouat A, Weitzenblum E, Krieger J, et al.. Association of chronic obstructive pulmonary disease and sleep apnea syndrome. *Am J Respir Crit Care Med*, 1995;151:82–6.

[88] Lopez-Acevedo MN, Torres-Palacios A, Elena Ocasio-Tascon M, Campos-Santiago Z, Rodriguez-

[89] tron W. Overlap syndrome: an indication for sleep studies?: a pilot study. Sleep Breath. 2009; 13(4):409–413.

[90] Bednarek M, Plywaczewski R, Jonczak L, Zielinski J. There is no relationship between chronic obstructive pulmonary disease and obstructive sleep apnea syndrome: a population study. Respiration. 2005; 72(2):142–149.

[91] Iber C, Ancoli-Israel S, Chesson AL, Quan SF. Thea AASM manual for the scoring of sleep and associated events. Rules, terminology, and technical specifications. Westchester, III, Illinois: American Academy of Sleep Medicine, 2007.

[92] The Global strategy for the diagnosis, management and prevention of COPD, 2011

[93] Guilleminault C, Tilkian A, Dement WC. The sleep apnea syndromes. *Ann Rev Med*, 1976;27:465–84.

[94] Leech JA, Onal E, Baer P, et al. Determinants of hypercapnia in occlusive sleep apnea syndrome. *Chest*, 1987;92:807–13.

[95] Chan CS, Bye PTP, Woolclock AJ, Sullivan Ce. Eucapnia and hypercapnia in patients with chronic airflow limitation. The role of upper airways. Am Rev Respir Dis 1990;141:861-865.

[96] Radwan L, Maszczyk Z, Koziorowski A, Koziej M, Cieslicki J, Sliwinski P, Zielinski J. Control of breathing in obstructive sleep apnoea and in patients with the overlap syndrome. Eur Respir J. 1995; 8(4):542–545.

[97] Chien MY, Wu YT, Lee Pl, Chang YJ, Yang PC. Inspiratory muscle dysfunction in patients with severe obstructive sleep apnea. Eur Respir J 2010;35:373-80.

[98] Yee BJ, Cheung J, Phipps P, Banerjee D, Piper AJ, Grunstein RR. Treatment of obesity hypoventilation syndrome and serum leptin. Respiration. 2006; 73(2):209–212.

[99] Sanner BM, Doberauer C, Konermann M, et al.. Pulmonary hypertension in patients with obstructive sleep apnea syndrome. *Arch Intern Med*, 1997;157:2483–7.

[100] Bady E, Achkar A, Pascal S, et alPulmonary arterial hypertension in patients with sleep apnoea syndrome. *Thorax*,.2000;55:934–9.

[101] Sajkov D, Wang T, Saunders NA, et al. Daytime pulmonary hemodynamics in patients with obstructive sleep apnea without lung disease. *Am J Respir Crit Care Med*, 1999;159:1518 26.

[102] Laks L, Lehrhaft B, Grunstein RR, et al. Pulmonary hypertension in obstructive sleep apnoea. *Eur Respir J*, 1995;8:537–41.

[103] Bradley TD.. Right and left ventricular functional impairment and sleep apnea. *Clin Chest Med*, 1992;13:459–79.

[104] Hawrylkiewicz I, Sliwinski P, Gorecka D, Plywaczewski R, Zielinski J. Pulmonary haemodynamics in patients with OSAS or an overlap syndrome. Monaldi Arch Chest Dis. 2004;61(3):148–152.

[105] Arias MA, Garcia-Rio F, Alonso-Fernandez A, Martinez I, Villamor J. Pulmonary hypertension in obstructive sleep apnoea: effects of continuous positive airway pressure: a randomized, controlled cross-over study. Eur Heart J. 2006; 27(9):1106–1113.

[106] Gami AS, Howard DE, Olson EJ, Somers VK. Day-night pattern of sudden death in obstructive sleep apnea. N Engl J Med. 2005; 352(12):1206–1214.

[107] Olmetti F, La Rovere MT, Robbi E, et al. Nocturnal cardiac arrhythmia in patients with obstructive sleep apnea. *Sleep Med*, 2008, 9:475-80.

[108] Chaouat A, Weitzenblum E, Krieger J, Krieger J, Sforza E, Hammad H, Oswald M, Kessler R. Prognostic value of lung function and pulmonary haemodynamics in OSA patients treated with CPAP. Eur Respir J. 1999; 13(5):1091–1096.

[109] Lavie P, Herer P, Lavie L. Mortality risk factors in sleep apnoea: a matched case-control study. J Sleep Res. 2007; 16(1):128–134.

[110] Lavie P, Herer P, Peled R, Berger I, Yoffe N, Zomer J, Rubin AH. Mortality in sleep apnea patients: a multivariate analysis of risk factors. Sleep. 1995; 18(3):149–157.

[111] Mermigkis C, Kopanakis A, Foldvary-Schaefer N, Golish J, Polychronopoulos V, Schiza S, et al. Health-related quality of life in patients with obstructive sleep apnoea and chronic obstructive pulmonary disease (overlap syndrome). Int J Clin Pract. 2007; 61(2):207–211.

[112] Ross R. Atherosclerosis--an infl ammatory disease. *N Engl J Med*, 1999;340:115–26.

[113] Hansson GK.Inflammation, atherosclerosis, and coronary artery disease. *N Engl J Med*, 2005;352:1685–95

[114] Agusti AG, Noguera A, Sauleda J, et al.. Systemic effects of chronic obstructive pulmonary disease. *Eur Respir J*, 2003;21:347–60.

[115] Yende S, Waterer GW, Tolley EA, et al. Infl ammatory markers are associated with ventilatory limitation and muscle dysfunction in obstructive lung disease in well functioning elderly subjects. *Thorax*, 2006; 61:10–6.

[116] Camilli AE, Robbins DR, Lebowitz MD. Death certifi cate reporting of confirmed airways obstructive disease. *Am J Epidemiol*, 1991;133:795–800.

[117] Sin DD, Man SF.Why are patients with chronic obstructive pulmonary disease at increased risk of cardiovascular diseases? The potential role of systemic infl ammation in chronic obstructive pulmonary disease. *Circulation*, 2003;107:1514–9.

[118] Nieto FJ, Herrington DM, Redline S, et alSleep apnea and markers of vascular endothelial function in a large community sample of older adults. *Am J Respir Crit Care Med*,. 2004;169:354–60.

[119] Jelic S, Bartels MN, Mateika JH, et al. Arterial stiffness increases during obstructive sleep apneas. *Sleep*, 2002;25:850–5.

[120] RidkerPM,Cushman M, Stamfer MJ,Tracy RP,Henekenes Ch. Inflammation, aspirin, and the risk of cardiovascular disease in apparently healthy men. N Engl. J Med, 1997;336:973-979.

[121] Yokoe T, Mingouchi K, Matsuo H et al. Elevated levels of C-reactive protein and IL-6 in patients with OSA are decreased after nasal continuous positive airway pressure. Circulation 2003;107:1129-34.

[122] Mehra R, Strfofer –Isser A, Kirchner HL, et al. Soluble IL-6 receptor: a marker of moderate to severe sleep related brething disorders.Arch intern Med 2006;166:1725-31.

[123] Man SF, Connett JE, Anthonisen NR, et al. C-reactive protein and mortality in mild to moderate chronic obstructive pulmonary disease. *Thorax*, 2006;61:849–53.

[124] Pinto-Plata VM, Mullerova H, Toso JF, et al. C-reactive protein in patients with COPD, control smokers and non-smokers. *Thorax*, 2006;61:23–8.

[125] Zamarron-Sanz C, Ricoy-Galbaldon J, Gude-Sampedro F, et al. Plasma levels of vascular endothelial markers in obstructive sleep apnea. *Arch Med Res*, 2006;37:552–5

[126] Ryan S, Taylor CT, McNicholas WT, et al. Slective activation of inflammatory pathways by intermittent hypoxia in OSA. Circulation 2005;112:2660-2667.

[127] Ryan S, Taylor CT, McNicholas WT, et al. Predictors of elevated NF-kB dependent genes in OSA. Am J Resp Crit Care Med,2006:174:824-830.

[128] Cesari M, Pennix BWJH, Newman AB, et al. Inflammatory markers and onset of cardiovascular events: results from the Health ABC Study. Circulation, 2003;108:2317-22.

[129] MacNee W. Oxidants/antioxidants and COPD. Chest 2000;117:303-317.

[130] Lavie L. Obstructive sleep apnea syndrome-an oxidative stress disorder. Sleep Med Rev 2003;7:35-51.

[131] Schulz R, Mahmoudi S, Hattar K et al. Enhanced release of superoxide from polymorphonuclear neutrophils in obstructive sleep apnea : impact oof continuous positive airway pressure therapy. Am J Respir Crit Care Med 2000;162:566-570.

[132] Droge W. Free radicals in the physiological control of cell function. Physiol Rev 2002;82:47-95.

[133] Gan WQ, Man SFP, Senthilselvan A, Sin DD. Association between chronic obstructive pulmonary disease and systemic inflammation : a systemic review and a meta-analysis. Thorax, 2004;59:574-80.

[134] Dyuogovskaya L, Polyakov A, lavie P, Lavie L. Delayed neutrophil apoptosis in patients with sleep apnea. Am J respire Crit Care med. 2008;177:544-554.

[135] Nieto FJ, Young TB,Lind BK, et al.Association of sleep disordered breathing, sleep apnea, and hypertension in a large community-based study Sleep Heart Health Study. JAMA, 2000;283:1829-36.

[136] Peppard PE, Young T, Palta M et al. Prospective study of the association between sleep disordered breathing and hypertension. N Engl J Med 2000;342:1378-84.

[137] Gottlieb DJ, Yenokyan G, Newman AB, et al.Prospective study of obstructive sleep apnea and incident coronary heart disease and heart failure. Circulation, 2010;122:352-360.

[138] Redline S, Yenokyan G, Gottlieb DJ, et al. Obstructive sleep apnea and hypopnea and incident stroke. Am J Respir Crit Care Med 2010;182:269-277.

[139] Peker Y, Hadner J, Kraiczi H, et al. Respiratory disturbamce index an independent predictor of mortality in coronary heart disease. Am J Respir Crit Care Med 2000;162:81-86.

[140] Drager LF, Bortolotto LA, Lorenzi MC, et al.Early signs of atherosclerosis in obstructive sleep apnea Am J Respir Crit Care Med 2005;172:613-618.

[141] Nieto FJ,Peppard PE, Young TB. Sleep disordered breathing and the meatobolic syndrome. WMJ 2009;108:263-265

[142] Wolk R, Somers VK. Sleep and metabolic syndrome. Exp Physiol 2007;92:67-78.

[143] Colt HG, Haas H, Rich GB. Hypoxemia vs sleep fragmentation as cause of excessive daytime sleepiness in obstructive sleep apnea. *Chest*, 1991;100:1542–8

[144] Seneviratne U, Puvanendran K. Excessive daytime sleepiness in obstructive sleep apnea: prevalence, severity, and predictors. *Sleep Med*, 2004;5:339–43.

[145] Saaresranta T, Irjala K, Aittokallio T, et al. Sleep quality, daytime sleepiness and fasting insulin levels in women with chronic obstructive pulmonary disease. *Respir Med*, 2005;99:856–63.

[146] Zamarron C, Gude F, Otero Y, et al. Symptoms of sleep apnea syndrome in the general population. *Arch Bronconeumol*, 1998;34:245–9.

[147] Pichel F, Zamarron C, Magan F, et al. Health-related quality of life in patients with obstructive sleep apnea: effects of long-term positive airway pressure treatment. *Respir Med*, 2004;98:968–76.

[148] O'Brien A, Whitman K. Lack of benefi t of continuous positive airway pressure on lung function in patients with overlap syndrome. *Lung*, 2005;183:389–404.

[149] Resta O, Foschino-Barbaro MP, Bonfi tto P, et al.. Prevalence and mechanisms of diurnal hypercapnia in a sample of morbidly obese subjects with obstructive sleep apnoea. *Respir Med*, 2000;94:240–6.

[150] Kessler R, Chaouat A, Weitzenblum E, et al.Pulmonary hypertension in the obstructive sleep apnoea syndrome: prevalence, causes and therapeutic consequences. *Eur Respir J*, 1996;9:787–94.

[151] Marin JM, Carrizo SJ, Vicente E, et al. Long-term cardiovascular outcomes in men with obstructive sleep apnoea-hypopnoea with or without treatment with continuous positive airway pressure: an observational study. *Lancet*,. 2005;365:1046–53.

[152] Bradley JM, Lasserson T, Elborn S, et al. A systematic review of randomized controlled trials examining the short-term benefit of ambulatory oxygen in COPD. Chest. 2007 Jan;131(1):278-85.

[153] Laaban JP, Chailleux E.. Daytime hypercapnia in adult patients with obstructive sleep apnea syndrome in France, before initiating nocturnal nasal continuous positive airway pressure therapy. *Chest*, 2005;127:710–15.

[154] Martin RJ, Bartelson BL, Smith P, et al. Effect of ipratropium bromide treatment on oxygen saturation and sleep quality in COPD. Chest 1999;115:1338-45.

[155] McNicholas WT, Calverley PM, Lee A, Edwards JC. Long-acting inhaled anticholinergic therapy improves sleeping oxygen saturation in COPD. Eur Respir J 2004;23:825-31.

[156] Mulloy E, McNicholas WT. Theophylline improves gas exchange during rest, exercise, and sleep in severe chronic obstructive pulmonary disease. Am Rev Respir Dis 1993;148:1030-6.

[157] Berry RB, Desa MM, Branum JP, Light RW. Effect of theophylline on sleep and sleep-disordered breathing in patients with chronic obstructive pulmonary disease. Am Rev Respir Dis 1991;143:245-50.

[158] Man GC, Champman KR, Ali SH, Darke AC. Sleep quality and nocturnal respiratory function with once-daily theophylline (Uniphyl) and inhaled salbutamol in patients with COPD. Chest 1996;110:648-53.

[159] Martin RJ, Pak J. Overnight theophylline concentrations and effects on sleep and lung function in chronic obstructive pulmonary disease. Am Rev Respir Dis 1992;145:540-4.

[160] Block AJ, Dolly FR, Slayton PC. Does flurazepam ingestion affect breathing and oxygenation during sleep in patients with chronic obstructive lung disease? Am Rev Respir Dis 1984;129:230-3.

[161] Girault C, Muir JF, Mihaltan F, et al. Effects of repeated administration of zolpidem on sleep, diurnal and nocturnal respiratory function, vigilance, and physical performance in patients with COPD. Chest 1996;110:1203-11.

[162] Ryan S, Doherty LS, Rock C, Nolan GM, McNicholas WT. Effects of salmeterol on sleepingoxygen saturation in chronic obstructive pulmonary disease. Respiration. 2010;79:475-81.

[163] Sposato B, Mariotta S, Palmiero G, Ricci A, Gencarelli G, Franco C. Oral corticosteroids can improve nocturnal isolated hypoxemia in stable COPD patients with diurnal PaO2 > 60 mmHg. Eur Rev Med Pharmacol Sci. 2007; 11(6):365–372.

[164] Weitzenblum E, Chaouat A, Charpentier C, et al. Sleep-related hypoxaemia in chronic obstructive pulmonary disease: causes, consequences and treatment. *Respiration*, 1997;64:187–93.

[165] Nocturnal Oxygen Therapy Trial Group. Continuous or nocturnal oxygen therapy in hypoxemic chronic obstructive lung disease: a clinical trial. Ann Intern Med. 1980; 93(3):391–398.

[166] Report of the Medical Research Council Working Party. Long term domiciliary oxygen therapy inchronic hypoxic cor pulmonale complicating chronic bronchitis and emphysema. Lancet. 1981; 1(8222):681–686.

[167] Fletcher EC, Donner CF, Midgren B, zielinski J, Levi-Valensi P, Braghiroli A, et al. Survival in COPD patients with a daytime PaO2 greater than 60 mm Hg with and without nocturnal oxyhemoglobin desaturation. Chest. 1992; 101(3):649–655.

[168] Gorecka D, Gorzelak K, Sliwinski P, et al. Effect of long-term oxygen therapy on survival in patients with chronic obstructive pulmonary disease with moderate hypoxaemia.Thorax 1997;52:674-9.

[169] Fletcher EC, Luckett RA, Goodnight-White S, et al. A double-blind trial of nocturnal supplemental oxygen for sleep desaturation in patients with chronic obstructive pulmonary disease and a daytime PaO2 above 60 mm Hg. Am Rev Respir Dis 1992;145:1070-6.

[170] Kolodziej MA, Jensen L, Rowe B, Sin D. Systematic review of noninvasive positive pressure ventilation in severe stable COPD. Eur Respir J 2007;30:293-306.

[171] Clinical indications for noninvasive positive pressure ventilation in chronic respiratory failure due to restrictive lung disease, COPD, and nocturnal hypoventilation--a consensus conference report. Chest 1999;116:521-34.

[172] McEvoy RD, Pierce RJ, Hillman D, Esterman A, Ellis EE, Catcheside PG, et al. Nocturnal noninvasive nasal ventilation in stable hyper-capnic COPD: a randomised controlled trial. Thorax. 2009; 64(7):561–566.

[173] Windisch W, Haenel M, Storre JH, Dreher M. High-intensity non-invasive positive pressure ventilation for stable hypercapnic COPD. Int J Med Sci. 2009; 6(2):72–76.

[174] Giles TL, Lasserson TJ, Smith BJ, et al. Continuous positive airways pressure for obstructive sleep apnoea in adults. *Cochrane Database Syst Rev*, 2006.

[175] Marshall NS, Barnes M, Travier N, et al. Continuous positive airway pressure reduces daytime sleepiness in mild to moderate obstructive sleep apnoea: a meta-analysis. *Thorax*, 2006;61:430–4.

[176] Haynes PL.. The role of behavioral sleep medicine in the assessment and treatment of sleep disordered breathing. *Clin Psychol Rev*, 2005;25:673–705.

[177] Morgenthaler TI, Kapen S, Lee-Chiong T, Alessi C, Boehlecke B, Brown T, et al. Practice parameters for the medical therapy of obstructive sleep apnea. Sleep. 2006; 29(8): 1031–1035.

[178] Sampol G, Sagales MT, Roca A, de la Calzada MD, Bofill JM, Morell F. Nasal continuous positive airway pressure with supplemental oxygen in coexistent sleep apnoea-hypopnoea syndrome and severe chronic obstructive pulmonary disease. Eur Respir J. 1996; 9(1):111–116

[179] Costa D, Toledo A, Silva AB, et al. Influence of noninvasive ventilation on exercise tolerance and respiratory muscle strength in COPD patients.Rev Lationo-am Enfermagem, 2006;14:378-82.

[180] Mezzanotte WS, Tangel DJ, Fox AM, Ballard RD, White DP. Nocturnal nasal continuous positive airway pressure in patients with chronic obstructive pulmonary disease: influence on waking respiratory muscle function. Chest. 1994; 106(4):1100–1108

[181] Mansfield D, Naughton MT. Effects of continuous positive airway pressure on lung function in patients with chronic obstructive pulmonary disease and sleep disordered breathing. Respirology. 1999; 4(4):365–370.

[182] Sforza E, Krieger J, Weitzenblum E, Apprill M, Lampert E, Ratamaharo J. Long-term effects of treatment with nasal continuous positive airway pressure on daytime lung function and pulmonary hemodynamics in patients with obstructive sleep apnea. Am Rev Respir Dis. 1990; 141(4 Pt 1): 866–870.

[183] Peker Y, Hedner J, Johansson A, Bende M. Reduced hospitalization with cardiovascular and pulmonary disease in obstructive sleep apnea patients on nasal CPAP treatment. Sleep. 1997; 20(8):645–653.

[184] Campos-Rodriguez F, Perez-Ronchel J, Grilo-Reina A, et al. Longterm effect of continuous positive airway pressure on BP in patients with hypertension and sleep apnea *Chest*, 2007;132:1847–52.

[185] Machado MC, Vollmer WM, Togeiro SM, Bilderback AL, Oliveira MV, Leitao FS, et al. CPAP and survival in moderate-to-severe obstructive sleep apnoea syndrome and hypoxaemic COPD. Eur Respir J. 2010; 35(1):132–137.

[186] Kushida CA, Littner MR, Hirshkowitz M, et al. Practice parameters for the use of continuous and bilevel positive airway pressure devices to treat adult patients with sleep-related breathing disorders. *Sleep*, 2006;29:375–80.

[187] Schafer H, Ewig S, Hasper E, et al.. Failure of CPAP therapy in obstructive sleep apnea syndrome: predictive factors and treatment with bilevel positive airway pressure. *Respir Med*, 1998;92:208–15.

[188] Sanders MH, Kern N.. Obstructive sleep apnea treated by independently adjusted inspiratory and expiratory positive airway pressures via nasal mask. *Chest*, 1990;98:317–24.

[189] Kakkar RK, Berry RB. Positive airway pressure treatment for obstructive sleep apnea. *Chest*, 2007;132:1057–72.

[190] Holanda MA, Fortaleza SCB, Alves de Almeida M, et al. Continuous positive airway pressure effects on regional lung aeration in patients with COPD: A high resolution CT scan study. Chest, 2010; 138:305-314.

Chapter 6

Chronic Obstructive Pulmonary Disease and Sleep Quality

Hatice Tel Aydin

Additional information is available at the end of the chapter

http://dx.doi.org/10.5772/57559

1. Introduction

Sleep is a basic physiological need for all humans. People need to sleep and rest enough for a healthy and productive life. However, some factors may prevent attainment of adequate sleep and rest. While some of these factors may cause transient alterations in an individual's sleep-rest routine, other factors can affect sleep chronically. Chronic systemic diseases are one of the most important factors that can affect the characteristics of people's sleep for a long-time period. Chronic diseases cause various sleep problems and impair sleep quality. One of the chronic systemic diseases that affects the sleep routine and sleep quality of people severely is Chronic Obstructive Pulmonary Disease (COPD).

COPD is an important health problem with an increasing prevalence and high morbidity and mortality rate all over the world. In the last 20 years, the increasing mortality rates related to COPD emphasize that COPD is a growing health problem [1]. WHO predicts that COPD will become the third leading cause of death worldwide by 2030 [2]. The Global Initiative for Obstructive Lung Disease (GOLD) characterizes COPD as "a preventable and treatable disease with some significant extra pulmonary effects that may contribute to the severity in individual patients. The pulmonary component of COPD is characterized by airflow limitation that is not fully reversible. The airflow limitation is usually progressive and associated with an abnormal inflammatory response of the lung to noxious particles or gases". [3]

COPD, which affects individuals multidimensionally, has severe consequences. The complaints of patients with COPD are not limited to the symptoms of dyspneoa, cough and phlegm production [4]. Although COPD is a disease affecting primarily the respiratory tract and lungs, it has many systemic effects and complications related to the cardiovascular system, musculoskeletal system, neurological system, nutrition, and metabolism [5,6].

COPD severely affects the social and psychological aspects of patients' lives as well as their physical health. Due to the changes of the disease process, COPD forces patients to make changes in their lifestyles. Due to the stress, anxiety, loss of control and independence, change of sense of self, and respiratory distress, patients experience important psychological alterations including serious fear of death and depression [4,7-9]. Patients with COPD have to change most of their daily activities due to dyspnoea, functional impairment, and fatigue. With increasing fatigue and dyspnoea, they adopt a sedentary lifestyle [4]. Many patients with COPD have poor sleep quality, especially those who have high anxiety and depression [10-12]. Shackell et al (2007) stated that the anxiety experienced due to dyspnoea affects the sleep quality of patients with COPD and the sleep quality has effects on physical and emotional functions [13]. COPD-related sleep disturbances play a role in its morbidity and adversely affect quality of life. Poor sleep quality could contribute to poor COPD-related outcomes such as exacerbations or even mortality risk [14].

2. Oxgen desaturation during sleep in COPD patients and sleep problems

Sleep is a physiological situation that occurs depending on the special functional organization of the central nervous system. Each individual feels the need to sleep later in the evening and sleeping occurs generally at night [15]. Normal sleeping is divided into non-rapid eye movement (NREM) and rapid eye movement (REM). NREM consists of three stages: N1, N2 and N3 (quiet sleep or delta sleep). Strong stimuli are required to wake up someone whose NREM stages proceed. REM has tonic and phasic components. REM sleep has a parasympathetically medicated tonic component and sympathetically mediated phasic component. The phasic component of REM sleep is characterized by skeletal muscle twitches, increased heart rate variability, pupil dilation, and increased respiratory rate [16-18]. During NREM sleep, the metabolic demand of the brain decreases and the blood flow throughout the entire brain progressively decreases [19-21].

In order to understand the effect of COPD on respiration during sleep, one should principally know the physiological changes occurring during the periods of regular sleep and wakefulness. While the respiratory system provides the oxygen that the body needs on one part, it helps remove the carbon dioxide produced by the body's metabolic processes on the other part. Arrangement of the functions of the respiratory system basically occurs through negative feedback [3]. Ventilation is normally controlled by a combination of two systems: a metabolic system responsible for the automatic changes directly related to gas exchange, and a behavioral system responsible for the voluntary changes originating from cortical and forebrain structures [22-23].

While metabolic rate decreases during sleep, responses to various chemical, mechanical, and cortical stimuli also decrease. The respiratory response to the changes observed in the partial oxygen and partial carbon dioxide pressures in the arterial blood differs significantly in comparison to the wakefulness period [24]. Especially during REM sleep, such physiological changes may affect gas exchange and lead to hypoventilation resulting in clinically significant hypoxemia and hypercapnia in patients with COPD [25].

The most pronounced hypoxemia occurs during the REM stage of sleep because of the generalized muscle hypotonia that accompanies this stage [26]. REM-associated hypoxemia can reach critically low levels, especially in patients with already borderline waking oxygenation, with potentially deleterious clinical consequences such as cardiac dysrhythmias, pulmonary hypertension, and polycythemia [21,26].

Sleep affects respiration through changes in control of the respiratory center, in airway resistance, and in muscle contractility. These changes which usually are not consequential in healthy people may cause problems in patients with COPD. The gas exchange which occurs during sleep in patients with COPD arises as a result of the nature of the disease [3,27]. In COPD, breathing against expiratory airflow obstruction becomes more difficult during sleep when there is reduced tidal volume, ineffective ventilation, and hypoxemia [28]. Patients with COPD experience the most profound hypoxemia and hypercapnia during REM sleep [26]. The oxygen desaturation which occurs during sleep in COPD may be greater than that which occurs during maximal exercise [29]. This desaturation predisposes to cardiac arrhythmias at night [28,30], pulmonary hypertension [28,31,32] and probably deaths during acute attacks [33].

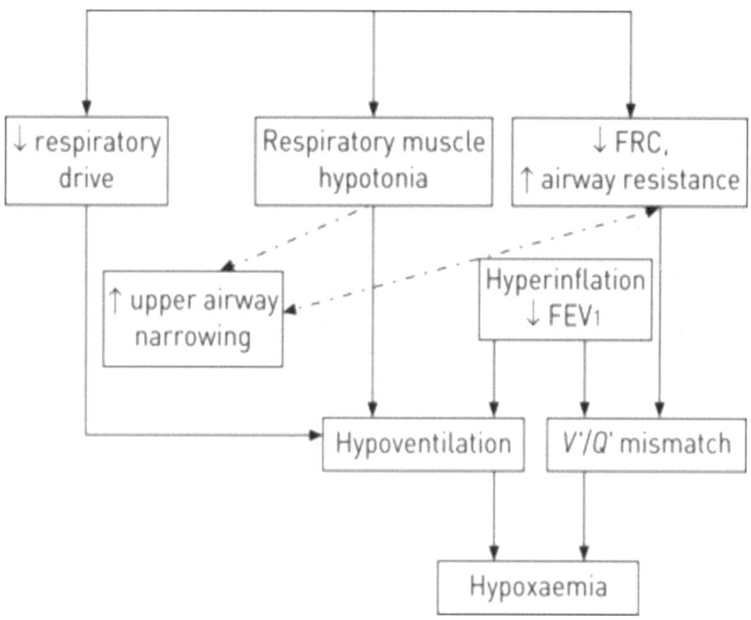

FRC=functional residual capacity; FEV_1=forced expiratory volume in 1 s; V'/Q'=ventilation/perfusion ratio;(McNicholas et al. Sleep disorders in COPD: the forgotten dimension. European Respiratory Review. 2013,22(129):365-375.)

Figure 1. Pathophysiology of sleep-related respiratory changes in chronic obstructive pulmonary disease.

COPD patients develop hypoxia and hypercapnia of varying degrees depending on the severity of their lung disease; hyperinflation occurs in the lungs due to air trapping and work of breathing increases [3]. Oxygen desaturation among the COPD patients is probably caused by physiologic hypoventilation that occurs during sleep precipitating a considerable decrease in the SaO_2 level of hypoxemic patients [28,34,35]. Hypoventilation during sleep is related to impairment of the respiratory center's response to chemical, mechanical and cortical stimuli [26,36, 37].

During sleep, ventilation/perfusion relationships are deranged. Especially in REM sleep, atony of accessory respiratory muscles develops decreasing functional residual capacity which further worsens ventilation/perfusion relationships, and hypoxemia intensifies. Decrease of intercostal muscle activity is important in patients with COPD who rely upon the use of accessory respiratory muscles to maintain respiration. Lung hyperinflation places the diaphragm, the only functioning respiratory muscle during REM sleep, at a mechanical disadvantage that also impairs oxygenation through alterations in ventilation/perfusion matching [26,37]. The compensatory efforts of the muscles that assist the diaphragm and hyperinflated lungs become inefficient after time [18,38] The diaphragm is at a mechanical disadvantage due to lung hyperinflation which adversely affects the contractile power of diaphragmatic muscle fibres (type I fibres). Such changes are of paramount importance as they restrict the effectiveness of the diaphragm during respiration [39,40]. In order to maintain respiratory effort, patients utilize accessory muscles in the chest, shoulder and abdomen. Due to atony, accessory muscles of respiration are unable to augment respiration during REM sleep which results in flattening of the diaphragm. Because the diaphragm is unable to contribute to ventilation during REM sleep, minute ventilation declines to half the daytime level. In addition, this reduction in ventilation is accompanied by deranged ventilation/perfusion (V/Q mismatch) and adequate gas exchange does not occur. As a result, arterial oxygen decreases and carbon dioxide increases. These derangements in gas exchange are more prominent among patients with COPD compared with the general population [21,38].

Drugs such as corticosteroids, methyl xanthenes and β-agonists which are used in the treatment of COPD also affect the sleep of the patient [41,42]. They can disrupt sleep and provoke sleeplessness irrespective of the severity of the patient's respiratory disease [3].

In patients with COPD, nocturnal desaturation and moderate hypoxemia are associated with an increase in pulmonary artery pressures [31,43,44]. In COPD patients, this hypoxemia associated rise in pulmonary arterial pressures is reversed with oxygen treatment [37]. In addition, in patients with COPD, premature ventricular contractions increase during sleep and oxygen treatment reduces their frequency [30].

The presence of other health problems that accompany COPD affects the occurrence and severity of sleep disorders. Patients with sleep apnea who do not have COPD experience rapid normalization of oxygen levels after apnea associated desaturations. However, in patients who suffer from both COPD and sleep apnea, apnea associated oxygen desaturation is more profound and longer because these patients are already hypoxic when the apnea begins. Therefore, patients with COPD are at risk for complications caused by chronic hypoxia like cor pulmonale and polycythemia [37].

Krachman et al summarized the potential consequences of changes in ventilatory control and respiratory muscle function during sleep in patients with chronic obstructive pulmonary disease (COPD) in Figure 2. [21]

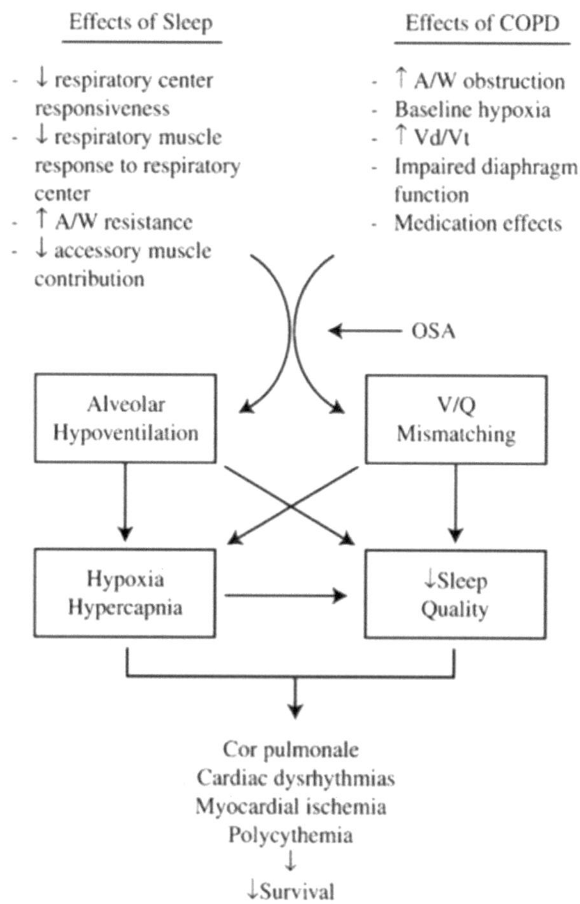

A/W=airways; OSA=obstructive sleep apnea. V/Q=ventilation/perfusion ratio. Vd/Vt=ratio of dead space volume to tidal volume.
(Krachman et al. Sleep abnormalities and treatment in emphysema. Proc Am Thorac Soc, 2008, 5(4):536-542)

Figure 2. Potential consequences of changes in ventilatory control and respiratory muscle function during sleep in patients with chronic obstructive pulmonary disease (COPD)

3. Evaluation of sleep and sleep quality in COPD patients

Many patients with COPD experience nocturnal respiratory symptoms which interrupt sleep. When the frequency and severity of night symptoms increase, sleep quality decreases [26]. Sleep quality in patients with COPD is decreased both subjectively and objectively. Indicators of poor sleep quality include the subjective complaints of difficulty falling and staying asleep, morning tiredness, early awakenings, and excessive daytime sleepiness [14,45, 46]. Cormick et al. asked patients with emphysema about their perception of sleep quality and found that 72% complained of daytime sleepiness, 32% reported impaired daytime concentration, and 28% complained of early morning headaches [14]. Sleeping problems seen in COPD patients are related to oxygen desaturation which occurs depending on the severity of the disease [37, 47]. During sleep, especially during REM, respiratory muscle function and the responsiveness of the respiratory centre to chemical stimulants decrease. Thus, COPD patients are at higher risk of developing nocturnal desaturation. Desaturation during sleep is considered a major determinant of disturbed sleep among COPD patients [48]. McSerry et al (2012) reported that sleep quality is poor in patients with severe COPD compared with individuals of similar age who do not have sleep apnea. Daytime hypoxaemia is independently associated with impaired sleep efficiency [49]. Kinsman et al. (1983) stated that disordered sleep is the third main complaint after dyspneoa and fatigue in patients with COPD and approximately half of the patients experience sleep disruption "always" or "generally always"[50]. Tel at al. (2006) determined that sleep quality is poor in patients with COPD and there is a significant relationship between the anxiety levels of patients and poor sleep quality [11]. Valipour et al. (2011) determined that compared with healthy people, patients with COPD experience more insomnia and sleep disorders [51].

Insomnia, nightmares, and somnulence are higher in patients with COPD than in the general population [52]. Nearly half of the patients with COPD stated that their quality of sleep was considerably impaired [37]. Valipour et al (2011) determined that insomnia, and sleep-maintenance difficulty occur frequently in patients with COPD [51]. Polysomnographic studies show that in patients with COPD, the sleep duration is shortened, arousals and awakenings occur frequently, and slow wave and REM sleep are shortened [14].

Poor quality of sleep in patients with COPD occurs as a result of many factors: age, severity of COPD, medications, underlying depression, and underlying sleep disorders [11,13,37,48]. George and Bayliff (2003) showed that the frequency of sleep disorders increases with the severity of the underlying pulmonary disease in COPD patients [41]. Pulmonary symptoms experienced by the patients also cause sleep disorders [53]. Omachi et al. (2012) found that sleep disorders are related to cough, dyspnoea and severity of illness in COPD patients. While many COPD patients suffer from the problem of excessive secretions, coughing to produce sputum/secretion results in interruptions in the sleep of the patients. Considering the sleep habits of the patients, most of them report that their sleep is frequently disrupted due to respiratory distress, cough and sputum production at night [54]. Using qualitative methods, Aydın Tel et al. (2012) showed that the majority of patients with COPD stated that their respiratory symptoms adversely affected their sleep [55].

Examples of patients' comments illustrating how their COPD affected their sleep include: Patient A *"Due to this disease, everything is problematic, including going to the toilet, having bath, dressing up, lying on the bed, sitting up and turning right and left. I become short of breath and I can do nothing."*

Patient B, *"Sometimes I have a stuffed throat and become short of breath during sleep and then wake up by fluttering. I can never sleep on my back, I always lie laterally. I sleep while sitting and sometimes, I fall while sleeping."* [55]. Many COPD patients prefer to sleep in a chair instead of lying supine in order to ease breathing and improve sleeping. This way of sleeping pulls the diaphragm downwards and relaxes the respiratory mechanism [3]. Thus, COPD patients frequently prefer this position to sleep more comfortably and soundly.

Sleep disorders are also closely associated with the fatigue experienced by COPD patients. Patients with sleep disorders suffer from daytime chronic fatigue and lethargy and, therefore, their life quality is poorer [14, 56]. Poor sleep quality leads to various dysfunctions in COPD patients by causing daytime excessive sleepiness and changing neuro-cognitive and psycho-motor wakefulness [25].

Although the exact impact of chronic sleep disorders on the pulmonary function of COPD patients is not known, interruptions in sleep may cause slight decreases in the forced vital capacity as well as at the forced expiratory volume in one second [57].

The most frequent sleep problems detected in patients with COPD are insomnia, waking up early in the morning, headache, and daytime sleepiness. Their prevalence varies between 30 % and 70 % in COPD patients [14, 45,52]. Klink et al. (1994) reported that 52.8% of COPD patients suffer from insomnia and daytime lethargy [58]. Subjective complaints related to sleep problems are accompanied by respiratory symptoms such as cough, dyspnoea, wheezing, and producing sputum [25]. Sleep disorders associated with COPD affect the quality of sleep deeply through multiple mechanisms. Omachi et al (2012) showed that sleep disorders experienced by COPD patients predict utilization of emergency services due to acute COPD exacerbations [54].

Successful COPD management requires consideration of all of the disease's effects on each person, not just from the perspective of COPD's main respiratory manifestations like dyspneoa, cough, and phlegm. Within this context, the relationship between pulmonary function and sleep shouldn't go unnoticed and a careful sleep history should be elicited from all patients with COPD. The first phase of effective disease management includes a diagnostic assessment of the patient and collecting the essential data to plan the treatment and care requirements accurately. Only successful disease management will eliminate the symptoms of COPD and improve a patient's clinical course. Hynnien et al. (2007) determined that anxiety, depression, and sleep disorders are associated with poor health perception by patients. According to their results, all patients should be assessed for anxiety, depression, sleep disorders, and daily functions irrespective of the severity/phase of their COPD [59]. Deficiencies in disease management result in the intensification of COPD symptoms, emergence of sleep disorders, significant changes in the cognitive functions, deterioration of the disease, and even death.

According to the results of the study conducted by Omachi et al. (2012), the relationship between sleep and pulmonary disorders in COPD patients is summarized in Figure 3 [54]. Seemingly, sleep disorders are experienced by all COPD patients and may lead to significant complications although their severities and intensities may be different. Thus, sleep habits of COPD patients and the factors affecting these habits should be assessed comprehensively [54].

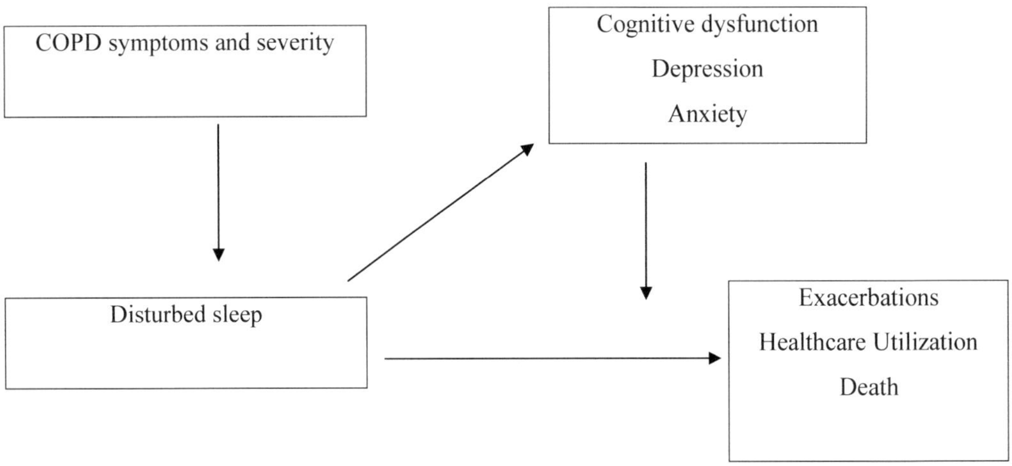

Figure 3. Omachi et al.(2012) Disturbed sleep among COPD patients is longitudinally associated with mortality and adverse COPD outcomes. Sleep Med, 2012, 13(5):476-483.

Most patients with COPD have poor sleep quality [11,36, 60,61]. Moreover, some studies suggest that in COPD patients, sleep quality is the most important health factor affecting quality of life. [36,62,63]. These results show that all COPD patients should be evaluated for symptoms of sleep disorders, snoring during sleep and potential sleep apnea syndrome symptoms like observable apneas [37]. In the clinical evaluation of COPD patients, questions to determine the sleep quality of patients and the potential existence of sleep apnea syndrome should be elicited.

Oxygen therapy, drug treatment, non-pharmacological approaches and sleep hygiene are the interventions recommended for COPD patients suffering from sleep disorders.

When discussing sleep problems in patients with COPD, the patient's respiratory symptoms should be discussed. Reduction in respiratory symptoms such as dyspnea and cough may be the initial management goals that will improve sleep quality [37]. When it is needed, nocturnal oxygen treatment should be provided and, as far as possible in patients with severe COPD, the use of hypnotics should be avoided [37]. The most important intervention is to prevent nocturnal hypoxemia [26]. Nocturnal oxygen treatment is suggested in cases of hypoxemia complications [37]. In a study of oxygen therapy on sleep quality Calverly et al. (1982) concluded that oxygen therapy increases REM sleep and sleep continuity and reduces sleep latency [64].

COPD medications may have varying effects on sleep quality. Theophylline [65] and anticholinergic medicines may ameliorate nocturnal desaturation and ipratropium increases sleep quality [66]. Ipratropium bromide enhances sleep quality, abrogates nocturnal oxygen desaturation, improves perceived sleep quality, and increases REM sleep duration without any effects on other sleep phases or total sleep duration [66]. On the other hand, while some studies examining the effect of Theophylline on sleep quality reported that it caused deterioration of sleep quality [65], other studies revealed that it had no effect on sleep quality [67-69].

Because of the potentional negative effects of benzodiazepines on ventilation, these medicines should be avoided in patients with COPD [70]. It is recommended not to use benzodiazepines in the patients with COPD as they may exacerbate the frequency, duration, and severity of nocturnal hypoxemia [71].

In patients with COPD, treatments that improve lung function and gas exchange should improve sleep quality and overall health [72]. In COPD patients, good sleep quality also contributes to better overall health of patients [73]. Soler et al. (2013) showed that pulmonary rehabilitation is effective in improving the sleep quality of patients with COPD [74]. Increased awareness by medical professionals of the sleep problems of patients with COPD is important, since the sleep quality has an effect on patients' quality of life. In addition to treatment approaches that improve lung function and help the symptoms of the disease to be brought under control such as pulmonary rehabilitation, sleep and sleep hygiene education will help COPD patients acquire a high quality sleep pattern and increase their sleep quality.

Like patients with any chronic disease, patients with COPD who have perceptions of poor health are likely to experience anxiety, depression, sleep disturbance, and problems with daily functioning. Lee et al. (2011) suggested that these findings show the need to screen routinely for sleep disturbance in patients with COPD and support the potential benefits of interventions to enhance self-efficacy and quality of sleep in reducing depression in COPD patients [75].

There are some studies examining the effectiveness of pulmonary rehabilitation in eliminating sleep disorders in COPD patients. Soler et al. (2013) showed that pulmonary rehabilitation produced significant improvements in life quality perceptions of patients in relation to dyspnoea, exercise tolerance, self-effectiveness and health while 19% of the patients had improved/advanced sleep quality. Soler et al. (2013) suggested that pulmonary rehabilitation may be an effective, non-pharmacologic treatment option for sleep problems in patients with COPD [74].

Most of the patients with COPD suffering from sleep problems report a lack of support from their physicians and few received advice for sleep problems [13]. Sleep problems in patients with COPD may need specific evaluation [6]. Assessment of the sleep problems of patients with COPD is an issue that should not be ignored during routine care. Sleep characteristics of the patient should be assessed. The impact on sleep duration and quality can be recorded using validated tools such as the Pittsburgh Sleep Quality Index [76].

Another approach is to measure the emergence of daytime symptoms, such as day time sleepiness or fatigue, related to sleep deprivation. Daytime sleepiness can be assessed by the Epworth Sleepiness Scale [77]. The St George's Respiratory Questionnaire includes one question about sleep disturbance caused by cough or breathlessness [6]. For assessment of the impact of night-time symptoms and sleep disturbance in COPD, the COPD and Asthma Sleep Impact Scale may be used [78]. The patient should be informed adequately about all the processes in order to engage his/her participation in the practices aimed at solving the sleep problems. As stress and anxiety due to a lack of information will affect sleep, patients should be provided with adequate and timely information.

Restlessness, anxiety, confusion, and sleeplessness experienced by the patients with COPD are common symptoms of hypoxia and hypoxemia. To detect these symptoms, consciousness level and mental status of the patient should be monitored routinely. Supporting the positions that will ease the respiration of the patient and changing the position, if necessary, will help the patient breathe more comfortably. Patients with COPD frequently prefer sleeping in an upright position instead of lying on their back [53].

Encouraging and supporting the patients to produce sputum will facilitate clearance of secretions and ease breathing. To improve sleep quality of patients with COPD, health professionals can recommend some interventions such as maintaining a regular sleep and wake schedule, establishing a regular relaxing bedtime routine, restricting their activities in bed to sleep and sex, not for other stimulating activities, creating a sleep environment that is cool, dark, and comfortable and avoiding caffeine in the hours before bedtime.

4. Conclusion

Sleep, a physiological necessity, is important for all people in order to attain physical, psychological, and emotional wellness. However, in some situations, sleep may be stressful for patients especially those with COPD. Sleep disorders experienced by COPD patients adversely affect their sleep quality. Although patients with COPD frequently experience sleep problems and their sleep quality is unsatisfactory, healthcare providers do not review regularly their sleep characteristics and quality. The routine examination of patients with COPD should include a review of sleep symptoms and sleep quality to ascertain the effects of sleep disturbances on their lives. Only through the active assessment of a comprehensive sleep history can sleep disorders be diagnosed and managed. Healthcare personnel who provide holistic care will assess patients' sleep problems and symptoms. This approach will help to diagnose sleep problems early, initiate appropriate interventions and management, and improve patients' wellness.

Author details

Hatice Tel Aydin

Cumhuriyet University Health Sciences Faculty, Sivas, Turkey

References

[1] Mannino DM. Epidemiology, prevelance, morbidity and mortality, and disease heterogeneity. Chest 2002;121(5) 121S-126S.

[2] Chronic Obstructive Pulmonary Disease(COPD). www.who.int/respiratory/copd/ (accessed 4 December 2013)

[3] Sharafkhaneh A, Jayaraman G, Kaleekal T, Sharafkhaneh H, Hirshkowitz M. Sleep disorders and their management in patients with COPD. Therapeutic Advances in Respiratory Disease 2009;3(6) 309-318.

[4] Kelly C, Lynes D. Psychological effects of chronic lung disease. Nursing Times 2008;104(47) 82-85.

[5] Andreassen H, Vestbo J. Chronic obstructive pulmonary disease as a systemic disease: an epidemiological perspectives. Eur Respir J Suppl 2003;46 2-4.

[6] Agusti AG. COPD a multicomponent disease: implications for management. Respir Med 2005;99(6):670-82.

[7] Willgoos T, Yohannes A, Goldbart J, Fatoye F. COPD and anxiety: is impact on patients' live. Nursing Times, 2011;107(15): http://www.nursingtimes.net/nursing-practice/clinical-zones/copd/copd-and-anxiety-its-impact-on-patients-lives/5028743.article(accessed 10 February 2012)

[8] Wilson I. Depression in the patient with COPD. International Journal of COPD 2006;1(1) 61–64.

[9] Mikkelsen RL, Middelboe T, Pisinger C, Stage KB. Anxiety and depression in patients with chronic obstructive pulmonary disease (COPD). A review. Nord J Psychiatry 2004; 58(1) 65-70.

[10] Suh S, Ellis RJ, Sollers JJ, Thayer JF, Yanh HC, Emery CF. The effect of anxiety on heart rate variability, depression, and sleep in Chronic Obstructive Pulmonary Disease. Journal of Psychosomatic Research 2013; 75-4(5) 407-413.

[11] Tel H, Tel H, Alp F. Sleep quality, anxiety and depression in patients with chronic obstructive pulmonary disease. Neurology Psychiatry and Brain Research 2006; 13(3) 131-134.

[12] Wong CJ, Goodridge D, Marciniuk DD, Rennie D. Fatigue in patients with COPD participating in a pulmonary rehabilitation program. International Journal of Chronic Obstructive Pulmonary Disease 2010; 5 319–326.

[13] Shackell BS, Jones RCM, Harding G, Pearse S, Campbell J. Am I going to see the next morning? A qualitative study of patients' perpectives of sleep in COPD. Primary Care Respiratory Journal 2007;16(6) 378-383.

[14] Cormick W, Olson LG, Hensley MJ, Saunders NA. Nocturnal hypoxaemia and quality of sleep in patients with chronic obstructive lung disease. Thorax 1986;41(11) 846-54.

[15] Rodenstein DO. Sleep disorders in patients with pulmonay disease. In. Pulmonary Rehabilitation Guidelines to Succes.(Eds. Hodgkin JE, Celli BR, Connors GL) Fourth Edition, Mosby Elsevier, 2009, p:417-431.

[16] Morrison AR. Coming to grips with a "new" state of consciousness: the study of rapid-eye-movement sleep in the 1960s. J Hist Neurosci. 2013;22(4):392-407.

[17] Tobaldini E, Nobili L, Strada S, Casali KR, Braghiroli A, Montano N. Heart rate variability in normal and pathological sleep. *Front Physiol*. 2013,16(4):294.

[18] Stevens MS, Benbadis SR. Normal sleep, sleep physiology, and sleep deprivation. emedicine.medscape.com/article/1188226-overview=a30(accessed 20 November 2013).

[19] Braun AR, Balkin TJ, Wesensten NJ, Oarsan RE, Varga M, Baldwin P, Selbie S, Belenky G, Hercovitch P. Regional cerebral blood flow throughout the sleep-wake cycle. An H2(15)O PET study. *Brain*. 1997,120 (7):1173-97.

[20] Desseilles M, Dang-Vu T, Schabus M, Sterpenich V, Maquet P, Schwartz S. Nueroimaging insights into the pathophysiology of sleep disorders. *Sleep*. 2008,31(6):777-94.

[21] Krachman S, Minai OA, Scharf SM. Sleep abnormalities and treatment in emphysema. Proc Am Thorac Soc, 2008, 5(4):536-542.

[22] Gay PC. Chronic Obstructive Pulmonary Disease and Sleep. Respiratory Care. 2004,49(1):39-51.

[23] McNicholas WT, Verbraecken J, Marin JM. Sleep disorders in COPD: the forgotten dimension. European Respiratory Review. 2013,22(129):365-375.

[24] Berthon-Jones M, Sullivan CE. Ventilatory and arousal responses to hypoxia in sleeping humans. Am Rev Respir Dis 1982;125 632-9.

[25] Ramar K. Sleep problems in chronic obstructive pulmonary disease. Tur Toraks Der 2008; 9 117-123.

[26] Ezzie ME, Parsons JP, Mastronarde JG. Sleep and Obstructive Lung Diseases. Sleep Med Clin 2008; 3(4) 505-515.

[27] McNicholas WT. Impact of sleep in COPD. Chest. 2000; 117(2 Suppl) 48S-53S.

[28] Douglas NJ. Sleep in patients with chronic obstructive pulmonary disease. Clin Chest Med 1998;19(1) 115-25.

[29] Mulloy E, McNicholas WT. Ventilation and gas exchange during sleep and exercise in patients with severe COPD. Chest 1996;109(2) 387–394.

[30] Tirlapur VG, Mir MA. Nocturnal hypoxemia and associated electrocardiographic changes in patients with chronic obstructive airways disease. N Engl J Med 1982; 306(3) 125–130.

[31] Levi-Valensi P, Weitzenblum E, Rida Z, Aubry P, Braghiroli A, Donner C, Aprill M, Zielinski J, Würtemberger G. Sleep-related oxygen desaturation and daytime pulmonary hemodynamics in COPD patients. Eur Resp J 1992; 5(5) 301–307.

[32] Fletcher EC, Luckett RA, Miller T, Costarangos C, Kutka N, Fletcher JG. Pulmonary vascular hemodynamics in chronic lung disease patients with and without oxyhemoglobin desaturation during sleep. Chest 1989; 95(4) 757–766.

[33] McNicholas WT, FitzGerald MX. Nocturnal death among patients with chronic bronchitis and emphysema. BMJ 1984; 289(6449) 878.

[34] Hudgel DW, Martin RJ, Capehart M, Johnson B, Hill P. Contribution of hypoventilation to sleep oxygen desaturation in chronic obstructive pulmonary disease. J Appl Physiol 1983; 55(3) 669–677.

[35] Fletcher E C, Miller J, Divine G W, Fletcher J G, Miller T. Nocturnal oxyhemoglobin desaturation in COPD patients with arterial oxygen tensions above 60 mm Hg. Chest 1987; 92(4) 604-8.

[36] Nunes DM, Mota RMS, Neto OLP, Pereira EDB, de Bruin VMS, de Bruin PFC. Impaired sleep reduces quality of life in chronic obstructive pulmonary disease. Lung 2009;187(3) 159-163.

[37] McNicholson W, McNee W, Celli BR. Management of stable COPD: Sleep. In Standards for the Diagnosis and Management of Patients with COPD. American Thorasic Society and European Thorasic Society 2004; 152-158.

[38] Common sense Respiratory "COPD". www.rotech.com/respiratory/documents/CSR-COPD(accessed 10 November 2013).

[39] Ottenheijm CA, Heunks LM, Dekhuijzen PN. Diaphragm muscle fiber dysfunction in chronic obstructive pulmonary disease: toward a pathophysiological concept. Am J Respir Crit Care Med 2007;175(12) 1233-40.

[40] Levine S, Kaiser L, Leferovich J, Tikunov B. Cellular adaptations in the diaphragm in chronic obstructive pulmonary disease. N Engl J Med 1997; 337(25) 1799-806.

[41] George CF, Bayliff CD. Management of insomnia in patients with chronic obstructive pulmonary disease. Drugs 2003;63(4) 379-87.

[42] Kutty K. Sleep and chronic obstructive pulmonary disease. Curr Opin Pulm Med 2004; 10(2) 104-12.

[43] Ballard RD, Clover CW, Suh BY. Influence of sleep on respiratory function in emphysema. Am J Respir Crit Care Med 1995;151(4) 945-51.

[44] Connaughton JJ, Catterall JR, Elton RA, Stradling JR, Douglas NJ. Do sleep studies contribute to the management of patients with severe chronic obstructive pulmonary disease? Am Rev Respir Dis 1988;138(2) 341-4.

[45] Bellia V, Catalano F, Scichilone N, Incalzi RA, Spatafora M, Vergani C, et al. Sleep disorders in the elderly with and without chronic airflow obstruction: the SARA study. Sleep 2003;26 318–323.

[46] Dodge R, Cline MG, Quan SF. The natural history of insomnia and its relationship to respiratory symptoms. Arch Intern Med 1995;155:1797–1800.

[47] Krachman SL, Chatila W, Martin UJ, Permut I, D'Alonzo GE, Gaughan JP, Sternberg AL, Ciccolella D, Criner GJ. Physiologic correlates of sleep quality in sever emphysema. COPD: Journal of Chronic Obstructive Pulmonary Disease 2011; 8(3) 182-188.

[48] De S. Subjective assessment of quality of sleep in chronic obstructive pulmonary disease patient and its relationship with associated depression. Lung India 2012; 29(4) 332-335.

[49] McSharry DG, Ryan S, Calverley P, Edwards JC, McNicholas WT. Sleep quality in chronic obstructive pulmonary disease. Respirology 2012;17(7) 1119-1124.

[50] Kinsman RA, Yaroush RA, Fernandes E, Dirks JF, Schocket M, Fukuhara J. Symptoms and experiences in chronic bronchitis and emphysema. Chest 1983; 83(5) 755-61.

[51] Valipour A, Lavie P, Lothaller H, Mikulic I, Burghuber OC. Sleep profile and symptoms of sleep disorders in patients with mild to moderate chronic obstructive pulmonary disease. Sleep Medicine 2011;12(4) 367-372.

[52] Klink M, Quan SF. Prevalence of reported sleep disturbances in a general adult population and their relationship to obstructive airways diseases. Chest 1987; 91 540-6.

[53] Sleep disorders. http://www.sleepfoundation.org/article/sleep-related-problems. (accessed 12 March 2013).

[54] Omachi TA, Blanc PD, Claman DM, Chen H, Yelin EH, Katz PP. Disturbed sleep among COPD patients is longitudianally associated with mortality and adverse COPD outcomes. Sleep Med 2012;13(5):476-483

[55] Aydın Tel H, Yıldız Tok F, Karagözoğlu Ş, Özden D. Hastaların Bakış Açısıyla Kronik Obstrüktif Akciğer Hastalığı ile Yaşamak: Fenomenolojik Çalışma. İ Ü F N Hem Derg 2012;20(3):177-183. (Aydın Tel H, Yıldız Tok F, Karagözoğlu Ş, Özden D. Living with Chronic Obstructive Pulmonary Disease from the perspective of patients: A phenomenological study. IUFN Nurs J 2012;20(3):177-183).

[56] Breslin E, Van der Schans C, Breubink S, et al. Perception of fatigue and quality of life in patients with COPD. Chest 1998; 114(4) 958–964.

[57] Phillips BA, Cooper KR, Burke TV. The effect of sleep loss on breathing in chronic obstructive pulmonary disease. Chest 1987;91(1) 29–32.

[58] Klink ME, Dodge R, Quan SF. The relation of sleep complaints to respiratory symptoms in the general population. Chest 1994;105 151–154.

[59] Hynninen MJ, Pallesen S, Nordhus IH. Factors affecting health status in COPD patients with co-morbid anxiety or depression. Int J Chron Obstruct Pulmon Dis 2007; 2(3) 323-8.

[60] Santos CEVG, Viegas CAA. Sleep pattern in patients with chronic obstructive pulmonary disease and correlation among gasometric, spirometric, and polysomnographic variables. J Pneumol 2003;29(2) 69-74.

[61] Fleetham J, West P, Mezon B, Conway W, Roth T, Kryger MH. Sleep, arousals and oxygen desaturation in chronic obstructive pulmonary disease. The effect of oxygen therapy. Am rev Respir Dis 1982;126(3) 429-433.

[62] Zohal MA, Yazdı Z, Kazemifar AM. Daytime sleepiness and quality of sleep in patients with COPD compared to control group. Global Journal of Health Science 2013; 5(3) 150-155.

[63] Scharf SM, Maimon N, Simon-Tuval T, Bernard-Scharf BJ, Reuveni H, Tarasuik A. Sleep quality predicts quality of life in chronic obstructive pulmonary disease. Internetional Journal of COPD 2011; 6(1) 1-12.

[64] Calverley PM, Brezinova V, Douglas NJ, Catterall JR, Flenley DC. The effect of oxygenation. Chest 1987;92(4) 604-608.

[65] Mulloy E, McNicholas WT. Theophylline improves gas exchange during rest, exercise and sleep in severe chronic obstructive pulmonary disease. Am Rev Respir Dis 1993; 148(4) 1030–1036.

[66] Martin RJ, Bartelson BL, Smith P, Hudgel DW, Lewis D, Pohl G, Koker P, Souhrada JF. Effect of ipratropium bromide treatment on oxygen saturation and sleep quality in COPD. Chest 1999;115(5) 1338–1345.

[67] Berry RB, Desa MM, Branum JP, Light RW. Effect of theophylline on sleep and sleep-disordered breathing in patients with chronic obstructive pulmonary disease. Am Rev Respir. Dis 1991;143 245-50.

[68] Man GC, Champman KR, Ali SH, Darke AC. Sleep quality and nocturnal respiratory function with once-daily theophylline (Uniphyl) and inhaled salbutamol in patients with COPD. Chest 1996;110 648-53.

[69] Martin RJ, Pak J. Overnight theophylline concentrations and effects on sleep and lung function in chronic obstructive pulmonary disease. Am Rev Respir Dis 1992;145 540-4.

[70] Steens R, Pouliot Z, Millar T, Kryger M, George C. Effects of Zolpidem and Triazolam on sleep and respiration in mild to moderate chronic obstructive pulmonary disease. Sleep 1993;16(4) 318–326.

[71] Block AJ, Dolly FR, Slayton PC. Does flurazepam ingestion affect breathing and oxygenation during sleep in patients with chronic obstructive lung disease? Am Rev Respir Dis 1984;129 230-3.

[72] Urbano F, Mohsenin V. Chronic obstructive pulmonary disease and sleep: The interaction. Panminerva Medica 2006; 48(4) 223-230.

[73] Mohsenin V. Sleep in Chronic Obstructive Pulmonary Disease. Sleep Medicine Clinics 2007; 2(1) 1-8.

[74] Soler X, Diaz-Piedra C, Ries AL. Pulmonary rehabilitation improves sleep quality in chronic lung disease. COPD. Journal of Chronic Obstructive Pulmonary Disease 2013; 10(2) 156-163.

[75] Lee H, Kim I, Lim Y, Jung HY, Park HK. Depression and sleep disturbance in patients with chronic obstructive pulmonary disease. Geriatr Nurs 2011; 32(6) 408-17.

[76] Backhaus J, Junghanns K, Broocks A. Et al. Test-retest reliability and valisdity of Pittsburgh Sleep Quality Index in primary insomnia. J Psychosom Res 2002;53 737-740.

[77] Johns MW. A new method for measuring daytime sleepiness: the Epworth Sleepines Scale. Sleep 1991;14 540-545.

[78] Pokrzywinski RF, Meads DM, McKenna SP, et al. Development and psychometric assessment of COPd and Asthma Sleep Impact Scale(CASIS). Health Quality Life Outcomes 2009;7, 98.

Chapter 7

Advances in Comprehensive Pulmonary Rehabilitation for COPD Patients

R. Martín-Valero, M.C. Rodríguez-Martínez,
R. Cantero-Tellez, E. Villanueva-Calvero and
F. Fernández-Martín

Additional information is available at the end of the chapter

http://dx.doi.org/10.5772/57563

1. Introduction

Physical inactivity (lack of exertional pursuits) is the fourth leading risk factor for mortality worldwide and contributes to 6% of all deaths. Only hypertension, smoking, and diabetes are associated with greater mortality [1]. In addition, nearly 5% of worldwide mortality is caused by excessive weight [2]. Numerous prospective, observational studies suggest that the least active and unfit people are at the greatest risk for developing a variety of chronic diseases [3]. Physical inactivity has been identified as an independent risk factor for cardiovascular disease, diabetes, hypertension, obesity, osteoporosis, colon, breast and other cancers, depression, anxiety and other illnesses [4].

Chronic Obstructive Pulmonary disease (COPD) is the most common chronic lung disease and is the fourth leading cause of death in the world. COPD has a high impact on patients′ wellbeing, health care utilization, and mortality [5] and causes a substantial and increasing economic and social burden [6, 7].

As COPD worsens and individuals experience increasing respiratory symptoms, a vicious cycle develops whereby activity declines, walking speed is reduced, fitness levels decline, and activities of daily living become too difficult to carry out, eventually causing disability and dependence [8]. Physical activity is reduced in severe COPD [9] but the level of activity in individuals with moderate COPD is less well studied. Hence, inactivity may not only be a manifestation of disease severity in COPD but may also contribute to disease progression [10]. In a recent study of the patterns of physical activity including the frequency, duration and intensity of episodes of physical activity, patients with COPD wore the SenseWear® armband accelerometer for eight consecutive days [11]. With increasing COPD severity, time in physical activity, proportion of time performing activities, and frequency of activity decreased. These objective outcomes provide the best measures of physical activity [12].

COPD is characterized by inexorably progressive, non-normalizing airflow limitation and the severity of obstruction correlates with its morbidity and mortality [5, 13]. Based upon the presence of oxidative stress, increased levels of circulating cytokines, and multiple nonpulmonary manifestations, COPD is increasingly being recognized as a systemic disorder [5]. Furthermore, COPD does not manifest in a homogeneous manner and many different subgroups or phenotypes are being recognized. The polysystemic manifestations and heterogeneity of clinical and inflammatory profile presentations of COPD have led to an expanded classification in the most recent GOLD guidelines that incorporate clinical manifestations including effects on physical activity and healthcare utilization or risk in addition to physiologic impairment [5]. This multifactorial classification is used to stage COPD severity and to guide and monitor treatment [5]. In addition, the clinical course of patients with COPD is marked by repetitive exacerbations and abnormal inflammatory response which further contribute to a downward spiral of physical activity [5, 14].

Decreased caloric intake leading to nutritional depletion occurs in about 20-35% of outpatients with COPD and up to 70% of patients with acute respiratory failure or waiting for lung transplantation [15]. Cachexia, defined as weight loss with disproportional fat-free mass wasting, occurs in about one-third of patients with COPD eligible for pulmonary rehabilitation and represents a cause of increased mortality independent of ventilatory limitation [16].

2. Biochemical changes

Many of the major pathophysiologic derangements in advanced COPD have been attributed to systemic inflammation [17]. Previous studies show that systematic inflammation is induced by inflammatory cytokines, such as tumor necrosis factor (TNF-α), interleukin (IL-6) and IL-8 [18, 19]. Fat-free mass (FFM) depletion marks the imbalance between tissue protein synthesis and breakdown that occurs in COPD [20]. These inflammatory cytokines and endocrine hormones contribute to the reduction in exercise tolerance and poor quality of life caused by skeletal myopathy in COPD patients [21]. Skeletal muscle dysfunction plays an important role in the symptoms and impairments in strength, endurance, and maximal exercise capacity experienced by patients [22].

Bronchiectasis, permanent damage and widening of one or more of the large connecting bronchi (airways), may occur in nearly one third of individuals with COPD [22]. Individuals with bronchiectasis have elevated levels of proinflammatory cytokines that are associated with decreased fat-free mass, increased proteolysis and worse respiratory function [22-24]. This chronic inflammation increases the levels of oxidative stress [25, 26]. Circulating (plasma) and intracellular biomarkers of oxidative stress are increased in patients with bronchiectasis compared with control subjects [25].

Decline in nutritional status is directly related to lung function outcomes and has been proposed as a predictor of morbidity and even mortality in patients with chronic respiratory diseases independent of the ventilatory limitation [15]. Furthermore, malnutrition is accompanied by a loss of diaphragmatic and structural skeletal muscle mass, as well as humoral and cellular dysfunction [15]. Anabolic stimulation through a combination of nutritional support and exercise appears to be the best approach to improving functional status [27]. A multicenter study of stable COPD patients with a body mass index of 22 kg/m^2 and a fat-free mass index of 16 showed that the consumption of oral nutritional supplements, rich in proteins (with 50% of whey protein) produced a significant improvement in quality of life [28]. A subsequent Cochrane Database meta-analysis showed that undernourished patients with COPD improved with nutritional supplementation [29]. Malnourished patients who received supplementation had significantly better maximum inspiratory pressures and maximum expiratory pressures [29].

Thus, impaired skeletal muscle function is a potentially remediable systemic manifestation of COPD [30]. These findings have implications for identification of drug targets aimed at improving muscle function in COPD [30]. Except for markers of myogenesis, molecular responses to resistance training are not tightly coupled to lean mass gains [30].

3. Management of comprehensive pulmonary rehabilitation

Pulmonary Rehabilitation (PR) has become a cornerstone in the management of patients with stable COPD in recent years [31]. Systematic reviews show large and important clinical effects of PR in these patients [32]. PR improves anxiety and depression in patients with COPD [33]. PR also reduces the number and duration of hospitalizations [34, 35]. In addition, physical training and chest physiotherapy in respiratory disease have long-term, durable benefits [36-38]. The components of PR vary widely but a comprehensive program includes smoking cessation, education, nutrition counseling, and exercise training [5].

3.1. Educational and nutritional management

All patients enrolled in PR should receive educational and nutritional interventions as part of an integrated care plan that seeks to achieve a normal nutritional status, either through natural diet or supplements [15, 39]. Nutrition depletion occurs by multiple mechanisms including energy imbalance, disuse atrophy of the muscles, hypoxemia, systemic inflammation and oxidative stress [15]. Each of these mechanisms may represent targets for nutritional intervention.

Patients with COPD are best managed through multimodal therapies delivered through an integrated healthcare system [40]. Dietary supplementation with whey may potentiate the effects of exercise training on exercise tolerance and quality of life in patients with COPD [41]. Use of a nutritional supplement containing anti-inflammatory whey peptide with exercise therapy in stable elderly COPD patients increased body weight, reduced markers of systemic inflammation, and improved exercise levels and respiratory health [17].

There is a clear need for adequately powered and controlled intervention and maintenance trials to establish the role of nutritional supplementation in the enhancement of exercise performance and training and wider management of the systemic features of COPD [40]. Hence, combination therapy, nutritional, pharmacologic, and physical training, may produce weight gain, increases in lean mass, respiratory muscle strength, exercise capacity, lung function, and respiratory health while reducing morbidity and mortality. Physiotherapy, occupational therapy, and medical treatment are individually adjusted to each patient's needs and requirements with the goal of improving current quality of life and these targets should be re-adjusted when patients opt for palliative care [42].

Although prior reviews did not provide evidence for the usefulness of nutritional supplementation therapy, more recent analyses concluded that nutritional supplemental therapy increased weight, fat free mass, exercise tolerance, and hand grip strength in undernourished patients with COPD [29, 43, 44]. High calorie nutrition therapy and L-carnitine supplementation may be beneficial whereas no effect is observed with additional creatine [45]. The duration and type of exercise may also affect PR results. Although both low and high intensity exercise training are beneficial for patients with COPD, higher intensity lower extremity exercise yields better physiologic improvement than lower intensity exercise [46]. PR programs that are 12 weeks or longer produce enhanced and more durable results than shorter programs [43, 46]. The benefits of PR tend to wane gradually over 12 to 18 months [43, 46].

3.2. Importance of exercise training

There are two different types of Physical Exercise Training for COPD patients: endurance and interval type training [47]. Endurance or continuous programmes include constant load and incremental load training. However, patients with symptoms of severe dysnea during exercises were incapable of performing high-intensity (70 to 80 % of the peak work rate) continuous type training. Interval training is recommended as an alternative to continuous training in patients with severe symptoms of dyspnoea during exercise due to an inability to sustain continuous training at the recommended intensities. During interval training short exercise bouts (30-180 seconds) are performed at high intensity (at least 70-80% of peak work rate). Recommended frequency of training is the same as with continuous training [47]. Finally, there is evidence that regular physical activity contributes to the primary and secondary prevention of several chronic diseases and is associated with a reduced risk of premature death [48].

Physical activity is defined as any bodily movement produced by the contraction of skeletal muscle that increases energy expenditure above a basal level [49]. Exercise therapy is defined as a subcategory of physical activity in which planned, structured, and repetitive bodily movements are performed to maintain or improve one or more attributes of physical fitness [49]. Physical fitness refers to the ability to carry out daily tasks with vigor and alertness without undue fatigue and with ample energy to enjoy leisure time pursuits and to meet unforeseen emergencies [49].

Physical activity is the strongest predictor of all-cause mortality in patients with COPD [50]. Nowadays, lack of physical activity is associated with the burden of chronic disease [51]. The low levels of Physical Activity (PA) generally observed in people with COPD may be due in part to the difficulties they experience as they attempt to perform daily activities that they need and want to perform [14]. Importantly, physical inactivity is potentially reversible [52].

There is strong evidence that community physiotherapy benefits health by promoting physical activity [8, 53]. Exercise prescribed by a physiotherapist can target directly any impairments contributing to activity limitations and requires the active participation of subjects in an individualized physical exercise program [53]. Exercise training can produce significant improvement in health related quality of life, exercise capacity, respiratory muscle strength, and exertional dyspnea in patients with COPD who have normal exercise capacity [54]. Hence, enrollment in a comprehensive Pulmonary Rehabilitation Program (PRP) that includes exercise training and dietary supplementation may benefit patients with COPD. PRP may be supported by motivational counseling [55]. Furthermore, physical activity is an attractive outcome measure for interventional studies in patients with COPD.

Both physical activity and daily exercise improve the health of COPD patients [10]. It is necessary to avoid a sedentary lifestyle and encourage them to perform physical activity and exercises [10]. The performance of regular physical activity by patients with COPD reduces the risk of both hospital admissions and all-cause and respiratory mortality [10]. It appears that patients with COPD have a significantly reduced duration, intensity, and number of daily physical activities when compared with healthy control subjects [56]. Hence, the recommendation that COPD patients be encouraged to maintain or increase their levels of regular physical activity should be considered in future research [10]. A Spanish research group developed a novel alternative to formal PRP that includes a walking training circuit in the city of Catalonia [57] that has been replicated in other cities such as Navarre [58] (Figure 1).

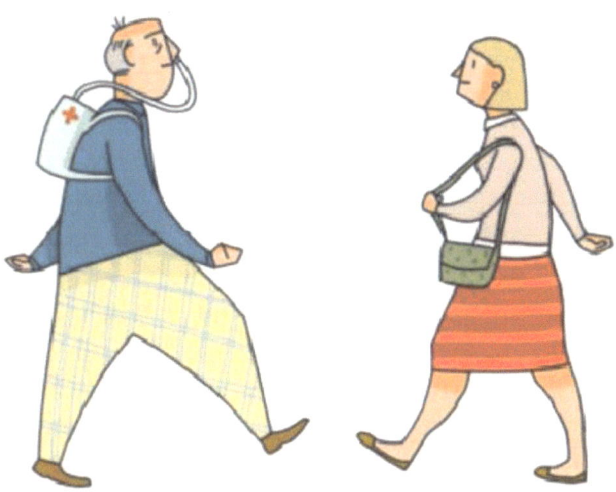

Figure 1. Walking circuits from "Walking Guide for COPD patients" [58]

3.3. Oxygen therapy

Oxygen theray is one of the therapies currently available to reduce COPD mortality [59]. Long-term oxygen therapy (LTOT) reduces pulmonary hypertension and improves survival in patients with COPD and resting hypoxemia (arterial partial pressure of oxygen ≤55 mmHg) [60].

The use of oxygen supplementation during exercise training for individuals with COPD is unclear [61]. Supplemental oxygen during exercise training improves functional outcomes such as symptoms, health-related quality of life, and ambulation [61]. However, there are no significant differences in maximal exercise outcomes, functional exercise outcomes (six-minute walk test), shuttle walk distance, health-related quality of life, or oxygenation status [61, 62].

COPD patients with low fat-free mass (FFM) have lower levels of oxidative stress with supplemental oxygen [63]. Patients with COPD are able to achieve a higher work rate during exercise training, which positively affects training results after several weeks [64]. It is generally recommended that COPD patients who are already hypoxaemic at rest should use oxygen during exercise, aiming at a rather arbitrary oxygen saturation of > 90% [64]. A review of the effect of oxygen in COPD patients with or without desaturation during exercise training concluded that hyperoxia has no clear effect on the results of exercise training in COPD patients with or without documented desaturation during exercise [64]. Only one study demonstrated a significant, and clinically relevant, improvement in higher work load during rehabilitation [65]. In conclusion, more studies are needed to define the role of supplemental oxygen in PR; for instance, on the oxygen concentration, intensity of exercise programmes, and its effects in different COPD phenotypes.

4. Measuring and improving the physical activity level in COPD patients?

Exercise tolerance is a well accepted clinical marker in COPD and provides information about disease stage, prognosis, functional capacity, and the effects of treatment [66]. The assessment of physical activity in healthy populations and in those with chronic diseases is challenging. Furthermore, physical activity is most accurately measured using objective tools such as accelerometer-based activity monitors [67]. In addition, other outcomes must be included, such as quadriceps and grip strength [68].

Physical activity monitors are frequently used to estimate levels of daily physical activity [69]. These devices use piezoelectric accelerometers, which measure the body´s acceleration, in one, two or three axes (uniaxial, biaxial or triaxial activity monitors). The signal can then be transformed into an estimate of energy expenditure using one of a variety of algorithms, or summarized as activity counts or vector magnitude units (reflecting acceleration) [69]. With the information obtained in the vertical plane or through pattern recognition, steps or walking time can also be derived from some monitors [69].

A systematic review identifies the available activity monitors that have been appropriately validated for use in assessing physical activity in these groups [70]. Forty monitors were tested in validation studies; 12 uniaxial, 3 biaxial, 16 triaxial accelerometers and 9 multisensor devices [70]. Furthermore, a recent study evaluated the validity and usability of six activity monitors in COPD patients against the double labelled water indirect calorimetry method [71]. The Actigraph GT3X and DynaPort MoveMonitor best explained the majority of the total energy expenditure variance not explained by total body water and showed the most significant correlations with activity energy expenditure [71].

Moreover, the Dynaport MiniMod and Actigraph GT3X discriminate best between different walking speeds [69]. Overall, these findings should guide the choice of valid activity monitors for research or for clinical use in patients with chronic diseases such as COPD. In a recent comparison, two types of accelerometer: the DynaPort and the Actiwatch were used in order to assess the level of physical activity [12] and compared with a multisensory armband device (SenseWear, BodyMedia; Pittsburgh, PA) [9]. The main finding of this pilot-study was the significant reduction in physical activity observed with each patient. The study provides evidence for a gradual reduction in daily physical activity levels with increasing GOLD stage, although the correlation between physical activity and lung function is weak [9].

5. Does the choice for inspiratory or expiratory muscle strength or endurance training matter?

COPD alters muscle structure and/or functional. Strength and endurance are the two main functional properties of both respiratory and peripheral muscles and reduction in either strength or endurance leads to muscle dysfunction. Strength mainly depends on muscle mass, and endurance is related to muscle fiber aerobic properties [72]. Muscle weakness is a relatively stable condition related to the loss of muscle strength which requires long-term therapeutic measures (training and/or nutritional interventions). In contrast, muscle fatigue is a temporary dysfunction related to endurance [73]. Many COPD patients experience muscle dysfunction and reduced muscle mass, primarily as a result of chronic immobilization [74]. Over the last decade, the potential use of resistance training for COPD has gained increasing attention.

A Cochrane Database Systematic Review showed that breathing exercises over four to 15 weeks improve functional exercise capacity in people with COPD compared to no intervention; however, there were no consistent and clear effects on dysnoea or health-related quality of life [75].

Muscle strength can be measured by the maximal inspiratory pressure (MIP) and maximal expiratory pressure (MEP) [76]. Inspiratory muscle training (IMT) provides breathing training together with resistance loading produced by a valve and is regarded as a mixture of strength and endurance training. IMT may improve inspiratory muscle strength, endurance, functional exercise capacity, dyspnoea, and quality of life. A question to be taken into account in the planning of a respiratory muscles training protocol in COPD patients would be to determine which is more important, inspiratory muscle strength training or endurance training. A meta-analysis showed that inspiratory muscle endurance training was less effective than respiratory muscle strength training [76]. Both types of training (strength and endurance) significantly improve the endurance of the muscles, but only strength training was able to significantly improve the MIP, the MEP and functional exercise capacity [76].

Although many resistance devices are available, the Threshold-IMT® is frequently used and produces loads of 7-41 cm H_2O. The devices produce a range of resistance levels, with lower resistance levels offered by the Threshold Inspiratory Muscle Trainer (Phillips Respironics, Murrysville, PA) and higher resistance levels offered by the POWERBreathe® (HaB International Ltd, Southam, Warwickshire, UK) and the PowerLung® (PowerLung, Houston, TX). The POWERBreathe® is only for inspiratory muscle training and has three models. The Light POWERbreathe® produces loads of 17-98 cm H_2O, the medium device delivers loads of 23-186 cm H_2O, and the heavy device achieves loads of 29-274 cm H_2O. The PowerLung® is for inspiratory and expiratory muscles training and has four models that produce varying levels of resistance [72].

The Orygen-Dual Valve® was designed and patented by researchers of Barcelona and allows both simultaneous and sequential dual training work (expiratory and inspiratory muscles) (Figure 2) [72]. The Orygen-Dual Valve® is a relatively cheap, portable, and easy to use piece of equipment that provides workloads up to 70 cm H_2O at a rate of 15-20 breaths/min [72].

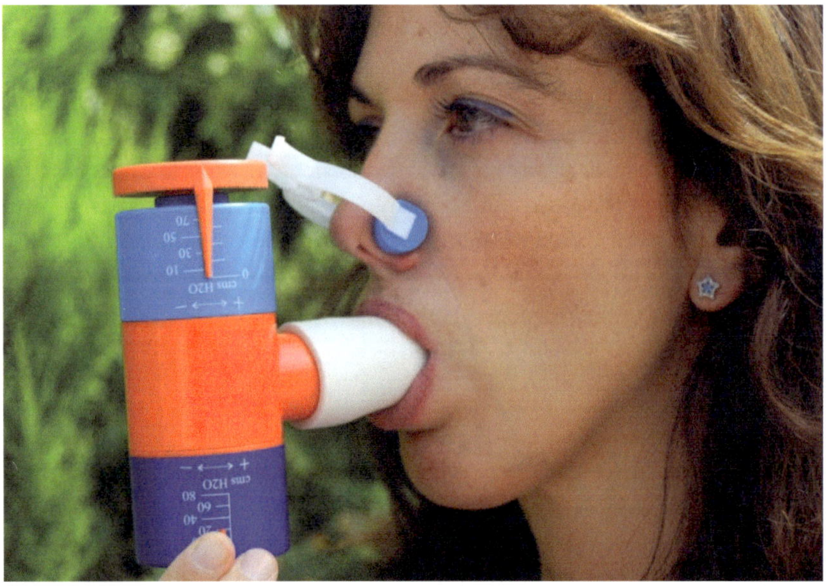

Figure 2. Martín-Valero, R. makes the rehabilitation programme with Orygen-Dual Valve®

High-intensity inspiratory muscle training improved inspiratory muscle function in subjects with moderate-to-severe COPD, producing significant reductions in dyspnoea and fatigue [77]. In addition, a 4-week supervised high-intensity respiratory training program in patients with COPD demonstrated functional improvements [78, 79]. The Orygen-Dual Valve® makes the rehabilitation programme more efficient than usual training as it requires fewer resources in terms of time and staff, and allows patients to acquire skills for further training outside the Hospital [68]. Furthermore, the hi-IMT achieves this result in a shorter time, which is an advantage for improving the efficiency of rehabilitation programmes within the public health system [72]. The training must be supervised by a therapist once a week during the first month.

The addition of high-intensity IMT to aerobic exercise produced incremental benefits in muscle weakness, cardiopulmonary function, and health-related quality of life in a randomized study of patients with chronic heart failure [80]. A multicenter randomized controlled trial is currently underway to determine whether the addition of IMT to a general exercise training program improves the distance walked in six minutes, health related quality of life, daily physical activity, and inspiratory muscle function in individuals with COPD and reduced inspiratory muscle strength [81].

6. What are the views and perceptions of people with COPD regarding a pumonary rehabilitacion?

Individuals with COPD people who complete a course of PR believe that ongoing structured exercise with professional and peer support assists them with continued regular exercise [82]. However, patients with COPD often encounter potential barriers to PR attendance including difficulties with travel to exercise venues, fluctuating health status with respiratory symptoms that impede physical activity, and psychological emotional effects including feelings of embarrassment [82, 83].

Many qualitative studies of PR in patients with COPD have been performed over the past decade to determine the impressions and opinions of PR participants. There are two main theories that have been used to analyse qualitative research [88, 89]. The first one is known as the grounded theory approach [90] and the second theory is the interpretative phenomenological analysis framework [88, 89, 91]. Qualitative research uses data collected from focus groups [82, 92], semi-structured interviews [87, 93, 94] or a combination of both methods [92, 95]. Some studies use triangulation research (96) or embed a qualitative study in a randomized controlled trial in order to explore patients' views on self-management [97]. The main areas of research were: the effect of people´s health status on exercise adherence [82], pain (85), and social relationships, such as social integration and social support [86].

It is necessary to increase strategies for self motivation among individuals with COPD [87]. Encouraging health behaviours is a key feature relating to PR participation including physical activity and smoking reduction or cessation [55]. Telephone delivery of health-mentoring is feasible and acceptable to individuals with COPD in primary care and may improve PR participation [55]. Telemonitoring of individuals with COPD enhanced self-management by improving patients' knowledge about their disease [97].

7. Occupational therapy in COPD

Patients with COPD may benefit from occupational therapy as well as physical therapy. However, there are few studies evaluating occupational therapy for individuals with COPD. A qualitative study suggested that occupational therapy may reduce breathlessness, improve mental outlook, and increase the confidence of individuals with COPD [84].

In the future, occupational therapists may be able to assess and provide rehabilitation interventions for patients with COPD [98]. Incorporation of occupational therapy in PR may increase patients' knowledge of COPD, elevate their sense of control, promote re-engagement in activities, reduce anxiety, and improve social engagement [98].

Theoretical and clinical occupational therapy supports a rehabilitation model based on continued participation in activities that are considered essential in the life of the person [99]. The respiratory symptoms of patients with COPD have an impact on activities of daily living. Occupational therapy interventions in patients with COPD aim to develop specific strategies to perform basic activities of daily living, and leisure activities, so that they involve the least possible waste of energy [100]. Through energy saving techniques, Occupational Therapy aims to reduce the patient's subjective respiratory distress. In activities of daily living training, patients learn to work efficiency and also learn economies of movement, minimizing the energy cost of dressing, personal hygiene, home care, leisure activities, shopping, and other activities related to the patients´ work [100]. Although simple, energy saving techniques require a learning process that is difficult to achieve outside of a multidisciplinary rehabilitation program [100].

Research into COPD's psychological effects on patients' ability to perform daily activities provides a wholistic approach to COPD and its consequences. The Occupational Therapy framework provides a basis for the design of a comprehensive PR intervention that addresses all aspects of a patient's life. Recent research shows that optimization of occupational performance improves the welfare of individuals with COPD [101]. Members of the patient's social network should not be excluded from these plans and interventions. Application of a family psychoeducational program based in training and information about COPD pathology including risk factors, habits that facilitate disease progression, specific strategies for handling the problems of daily life, and how to face the difficulties in occupational performance for each stage of the disease may empower the patient's friends and family to assist with rehabilitation [102]. An initial interview with the patient, family, and friends is the initial step to developing a comprehensive PR program that includes all members of the patients' social network [103].

8. Conclusion

In conclusion, a multidimensional therapeutic approach is recommended for developing a comprehensive pulmonary rehabilitation program for patients with COPD. Critical elements of PR include optimization of pharmacologic and nonpharmacologic management, exercise,

http://dx.doi.org/10.5772/57563

physical activity, ventilatory support, nutritional, and occupational therapy interventions. In addition, there is a need for new models for pulmonary rehabilitation which allow all program components to be delivered at home, with proven clinical outcomes and low costs [104]. It is possible that undertaking pulmonary rehabilitation within the home environment may promote more effective integration of exercise routines into daily life over the longer term with greater adherence to exercise [104]. In fact, home-based exercise programs achieve equivalent clinical outcomes and are cost effective compared with hospital-based programs. The decentralization of pulmonary rehabilitation increases the options for its provision and may assist in overcoming the most frequently identified barriers to pulmonary rehabilitation [104].

Author details

R. Martín-Valero, M.C. Rodríguez-Martínez, R. Cantero-Tellez, E. Villanueva-Calvero and F. Fernández-Martín

Faculty Health Sciences, Department Psychiatry and Physiotherapy, Málaga University, Spain

References

[1] Global Health risks: mortality and burden of disease atributable to selected major risks. Geneva: Organización Mundial de la Salud; 2009.

[2] Estadísticas Sanitarias Mundiales 2011. 2011; Available at: http://www.who.int/whosis/whostat/ES_WHS2011_Full.pdf. Accessed 03/01, 2012.

[3] Haskell WL, Blair SN, Hill JO. Physical activity: health outcomes and importance for public health policy. Prev Med 2009;49(4):280-282.

[4] Haskell WL, Lee IM, Pate RR, Powell KE, Blair SN, Franklin BA, et al. Physical activity and public health: updated recommendation for adults from the American College of Sports Medicine and the American Heart Association. Med Sci Sports Exerc 2007 Aug;39(8):1423-1434.

[5] Global Initiative for Chronic Obstructive Lung Disease (GOLD). Global Strategy for the Diagnosis, Management, and Prevention of Chronic Obstructive Pulmonary Disease. 2013.

[6] Lopez AD, Shibuya K, Rao C, Mathers CD, Hansell AL, Held LS, et al. Chronic obstructive pulmonary disease: current burden and future projections. Eur Respir J 2006 Feb;27(2):397-412.

[7] Mathers CD, Loncar D. Projections of global mortality and burden of disease from 2002 to 2030. PLoS Med 2006 Nov;3(11):e442.

[8] Wittink H, Engelbert R, Takken T. The dangers of inactivity; exercise and inactivity physiology for the manual therapist. Man Ther 2011 Jun;16(3):209-216.

[9] Troosters T, Sciurba F, Battaglia S, Langer D, Valluri SR, Martino L, et al. Physical inactivity in patients with COPD, a controlled multi-center pilot-study. Respir Med 2010 Jul;104(7):1005-1011.

[10] Garcia-Aymerich J, Lange P, Benet M, Schnohr P, Anto JM. Regular physical activity reduces hospital admission and mortality in chronic obstructive pulmonary disease: a population based cohort study. Thorax 2006 Sep;61(9):772-778.

[11] Donaire-Gonzalez D, Gimeno-Santos E, Balcells E, Rodriguez DA, Farrero E, Batlle JD, et al. Physical activity in COPD patients: patterns and bouts. Eur Respir J 2012 Dec 20.

[12] Stuart Albert P. Physical Activity Monitoring in COPD patients. University of Liverpool 2012.

[13] Mannino DM, Reichert MM, Davis KJ. Lung function decline and outcomes in an adult population. Am J Respir Crit Care Med 2006 May 1;173(9):985-990.

[14] ZuWallack R. How are you doing? What are you doing? Differing perspectives in the assessment of individuals with COPD. COPD 2007 Sep;4(3):293-297.

[15] Aniwidyaningsih W, Varraso R, Cano N, Pison C. Impact of nutritional status on body functioning in chronic obstructive pulmonary disease and how to intervene. Curr Opin Clin Nutr Metab Care 2008 Jul;11(4):435-442.

[16] Schols AM, Soeters PB, Dingemans AM, Mostert R, Frantzen PJ, Wouters EF. Prevalence and characteristics of nutritional depletion in patients with stable COPD eligible for pulmonary rehabilitation. Am Rev Respir Dis 1993 May;147(5):1151-1156.

[17] Sugawara K, Takahashi H, Kashiwagura T, Yamada K, Yanagida S, Homma M, et al. Effect of anti-inflammatory supplementation with whey peptide and exercise therapy in patients with COPD. Respir Med 2012 Nov;106(11):1526-1534.

[18] Schols AM, Buurman WA, Staal van den Brekel AJ, Dentener MA, Wouters EF. Evidence for a relation between metabolic derangements and increased levels of inflammatory mediators in a subgroup of patients with chronic obstructive pulmonary disease. Thorax 1996 Aug;51(8):819-824.

[19] Broekhuizen R, Wouters EF, Creutzberg EC, Schols AM. Raised CRP levels mark metabolic and functional impairment in advanced COPD. Thorax 2006 Jan;61(1):17-22.

[20] Baldi S, Aquilani R, Pinna GD, Poggi P, De Martini A, Bruschi C. Fat-free mass change after nutritional rehabilitation in weight losing COPD: role of insulin, C-reactive protein and tissue hypoxia. Int J Chron Obstruct Pulmon Dis 2010 Feb 18;5:29-39.

[21] Agusti AG, Sauleda J, Miralles C, Gomez C, Togores B, Sala E, et al. Skeletal muscle apoptosis and weight loss in chronic obstructive pulmonary disease. Am J Respir Crit Care Med 2002 Aug 15;166(4):485-489.

[22] Vendrell M, de Gracia J, Olveira C, Martinez MA, Giron R, Maiz L, et al. Diagnosis and treatment of bronchiectasis. Spanish Society of Pneumology and Thoracic Surgery. Arch Bronconeumol 2008 Nov;44(11):629-640.

[23] Fuschillo S, De Felice A, Balzano G. Mucosal inflammation in idiopathic bronchiectasis: cellular and molecular mechanisms. Eur Respir J 2008 Feb;31(2):396-406.

[24] Olveira G, Olveira C, Gaspar I, Porras N, Martin-Nunez G, Rubio E, et al. Fat-free mass depletion and inflammation in patients with bronchiectasis. J Acad Nutr Diet 2012 Dec;112(12):1999-2006.

[25] Olveira G, Olveira C, Dorado A, Garcia-Fuentes E, Rubio E, Tinahones F, et al. Cellular and plasma oxidative stress biomarkers are raised in adults with bronchiectasis. Clin Nutr 2013 Feb;32(1):112-117.

[26] Wood LG, Garg ML, Simpson JL, Mori TA, Croft KD, Wark PA, et al. Induced sputum 8-isoprostane concentrations in inflammatory airway diseases. Am J Respir Crit Care Med 2005 Mar 1;171(5):426-430.

[27] Schols A. Nutritional modulation as part of the integrated management of chronic obstructive pulmonary disease. Proc Nutr Soc 2003 Nov;62(4):783-791.

[28] Planas M, Alvarez J, Garcia-Peris PA, de la Cuerda C, de Lucas P, Castella M, et al. Nutritional support and quality of life in stable chronic obstructive pulmonary disease (COPD) patients. Clin Nutr 2005 Jun;24(3):433-441.

[29] Ferreira IM, Brooks D, White J, Goldstein R. Nutritional supplementation for stable chronic obstructive pulmonary disease. Cochrane Database Syst Rev 2012 Dec 12;12:CD000998.

[30] Constantin D, Menon MK, Houchen-Wolloff L, Morgan MD, Singh SJ, Greenhaff P, et al. Skeletal muscle molecular responses to resistance training and dietary supplementation in COPD. Thorax 2013 Mar 27.

[31] Puhan MA, Gimeno-Santos E, Scharplatz M, Troosters T, Walters EH, Steurer J. Pulmonary rehabilitation following exacerbations of chronic obstructive pulmonary disease. Cochrane Database Syst Rev 2011 Oct 5;(10):CD005305. doi(10):CD005305.

[32] Gosselink R, De Vos J, van den Heuvel SP, Segers J, Decramer M, Kwakkel G. Impact of inspiratory muscle training in patients with COPD: what is the evidence? Eur Respir J 2011 Feb;37(2):416-425.

[33] Bhandari NJ, Jain T, Marolda C, ZuWallack RL. Comprehensive pulmonary rehabilitation results in clinically meaningful improvements in anxiety and depression in patients with chronic obstructive pulmonary disease. J Cardiopulm Rehabil Prev 2013 Mar-Apr;33(2):123-127.

[34] Osadnik CR, McDonald CF, Jones AP, Holland AE. Airway clearance techniques for chronic obstructive pulmonary disease. Cochrane Database Syst Rev 2012 Mar 14;3:CD008328.

[35] Flude LJ, Agent P, Bilton D. Chest physiotherapy techniques in bronchiectasis. Clin Chest Med 2012 Jun;33(2):351-361.

[36] Lee AL, Cecins N, Hill CJ, Holland AE, Rautela L, Stirling RG, et al. The effects of pulmonary rehabilitation in patients with non-cystic fibrosis bronchiectasis: protocol for a randomised controlled trial. BMC Pulm Med 2010 Feb 2;10:5.

[37] Murray MP, Pentland JL, Hill AT. A randomised crossover trial of chest physiotherapy in non-cystic fibrosis bronchiectasis. Eur Respir J 2009 Nov;34(5):1086-1092.

[38] Mandal P, Sidhu MK, Kope L, Pollock W, Stevenson LM, Pentland JL, et al. A pilot study of pulmonary rehabilitation and chest physiotherapy versus chest physiotherapy alone in bronchiectasis. Respir Med 2012 Dec;106(12):1647-1654.

[39] Olveira G, Olveira C, Fernández-García JC, Espildora F. Soporte nutricional en el paciente con patología pulmonar, enfermedad pulmonar obstructiva crónica y fibrosis quística. In: Bellido D, De Luis D, editor. Manual de Metabolismo y Nutrición. ; 2009. p. 455-470.

[40] van de Bool C, Steiner MC, Schols AM. Nutritional targets to enhance exercise performance in chronic obstructive pulmonary disease. Curr Opin Clin Nutr Metab Care 2012 Nov;15(6):553-560.

[41] Laviolette L, Lands LC, Dauletbaev N, Saey D, Milot J, Provencher S, et al. Combined effect of dietary supplementation with pressurized whey and exercise training in chronic obstructive pulmonary disease: a randomized, controlled, double-blind pilot study. J Med Food 2010 Jun;13(3):589-598.

[42] Ringbaek T, Wilcke T. Rehabilitation and palliative care of patients with severe COPD must be integrated. Ugeskr Laeger 2013 Apr 29;175(18):1277-1280.

[43] Ferreira IM, Brooks D, Lacasse Y, Goldstein RS, White J. Nutritional supplementation for stable chronic obstructive pulmonary disease. Cochrane Database Syst Rev 2005 Apr 18;(2)(2):CD000998.

[44] Collins PF, Stratton RJ, Elia M. Nutritional support in chronic obstructive pulmonary disease: a systematic review and meta-analysis. Am J Clin Nutr 2012 Jun;95(6): 1385-1395.

[45] Itoh M, Tsuji T, Nemoto K, Nakamura H, Aoshiba K. Undernutrition in patients with COPD and its treatment. Nutrients 2013 Apr 18;5(4):1316-1335.

[46] Ries AL. Pulmonary rehabilitation: summary of an evidence-based guideline. Respir Care 2008 Sep;53(9):1203-1207.

[47] Martín-Valero R, Cuesta-Vargas AI, Labajos-Manzanares MT. Types of Physical Exercise Training for COPD patients. In: Kian-Chung Ong, editor. Chronic Obstructive Pulmonary Disease-Current Concepts and Practice Croacia: Intechweb.org; 2012. p. 351-374.

[48] Warburton DE, Nicol CW, Bredin SS. Health benefits of physical activity: the evidence. CMAJ 2006 Mar 14;174(6):801-809.

[49] Caspersen CJ, Powell KE, Christenson GM. Physical activity, exercise, and physical fitness: definitions and distinctions for health-related research. Public Health Rep 1985 Mar-Apr;100(2):126-131.

[50] Waschki B, Kirsten A, Holz O, Muller KC, Meyer T, Watz H, et al. Physical activity is the strongest predictor of all-cause mortality in patients with COPD: a prospective cohort study. Chest 2011 Aug;140(2):331-342.

[51] Scarborough P, Bhatnagar P, Wickramasinghe KK, Allender S, Foster C, Rayner M. The economic burden of ill health due to diet, physical inactivity, smoking, alcohol and obesity in the UK: an update to 2006-07 NHS costs. J Public Health (Oxf) 2011 Dec;33(4):527-535.

[52] Waschki B, Spruit MA, Watz H, Albert PS, Shrikrishna D, Groenen M, et al. Physical activity monitoring in COPD: compliance and associations with clinical characteristics in a multicenter study. Respir Med 2012 Apr;106(4):522-530.

[53] Taylor NF, Dodd KJ, Shields N, Bruder A. Therapeutic exercise in physiotherapy practice is beneficial: a summary of systematic reviews 2002-2005. Aust J Physiother 2007;53(1):7-16.

[54] Lan CC, Chu WH, Yang MC, Lee CH, Wu YK, Wu CP. Benefits of pulmonary rehabilitation in patients with COPD with normal exercise capacity. Respir Care 2013 Jan 3.

[55] Walters JA, Cameron-Tucker H, Courtney-Pratt H, Nelson M, Robinson A, Scott J, et al. Supporting health behaviour change in chronic obstructive pulmonary disease with telephone health-mentoring: insights from a qualitative study. BMC Fam Pract 2012 Jun 13;13:55-2296-13-55.

[56] Vorrink SN, Kort HS, Troosters T, Lammers JW. Level of daily physical activity in individuals with COPD compared with healthy controls. Respir Res 2011 Mar 22;12:33-9921-12-33.

[57] Arbillaga-Etxarri A, Gimeno-Santos J, Vilaró J, Vall-Casas J, García-Aymerich J. Diseño de Circuitos para el entrenamiento urbano en pacientes con Enfermedad Pulmo-

nar Obstructiva Crónica (EPOC). Archivos de Bronconeumologia 2013;Libro de Abstract 46 Congreso Nacional de SEPAR:74-75.

[58] El Gobierno de Navarra y la Universidad Pública de Navarra. Guía de paseos por Pamplona para pacientes con EPOC. 2013.

[59] Bártholo TP, Gomes MM, Noronha Filho AJ. DPOC-o impacto da oxigenoterapia domiciliar no tratamento. Pulmao 2009;1(1):79-84.

[60] Jindal SK, Agarwal R. Long-term oxygen therapy. Expert Rev Respir Med 2012 Dec; 6(6):639-649.

[61] Nonoyama ML, Brooks D, Lacasse Y, Guyatt GH, Goldstein RS. Oxygen therapy during exercise training in chronic obstructive pulmonary disease. Cochrane Database Syst Rev 2007 Apr 18;(2)(2):CD005372.

[62] Cedano S, Bettencourt AR, Traldi F, Machado MC, Belasco AG. Quality of life and burden in carers for persons with Chronic Obstructive Pulmonary Disease receiving oxygen therapy. Rev Lat Am Enfermagem 2013 Jul-Aug;21(4):860-867.

[63] van Helvoort HA, Heijdra YF, Heunks LM, Meijer PL, Ruitenbeek W, Thijs HM, et al. Supplemental oxygen prevents exercise-induced oxidative stress in muscle-wasted patients with chronic obstructive pulmonary disease. Am J Respir Crit Care Med 2006 May 15;173(10):1122-1129.

[64] Wijkstra PJ, Wempe JB. New tools in pulmonary rehabilitation. Eur Respir J 2011 Dec;38(6):1468-1474.

[65] Emtner M, Porszasz J, Burns M, Somfay A, Casaburi R. Benefits of supplemental oxygen in exercise training in nonhypoxemic chronic obstructive pulmonary disease patients. Am J Respir Crit Care Med 2003 Nov 1;168(9):1034-1042.

[66] Rasekaba T, Lee AL, Naughton MT, Williams TJ, Holland AE. The six-minute walk test: a useful metric for the cardiopulmonary patient. Intern Med J 2009 Aug;39(8): 495-501.

[67] Pitta F, Troosters T, Probst VS, Spruit MA, Decramer M, Gosselink R. Quantifying physical activity in daily life with questionnaires and motion sensors in COPD. Eur Respir J 2006 May;27(5):1040-1055.

[68] Cortopassi F, Divo M, Pinto-Plata V, Celli B. Resting handgrip force and impaired cardiac function at rest and during exercise in COPD patients. Respir Med 2011 May; 105(5):748-754.

[69] Van Remoortel H, Raste Y, Louvaris Z, Giavedoni S, Burtin C, Langer D, et al. Validity of six activity monitors in chronic obstructive pulmonary disease: a comparison with indirect calorimetry. PLoS One 2012;7(6):e39198.

[70] Van Remoortel H, Giavedoni S, Raste Y, Burtin C, Louvaris Z, Gimeno-Santos E, et al. Validity of activity monitors in health and chronic disease: a systematic review. Int J Behav Nutr Phys Act 2012 Jul 9;9:84-5868-9-84.

[71] Rabinovich RA, Louvaris Z, Raste Y, Langer D, Remoortel HV, Giavedoni S, et al. Validity of physical activity monitors during daily life in patients with COPD. Eur Respir J 2013 Feb 8.

[72] Marco E, Ramirez-Sarmiento AL, Coloma A, Sartor M, Comin-Colet J, Vila J, et al. High-intensity vs. sham inspiratory muscle training in patients with chronic heart failure: a prospective randomized trial. Eur J Heart Fail 2013 Aug;15(8):892-901.

[73] Gea J, Casadevall C, Pascual S, Orozco-Levi M, Barreiro E. Respiratory diseases and muscle dysfunction. Expert Rev Respir Med 2012 Feb;6(1):75-90.

[74] Strasser B, Siebert U, Schobersberger W. Effects of resistance training on respiratory function in patients with chronic obstructive pulmonary disease: a systematic review and meta-analysis. Sleep Breath 2013 Mar;17(1):217-226.

[75] Holland AE, Hill CJ, Jones AY, McDonald CF. Breathing exercises for chronic obstructive pulmonary disease. Cochrane Database Syst Rev 2012 Oct 17;10:CD008250.

[76] Gosselink R, De Vos J, van den Heuvel SP, Segers J, Decramer M, Kwakkel G. Impact of inspiratory muscle training in patients with COPD: what is the evidence? Eur Respir J 2011 Feb;37(2):416-425.

[77] Hill K, Jenkins SC, Philippe DL, Cecins N, Shepherd KL, Green DJ, et al. High-intensity inspiratory muscle training in COPD. Eur Respir J 2006 Jun;27(6):1119-1128.

[78] Mota S, Guell R, Barreiro E, Solanes I, Ramirez-Sarmiento A, Orozco-Levi M, et al. Clinical outcomes of expiratory muscle training in severe COPD patients. Respir Med 2007 Mar;101(3):516-524.

[79] Ramirez-Sarmiento A, Orozco-Levi M, Guell R, Barreiro E, Hernandez N, Mota S, et al. Inspiratory Muscle Training in Patients with Chronic Obstructive Pulmonary Disease: Structural Adaptation and Physiologic Outcomes. Am J Respir Crit Care Med 2002 December 1;166(11):1491-1497.

[80] Laoutaris ID, Adamopoulos S, Manginas A, Panagiotakos DB, Kallistratos MS, Doulaptsis C, et al. Benefits of combined aerobic/resistance/inspiratory training in patients with chronic heart failure. A complete exercise model? A prospective randomised study. Int J Cardiol 2013 Sep 1;167(5):1967-1972.

[81] Charususin N, Gosselink R, Decramer M, McConnell A, Saey D, Maltais F, et al. Inspiratory muscle training protocol for patients with chronic obstructive pulmonary disease (IMTCO study): a multicentre randomised controlled trial. BMJ Open 2013 Aug 5;3(8):10.1136/bmjopen-2013-003101.

[82] Hogg L, Grant A, Garrod R, Fiddler H. People with COPD perceive ongoing, structured and socially supportive exercise opportunities to be important for maintaining

an active lifestyle following pulmonary rehabilitation: a qualitative study. J Physiother 2012;58(3):189-195.

[83] Hayton C, Clark A, Olive S, Browne P, Galey P, Knights E, et al. Barriers to pulmonary rehabilitation: characteristics that predict patient attendance and adherence. Respir Med 2013 Mar;107(3):401-407.

[84] Norweg A, Bose P, Snow G, Berkowitz ME. A pilot study of a pulmonary rehabilitation programme evaluated by four adults with chronic obstructive pulmonary disease. Occup Ther Int 2008;15(2):114-132.

[85] Lohne V, Heer HC, Andersen M, Miaskowski C, Kongerud J, Rustoen T. Qualitative study of pain of patients with chronic obstructive pulmonary disease. Heart Lung 2010 May-Jun;39(3):226-234.

[86] Halding AG, Wahl A, Heggdal K. 'Belonging'. 'Patients' experiences of social relationships during pulmonary rehabilitation. Disabil Rehabil 2010;32(15):1272-1280.

[87] Arnold E, Bruton A, Ellis-Hill C. Adherence to pulmonary rehabilitation: A qualitative study. Respir Med 2006 Oct;100(10):1716-1723.

[88] Taylor SJ, Bogdan R. Introducción a los métodos cualitativos de investigación. 1ª Paidos ed. Barcelna; 1998.

[89] Denzin NK and Lincoln Y. Handbook of Qualitative Research. California: Sage: Thousand Oaks; 1994.

[90] Charmaz K. Constructing grounded theory: a practical guide through qualitative analysis. Sage ed. London; 2006.

[91] Bulley C, Donaghy M, Howden S, Salisbury L, Whiteford S, Mackay E. A prospective qualitative exploration of views about attending pulmonary rehabilitation. Physiother Res Int 2009 Sep;14(3):181-192.

[92] Cleland J, Moffat M, Small I. A qualitative study of stakeholder views of a community-based anticipatory care service for patients with COPD. Prim Care Respir J 2012 Sep;21(3):255-260.

[93] Hamilton S, Huby G, Tierney A, Powell A, Kielmann T, Sheikh A, et al. Mind the gap between policy imperatives and service provision: a qualitative study of the process of respiratory service development in England and Wales. BMC Health Serv Res 2008 Dec 4;8:248-6963-8-248.

[94] Williams V, Bruton A, Ellis-Hill C, McPherson K. The effect of pulmonary rehabilitation on perceptions of breathlessness and activity in COPD patients: a qualitative study. Prim Care Respir J 2010 Mar;19(1):45-51.

[95] Jones P, Harding G, Wiklund I, Berry P, Leidy N. Improving the process and outcome of care in COPD: development of a standardised assessment tool. Prim Care Respir J 2009 Sep;18(3):208-215.

[96] Keating A, Lee AL, Holland AE. Lack of perceived benefit and inadequate transport influence uptake and completion of pulmonary rehabilitation in people with chronic obstructive pulmonary disease: a qualitative study. J Physiother 2011;57(3):183-190.

[97] Fairbrother P, Pinnock H, Hanley J, McCloughan L, Sheikh A, Pagliari C, et al. Exploring telemonitoring and self-management by patients with chronic obstructive pulmonary disease: A qualitative study embedded in a randomized controlled trial. Patient Educ Couns 2013 May 3.

[98] Chan SC. Chronic obstructive pulmonary disease and engagement in occupation. Am J Occup Ther 2004 Jul-Aug;58(4):408-415.

[99] American Occupational Therapy Association. Occupational Therapy framework: Domain and process (2nd ed.). Am J Occup Ther, 2008;62:625-683.

[100] Fraguas Cerezo, MP. Terapia ocupacional en rehabilitación respiratoria. Ter ocup: Rev APETO, 2003; 31: 2-4.

[101] Morgan DD, White KM. Occupational therapy interventions for breathlessness at the end of life. Am J Occup Ther, 2011;65(4):428-36.

[102] Coll Artés, R. Estrategias para el manejo de los problemas de la vida diaria: Terapia Ocupacional, soporte psicosocial y sexualidad. En: Güell Rous R, de Lucas Ramos P (eds.). Rehabilitación respiratoria. Medical & Marketing Comunications. Madrid, 1999.p 217-31.

[103] Ngo L, Latham NK, Jette AM, Soukup J, Lezzoni LI. Use of physical and occupational therapy by Medicare beneficiaries within five conditions: 1994-2001. Am J Phys Med Rehabil, 2009;88(4):308-321.

[104] Holland AE, Mahal A, Hill CJ, Lee AL, Burge AT, Moore R, et al. Benefits and costs of home-based pulmonary rehabilitation in chronic obstructive pulmonary disease-a multi-centre randomised controlled equivalence trial. BMC Pulm Med 2013 Sep 8;13:57-2466-13-57.